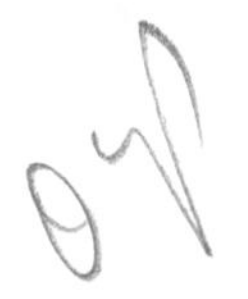

# Praise for the second edition of *Beyond Burnout: Overcoming Stress in Nursing & Healthcare for Optimal Health & Well-Being*

*"This book came at the perfect time! As healthcare leaders around the world continue to search for solutions to an ever-growing list of problems, this book clearly states the burnout issues we face and offers a wide variety of thoughtful and evidence-based solutions and strategies. The information is very helpful, and it's just nice to know so many others have similar challenges."*

–Trenda Ray, PhD, RN, NEA-BC
Chief Nursing Officer
Associate Vice Chancellor for Patient Care Services
Clinical Assistant Professor, UAMS College of Nursing

*"Another edition of renewable energy reminding us to be our best! This book takes us on a journey through stress, burnout, and post-traumatic stress and sparks innovative solutions. This book reminds us that people are our most valuable asset, and we must use our relationships, communication skills, and knowledge with intention to create psychologically safe environments. I loved the 'senseless acts of beauty' reference. Such a great way to reinforce the art and science of nursing!"*

–Kristin Christophersen, DNP, MBA, RN, NEA-BC, CENP, CPHQ, CLSSGB, FACHE
Healthcare Executive and Owner, VitalNow LLC

"Beyond Burnout *is a deeply informative nursing guide and resource for nursing and healthcare professionals. The topic of burnout is critically relevant in the healthcare industry, and Dr. Suzanne Waddill-Goad not only addresses its impact on nursing but also provides real-time tools to reframe and harness the impact of stress."*

–Kristin Jones Mensonides, MHA, MLS, FACHE
Executive Director, Integrated Service Lines, UC Davis Health

"Beyond Burnout *by Suzanne Waddill-Goad is a timely analysis for academics, managers, and hospital administrators. This unique collection of past and current perspectives explores staffing and interpersonal issues leading to burnout and stress. Comprehensive and thought-provoking, this is a research-based assessment of a real problem affecting every participant in the healthcare system from CEO to patient."*

–Elizabeth Sweeney, MSN, FNP-C, ARNP
Emergency Department/Urgent Care Nurse Practitioner

"Beyond Burnout *is timely, relevant, and critical to understanding the stressors that plague healthcare today. The tangible wisdom weaved throughout is a lifeline for nursing that can be applied to stabilize and strengthen work environments. This book is a road map to help get there."*

–Cindi M. Warburton, DNP, FNP
Executive Director, Northwest Organization of Nurse Leaders

"Beyond Burnout: Overcoming Stress in Nursing & Healthcare for Optimal Health & Well-Being *is one of the most timely resources for every nurse at any season in their career. Record high rates of burnout and nurse turnover are prevalent across the industry. Suzanne Waddill-Goad includes a reflection on the global pandemic and how it has not only fundamentally changed society but also exponentially exacerbated an existing crisis among healthcare workers and nurses in particular. The emphasis on health and wellness in this second edition underscores the importance of self-care and advocacy with tangible pearls from a trusted nurse leader."*

–Kim Tucker, PhD, RN, CNE
Director for Nursing Programs, Columbia Basin College

*"In 1979 when I started my career, there was a nursing shortage, and working the night shift was very stressful. Fast forward to 2023. There are opportunities for registered nurses that did not exist in 1979. The passion for the profession is the same, and we are still in a nursing shortage, but this time it's different. How can our profession assist our nurses to cope with the stressors that are causing burnout and the desire to leave the bedside? I have known Dr. Waddill-Goad for over 10 years. Suzanne has an extensive career in the business of healthcare both as a healthcare executive and a successful entrepreneur. Her book is an important one, as nurse burnout is in the news daily."*

–Pamela D. Hardesty, PhD, RN
Clinical Professor, College of Nursing
University of Tennessee, Knoxville

SECOND EDITION

# BEYOND BURNOUT

*overcoming* stress *in nursing & healthcare for optimal health & well-being*

Suzanne Waddill-Goad, DNP, MBA, BSN, RN, CEN, CHC

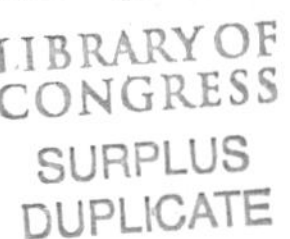


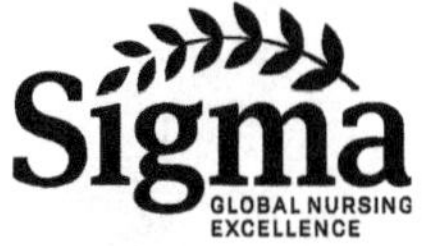

*Sigma Theta Tau International Honor Society of Nursing (Sigma) is a nonprofit organization whose mission is developing nurse leaders anywhere to improve healthcare everywhere. Founded in 1922, Sigma has more than 135,000 active members in over 100 countries and territories. Members include practicing nurses, instructors, researchers, policymakers, entrepreneurs, and others. Sigma's more than 540 chapters are located at more than 700 institutions of higher education throughout Armenia, Australia, Botswana, Brazil, Canada, Chile, Colombia, Croatia, England, Eswatini, Finland, Ghana, Hong Kong, Ireland, Israel, Italy, Jamaica, Japan, Jordan, Kenya, Lebanon, Malawi, Mexico, the Netherlands, Nigeria, Pakistan, Philippines, Portugal, Puerto Rico, Scotland, Singapore, South Africa, South Korea, Sweden, Taiwan, Tanzania, Thailand, the United States, and Wales. Learn more at www.sigmanursing.org.*

Sigma Theta Tau International
550 West North Street
Indianapolis, IN, USA 46202

To request a review copy for course adoption, order additional books, buy in bulk, or purchase for corporate use, contact Sigma Marketplace at 888.654.4968 (US/Canada toll-free), +1.317.687.2256 (International), or solutions@sigmamarketplace.org.

To request author information, or for speaker or other media requests, contact Sigma Marketing at 888.634.7575 (US/Canada toll-free) or +1.317.634.8171 (International).

**ISBN:** 9781646480753
**EPUB ISBN:** 9781646480777
**PDF ISBN:** 9781646480760
**MOBI ISBN:** 9781646480890

Library of Congress Control Number: 2023003549

First Printing, 2023

**Publisher:** Dustin Sullivan
**Acquisitions Editor:** Emily Hatch
**Development Editor:** Meaghan O'Keeffe
**Cover Designer:** Rebecca Batchelor
**Interior Design/Page Layout:** Rebecca Batchelor
**Indexer:** Larry D. Sweazy

**Managing Editor:** Carla Hall
**Publications Specialist:** Todd Lothery
**Project Editor:** Todd Lothery
**Copy Editor:** Erin Geile
**Proofreader:** Todd Lothery

# DEDICATION

A Taoist proverb states, "No one can see their reflection in running water. It is only in still water that we can see." Now that the world is emerging from a global pandemic, we must take pause to acknowledge what we've been through, where we are, and what needs to change to ensure a prosperous future.

This book is dedicated to all the healthcare heroes who survived the last few years of turmoil, chaos, stress, fatigue, and burnout during the recent COVID-19 pandemic. It taught us all many valuable lessons. Now, it's time to thrive, both in our personal and professional lives, putting to work our lessons learned.

I am truly grateful for those I've met in my healthcare travels, whose influence has shaped who I am as a nurse and a person. Their influence has been invaluable. I've been from coast to coast in the United States, helping others over the last two decades, and I am thankful for the countless opportunities the profession of nursing has provided me.

# ACKNOWLEDGMENTS

This book would not have been possible without four dedicated nurse colleagues who were committed to this project as contributors: Dr. Debra Buck, Dr. Holly Langster, Dr. Rusty McNew, and Dr. James Reedy. They are all accomplished nurse leaders in their varied disciplines. Their expertise, perspective, and guidance have made the final product better.

My family, friends, and colleagues provided encouragement to write this revised edition. They knew by watching my journey from afar and having their own experiences with the recent pandemic that the next chapter in this story needed to be told. Onward!

# ABOUT THE AUTHOR

**Suzanne Waddill-Goad, DNP, MBA, BSN, RN, CEN, CHC,** is President and Principal Consultant of Suzanne M. Waddill-Goad & Company, Inc. She began her journey in healthcare nearly 45 years ago and has spent her entire professional career working solely in the healthcare industry. Before she became self-employed, she held positions in various healthcare settings as a respiratory therapy technician, medical records clerk, transcriptionist, staff nurse, charge nurse, nursing supervisor, director of quality improvement, clinical educator, operations improvement coordinator, and chief nursing officer/assistant administrator.

Waddill-Goad holds a bachelor of science in nursing from the University of Colorado, a master of business administration from City University of Seattle, and a doctor of nursing practice in executive leadership from American Sentinel University. Her clinical practice spanned two decades in critical care and emergency nursing. Her graduate study was focused in the areas of managerial and executive leadership. In addition, she holds an executive education certificate as a Black Belt in Lean Six Sigma from The Ohio State University Fisher College of Business and retains clinical certification in emergency nursing.

Waddill-Goad's consulting practice has specialized in operational improvement and leadership development. During the last 20 years, she has assisted clients in multiple states to achieve operational improvements in leadership, quality, safety, regulatory compliance, risk reduction, finance, and customer service via consulting and/or interim leadership assignments. She has demonstrated success in developing new programs and leading teams with innovative ideas to their intended targets.

In 2014, she received an academic appointment as an Assistant Clinical Professor in the College of Nursing at the University of Tennessee. She worked on nursing program development and taught in the collaborative Executive Education Healthcare Program at the University of Tennessee Haslam College of Business until she relocated to the West Coast.

In 2021, Waddill-Goad completed the Institute for Integrative Nutrition's Health Coaching Program. And during 2022, she completed the curriculum and certification as an evidence-based Certified Health Coach (CHC) from the National Society of Health Coaches. In addition to her doctoral research on leadership fatigue, with a renewed interest in health and well-being she has expanded her business offerings to speaking, coaching, and consulting, specifically related to health, well-being, and peak human performance. She lives with her husband in the Washington State wine country.

# CONTRIBUTING AUTHORS

**Debra Buck, DNP, MSN, RN,** is part of the nursing faculty of Kellogg Community College, Spring Arbor University, and Walden University. She began her nursing career directly out of high school, graduating with an associate degree from a local community college. She worked in critical care and the emergency department for 14 years, transitioning to home care. During her time in home care, she completed her BSN from the University of Michigan.

After several years working in the community, Buck returned to the hospital setting as a nurse recruiter. During her tenure, she made the decision to obtain a master of science in nursing with the goal of teaching nursing. Prior to completing her MSN, she returned to the emergency department as a clinical manager, during which she was instrumental in the department's adoption of an electronic medical record as part of a hospital-wide initiative. After the completion of her MSN, Buck was approached by a colleague with an opportunity to teach at the BSN level for a local college. Developing the curriculum for a community nursing course launched her career in the world of academia. After she began teaching, the opportunity arose to become the Director of Student Health Services for a local liberal arts college. This position allowed her to better accommodate her teaching schedule while becoming immersed in the college life.

Buck made the decision to obtain a DNP in executive leadership to allow her the opportunity to teach at all levels. She completed her degree in 2014. Since then, she has been teaching at the ADN, BSN, and MSN levels. She teaches courses in the areas of nursing ethics, leadership, health policy, nursing research methods, community nursing, and medical informatics at the undergraduate and graduate levels. She is currently working with ADN students in the program she initially graduated from, teaching psychiatric nursing and leadership as well as fundamentals in the clinical setting.

**Holly Jo Langster, DNP, MHA, MSN, BSN, FNP-C, HCA, CENP, CPHQ,** is an Assistant Professor at the University of Central Arkansas. She is a small-town girl from central Illinois who selected nursing as a career three years after high school graduation. The profession of nursing has allowed Langster to advance and grow her career in a variety of different ways, experiencing several venues of the profession and applying that ever-expanding knowledge to each new adventure. When passionate about nursing, nothing is unachievable.

Langster has worked in many nursing fields—including medical/surgical, emergency department, and cardiac nursing—and thrives on challenge, new opportunities, discovery, program development, and executive nursing leadership. As a family nurse practitioner, she specialized in breast cancer. Administratively, she has worked in executive nursing and leadership for at least a decade. Finally, as a faculty member at the University of Central Arkansas School of Nursing, Langster educates future DNP-level family practice nurse practitioners. Legal nurse consulting has been an ongoing sideline career, as she works to assist the healthcare industry in defense against false accusations of mistreatment or neglect.

Langster holds a doctor of nursing practice in executive leadership from American Sentinel University, a master's in healthcare administration from Southern Illinois University, a master's in nursing as a family nurse practitioner from the University of Illinois-Chicago, a bachelor of science in nursing from Bradley University, and a nursing diploma from Methodist Medical Center School of Nursing. She is board certified as a family nurse practitioner, as an executive nursing leader, and in healthcare quality. She is the widow of an emergency department physician who she claims was the best ED physician who ever existed, and the proud mother of Lucas. Langster is the daughter of an RN, the granddaughter of an LPN, and the great granddaughter of the town midwife (she isn't sure there was actually training for that back then).

**Rusty McNew, DNP, MLS, RN, CENP,** is an established health system leader with significant experience in healthcare operations, performance improvement, regulatory and accreditation, and medical error prevention. Most recently, he served as the system Chief Nursing Officer of United Surgical Partners International, responsible for the nursing vision, quality, patient safety strategy, and clinical performance for hospitals and ambulatory surgery centers.

Prior to joining United Surgical Partners International, McNew served as the corporate Vice President for Quality and Patient Safety at Tenet Healthcare, where he led the delivery of safe, quality nursing and clinical care, clinical research, healthcare regulatory and accreditation programs, and the enterprise clinical auditing processes. Before that he held multiple leadership roles at the Parkland Health and Hospital System and worked as a registered nurse in the intensive care units, operating suites, and Level I Trauma emergency departments.

McNew has published 22 editions of the *Emergency Department Compliance Manual* with Aspen Publishing (now Wolters Kluwer). He also co-chaired the Homeland Security Healthcare Sector Coordinating Council and was a member of the Homeland Security Healthcare and Public Sector Clinical Infrastructure Partnership Advisory Council. McNew earned a doctor of nursing practice degree from American Sentinel University, a master of liberal arts from Southern Methodist University, and a bachelor of science in nursing from the University of Texas at Arlington. He is also a Certified Executive Nurse Professional from the American Organization of Nurse Leaders.

**James C. Reedy, DNP, MBA, MHA, RN, NEA-BC, CPHQ, CHFP, FACHE,** is a tenured nursing executive leader and a co-chair for the Northwest Organization for Nurse Leaders Leadership Commission. He has served in the role of Chief Nursing Officer within St. Charles Health System and Sutter Health, as a Neuroscience Service Line Director at Sutter Health and SSM Healthcare, and as Manager of the Neuroscience and Abdominal Transplant Intensive Care Unit for St. Louis University Hospital.

Clinically, Reedy was initiated into healthcare early on as a lifeguard and instructor for multiple Red Cross classes and trained as an EMT before beginning his storied nursing career. As a clinical nurse, he was proud to have learned the core values of teamwork and evidence-based practice working in trauma and surgical intensive care, emergency departments, and various intensive care specialties at St. Louis University Hospital, New York University–Tisch Hospital, and Barnes-Jewish Hospital. Working with colleagues, he achieved system standardization in areas such as quality, safety, growth, and affordability, and merging Lean, Six Sigma, shared governance, and the nursing process to amplify frontline nurses' engagement to meet organizational goals.

Reedy received his undergraduate nursing degree from St. Louis University School of Nursing; a master's degree in both health and business administration from Webster University's George Herbert Walker School of Business and Technology; and a doctor of nursing practice focused on health systems executive leadership from the University of Pittsburgh's School of Nursing.

Reedy's husband is an award-winning leader in the advancement of population health for diverse and high needs populations in Southern California. Reedy believes that nurses are the key to creating tomorrow's functional healthcare system, but to get there they must embrace innovation and technology and lean into caring differently: at the bedside, in the clinic, in the home, as leaders, and at the boardroom table. Reedy will serve on the Leadership Succession Committee for Sigma Theta Tau's Eta Chapter.

# ADDITIONAL BOOK RESOURCES

A companion workbook is available for sale from Sigma Marketplace and other online retailers. Follow this link or QR code to purchase directly from Sigma:

https://www.sigmamarketplace.org/workbook-for-beyond-burnout-second-edition

For a sample chapter and other free resources for this book, follow the URL below to the Sigma Repository or use the QR code.

https://sigma.nursingrepository.org/handle/10755/23016

# TABLE OF CONTENTS

# FOREWORD

For over 35 years I have had the pleasure of working in the US healthcare industry. During that time, I have met many caring professionals, none more impactful than my friend Dr. Suzanne Waddill-Goad. She is a role model leader. She stepped in to lead nursing in several of the hospitals I was responsible for, during times of change, stress, and need. She continues demonstrating her leadership by bringing together some of the nation's thought leaders of the nursing profession. Collectively, they have taken a thorough and thoughtful look at the conditions facing healthcare and the impact these conditions and the COVID-19 pandemic have had on caregivers. They have prescribed pragmatic solutions for our heroes to not only survive stress but also find a path to thrive.

In her latest book, *Beyond Burnout,* Dr. Waddill-Goad highlights the impact of the altruistic virtues of nursing—caring and compassion. These virtues were brought into clear focus by the worldwide crisis of the pandemic. In the early days of the pandemic, all of us realized that these virtues were often the only remedy we had to a deadly virus. Nurses stepped into the forefront of the crisis, and their role—never more vital—seemed to be the only answer for suffering patients and families. Nurses and all other caregivers were the front lines of defense. They absorbed the stress, pain, and uncertainly for us all, while we waited for scientific innovation. This is not the first time in our history when this has been true; in fact, the art and science of nursing has been and will always be the glue that holds the care-delivery system together.

*Beyond Burnout* is a vital and timely update for the heroes of our healthcare system. The healthcare industry needs to pay attention to the environment we have created. We must work together to re-recruit the millions of people who are considering healthcare as a career path and those who have chosen healthcare as their profession. *Beyond Burnout* is a practical guide for how to understand and cope with the stress that caring for people can create but also offers vital methods for identifying and moving toward optimal personal health. These messages have never been more important than now. The call for leaders to recognize the need to promote caregiver wellness is essential. My hope for us all is that we harness the lessons learned from the pandemic and use them as lights to guide the path forward for the next generation of caregivers.

*Beyond Burnout* provides an instructive collection of wisdom for leaders, caregivers, students, and patients. Dr. Waddill-Goad supplies expert advice, enlivened by personal examples in an easy-to-read format that has become an indispensable standard. This guide will support everyone combating stress and help them find ways to move past it so that they can create a life in which they enjoy serving others and also enhance their ability to thrive. Enjoy.

–Grant Davies
President and CEO, Solis Mammography
Addison, Texas
Former hospital executive and Joint Commission board member

# INTRODUCTION

## HEALTHCARE: AN ALTRUISTIC ENDEAVOR

Why write a book about stress, fatigue, and burnout . . . and then one about moving beyond it? The author and the contributors have well over 150 years of collective practice and have lived through a broad range of experiences, some good and some not so good. Since the first edition of this book was written, we've now experienced a global pandemic, escalated shortages of all types of personnel, supply chain challenges, and more. So, would each of the writers of this book choose nursing all over again? Absolutely!

Nursing has been a fabulous career choice; it offers diversity, flexibility, entrepreneurism, innovation, a true sense of satisfaction, and a nice lifestyle. Nurses are generally people who exhibit traits of caring, nurturing, and altruism. They are just good people to be around. Although the writers' journeys have been diverse, their reasons for becoming a nurse are very similar—to help others. Today, they each serve in different roles: One is a healthcare consultant and interim nurse leader; one is a nurse educator; one is an executive nurse leader; one is a risk, quality, and legal nurse consultant; and one is a nurse practitioner. They all work in assorted practice environments, but their mission is still the same—to truly help others.

The good thing is, helping others never gets old. What does wear on any healthcare provider's psyche is the environment. Adverse stimuli can be both internal and external: regulatory and policy changes, leadership influences, operational initiatives, industry mandates, customer expectations, the pace of change, publicly reported data, quality metrics, colleague relationships, public pressure, public perception, global uncertainty, and the list goes on.

This book explores those influences and discusses how they affect stress, fatigue, and burnout. The most important offerings from this book (the "Practice Pearls") are suggested strategies for fresh thinking, techniques to harness and manage overwhelming stress, and ways to set new priorities to care for yourself to move beyond burnout. Healthcare workers need to be encouraged to prioritize self-care and recovery time to promote their own health and well-being. We know they experience more stress than the wider working population and can find little respite from this reality. And this has certainly been amplified as evidenced by all the recent media coverage regarding the global pandemic and its deleterious effects on the nursing and healthcare workforce. The upside? It exposed the good, the bad, and the ugly of choosing a career in nursing and healthcare. Now it's time to get to work on how to move beyond what has happened in the past and plan for a brighter future!

Both the brain and body need downtime for optimal human performance. Stress and fatigue do affect safety and quality, and we can no longer push ourselves to the brink. We need "renewable" energy to be at our personal and professional best; we need to be mindful and think intentionally; and we need to perform in the best interest of ourselves as well as others. Much of the content in this book is applicable to many professions beyond nursing—other healthcare providers, those in any service profession, and more.

## STRESS, FATIGUE, AND BURNOUT IN NURSING

What is causing nurses' stress? Back in 2015, the American Holistic Nurses Association listed staffing (or the lack thereof), schedules (rotating), long shifts (often back to back), fatigue (both mental and physical), excessive noise in the workplace, workload (too much to do), time pressures (not enough time to get the work done), difficult colleagues (teamwork or the lack of), supervisors (not qualified for the role and/or not supportive of staff needs), challenging patients and families (sicker patients and families with unrealistic expectations), a lack of control in the work environment (mandates driven by others), role conflict, ambiguity, inadequate resources of all types, floating to new work areas with little or no orientation, underuse of talent, exposure to toxic substances, and the potential to experience hostility or violence (by patients, visitors, or coworkers), to name a few. Although this is not an exhaustive list of the challenges nurses and healthcare workers face, it a fairly comprehensive list of what might qualify as daily stressors in the work environment. And I'm afraid not much has changed eight years later. Honestly, the situation has only been compounded by poor communication structures and resource availability in the last three years.

A survey released in October 2021 by the American Nurses Foundation cited findings from 9,500 nurses related to their mental health and wellness. Nearly one-third rated their mental health as unhealthy, 75% said they felt stressed, 69% were frustrated, and 62% felt overwhelmed (ANA Enterprise, 2021). In addition, nearly one-half of all the survey respondents answered "yes" when asked about the effects of COVID-19 in relation to experiencing extremely stressful, disturbing, or traumatic events. Many said they intended to leave their positions within the next six months, citing work as negatively affecting their health and well-being, as well as insufficient staffing. Many of these problems have been long-standing in the nursing and healthcare industries and are clearly continuing to take a toll.

Why are nurses burning out? Three out of four nurses cited the effects of stress and overwork as a top health concern in a 2011 survey by the American Nurses Association (ANA); the ANA attributed problems of fatigue and burnout to what seems to be a chronic nursing shortage (ANA, 2011). More recent research has found nurses working shifts longer than eight to nine hours were two-and-a-half times more likely to experience burnout (Gupta, 2015). And a 2012 study by Stimpfel et al. revealed that nurses underestimate their own recovery time from long, intense clinical engagements and that consolidating challenging work into shorter time frames may not be a sustainable strategy to attain work-life balance. We now know the global COVID-19 pandemic only exacerbated what was already occurring for at least the last decade in the majority of healthcare work environments.

In addition, researchers at the University of Akron (Dill and Erickson) found in 2014 that nurses who are primarily motivated by the desire to help others, rather than enjoyment of work, were more likely to burn out (American

Sociological Association, 2014). Could we be our own worst enemies? Should education and awareness about the potential for burnout begin in formal nursing training? Should selection criteria to become a nurse include an assessment for motivation and the potential to burn out? Could we change our current trajectory if both of these were strongly considered in the selection of who should become a nurse?

Nurses are qualitative experts; we are constantly gathering information on a daily basis. What we have not been quite as good at is collecting formal data, analyzing it, and sharing evidence in our practice environments. Hence, some of the dated information in the nursing literature. If nurses were able to use the information they collect more effectively or on a real-time basis, could it decrease the potential for burnout?

The pandemic certainly challenged our practice norms. Change was coming nearly hourly about what we should be doing via the Centers for Disease Control; other state and federal regulatory agencies; corporate, system, and local-level leadership; as well as the boots on the ground. It showed the creativity that staff could bring to a real challenge. If nurses were allowed more autonomy in overall role design—assessing job fit, analyzing systems affecting their work, given training for optimal interpersonal relationships, and learning about the consequences of stress—is it plausible that burnout could be lessened and maybe entirely avoided?

I've always felt that nurses are the backbone of healthcare. No healthcare organization can be effectively run without them. So, what are the responsibilities of nurses, other healthcare workers, and leaders collaboratively for the future in relation to stress, fatigue, and burnout in nursing and other healthcare professions?

## PRACTICE PEARLS

- Know the signs and most common causes of burnout.
- Design or improve systems known to cause stress.
- Create a campaign of cultural awareness regarding the risks of burnout.

## WHY CHOOSE NURSING OR A CAREER IN HEALTHCARE?

Nursing and other healthcare professions are more than a job. Healthcare attracts those who value compassion and want to do greater good in the world. Many say it is a calling because it provides a platform for making a difference in other people's lives. The wide range of experiences that healthcare providers encounter from birth to death can be both painful and joyous—with every emotion in between.

The profession provides endless options to practice in a variety of healthcare settings. Specifically, a career in nursing provides the flexibility to choose from an array of options different from most other career choices. Nursing allows you to enter and exit the profession, work more or less than full time, work in nontraditional settings, have around-the-clock hours, and have fluid movement between types of healthcare milieus and patient populations. Many other professions inside and outside of healthcare aren't quite as flexible.

Healthcare offers ample time during a lifelong career to learn new skills for advancement. A multitude of possibilities exist for a nonlinear career track in various areas of specialty practice, both clinical and non-clinical. Additionally, a variety of educational options exist for continual learning in all sorts of relevant areas. Educational opportunities include both formal and informal coursework. This array of choices is appealing to many choosing a first or alternate career. And the choice of a career, specifically in nursing, often allows a planned or intentional approach to work-life balance. Sometimes moving to a new area or learning something new is just what the doctor ordered to combat stress, fatigue, and burnout. It provides an opportunity for a refresh!

Nursing is also both art and science; the profession has the capacity to capture a person's soul through experiences that may be singular in nature or that combine physical, mental, emotional, and spiritual encounters. Many of these encounters will leave a lasting impression. They will not only shape a nurse's professional practice journey but can also add positive value to a nurse's life as a whole. Many others who work in healthcare feel the same. From those cleaning patient rooms to medical providers to nutrition staff to ancillary clinical providers, nearly everyone has the same mission to help others and make a positive impact on a person's life.

Traditional nursing and medical practices are founded in science. Evidence-based care and compensable quality metrics are changing the practice of nursing and medicine (albeit slowly). We now have more industry best practices guiding patient care decision-making. While nurses have always been concerned about patient outcomes, responsibility has escalated, and now accountability lies in the hands of those providing direct care. This comes with both risk and reward for any healthcare provider.

Healthcare leaders' contributions to direct care include advanced educational preparation and the obligation to provide or ensure available resources—people, space, supplies, and equipment—for optimal care delivery. As the healthcare environment has become more fiscally challenged, this is often much more complicated than it appears. Staffing shortages, drug recalls, equipment back orders, supply chain mishaps, escalating costs of care, and space challenges often inhibit smooth transitions of care and efficient work processes. The resulting stress, especially for nurse leaders, can be quite overwhelming, as job expectations have drastically changed in recent years.

While nurses are qualified to use their ability to influence others' choices about health promotion and treatment of illness, they also need to care for themselves. They are often viewed by the public as experts and are the most revered profession with the highest levels of perceived honesty and ethical standards (Riffkin, 2014). This standing in the public eye has been demonstrated for decades and provides a respected voice to lead the future of healthcare; however, nurses must lead first by example.

A radical change in thinking is required; the old-style thinking of treatment of illness needs to be replaced with mindful intention for optimal health. Part of being mindful relative to health is prevention and adopted action to be healthy. Actions always speak louder than words. Daily decisions add up. No change ever comes from continuing on the same path—good, bad, or otherwise. And small changes in lifestyle habits can yield big differences in health or well-being outcomes.

Nursing also provides a stage to observe a variety of ethnic and cultural healing practices firsthand. Nurses play an important part of assisting others and their families through challenging health and psychosocial situations. The profession offers exceptional but often test-laden circumstances to be thoughtfully navigated on a daily basis. Boredom is seldom used to describe a day in a nurse's life. Each day offers a distinct experience, generally in the presence of newly introduced people.

The number of registered nurses in the US is estimated to be just over 3 million (US Bureau of Labor Statistics, 2020). In addition, the US Bureau of Labor Statistics *Occupational Outlook Handbook's* estimate for growth from 2020–2030 is only slightly above the average of all professions (8%), with nursing at a projected growth rate of 9%. This likely will become more problematic as the population ages and the need for medical services continues to rise in the currently designed system.

The median income for nursing, stated to be $77,600, is higher than most other professions, and the nursing profession can be entered with minimal academic preparation of an associate degree (US Bureau of Labor Statistics, 2020). However, many associate program requirements or prerequisites nearly equal a bachelor's degree, which is becoming a preferred entry requirement by many employers.

As also described in the *Occupational Outlook Handbook* (2020), the outpatient arena of healthcare encounters continues to grow, with technological advancement over recent years creating a shift in the traditional hospital-type acute care setting. This has seemingly been a good idea if patients are able to meet the downscaled criteria for this type of setting for their care. It has also expanded the non-acute care choices for all healthcare providers to choose a multitude of new career options. The outpatient setting also offers a number of other corollary benefits, including more traditional work hours without required weekend and holiday commitments. However, hospitals continue to occupy the top spot where nurses work at 61%.

### PRACTICE PEARLS

- Nursing provides a flexible and rewarding career.
- Nurses have the ability to make a stable living wage.
- Nurses have many opportunities to continue learning and to change practice among specialties.

## ADVANCES IN TECHNOLOGY

While the process of nursing has essentially remained the same for centuries, the practice of care delivery has changed significantly in recent decades. Research advances in medical care and treatment delivery have spurred new technology essentially focused on automation. Much of the healthcare delivery system can be or is sequenced and repetitive. This has facilitated the creation and use of new medical devices, improved safety, and driving more precise, predictable clinical outcomes. Examples include robotic surgery, high-tech implantable devices, newly developed pharmaceuticals, smart technology for medical equipment such as infusion pumps, and better beds, among many others.

Beginning in 2009, with the aim of improving healthcare processes through the use of health information technology, the US government promulgated use of electronic health records (EHR), where providers of the services were incentivized for adoption (Centers for Medicare & Medicaid Services, 2014; Slight et al., 2015). The improvement in access to timely medical information for emergent situations, or as people are transient and mobile in today's society, has benefited both patients and their caregivers by having the necessary information available to allow the best, informed choices at the time for their care. However, the effects on overall quality and safety remain uncertain (Slight et al., 2015).

Electronic access to information for nurses to make care decisions for patients is essential (Kelley et al., 2011). A multitude of nursing publishers have now made traditional texts, policies, procedures, and diagnostic tools immediately available via electronic means. This real-time information accessibility assists nurses and other caregivers in making sound care decisions for their assigned patient population. More recent graduates of nursing and other healthcare education programs may never have used paper documentation, reference manuals, or printed books to access information; electronic access is the only system they know.

The advent of social media has presented both benefits and challenges for the nursing and healthcare industries. The immediacy of information may be a benefit; however, the commitment to confidentiality and privacy can often be challenging—so much so that the National Council of State Boards of Nursing issued a 2018 publication on the do's and don'ts of using social media so that nurses don't inadvertently breach a patient's trusted health information.

Most organizations set policy regarding the use of social media, appropriate personal and professional cell-phone usage, and photography or video with a strict set of parameters not to be violated (for patient privacy) without extremely adverse consequences. All healthcare providers must use caution not to breach the trust of patient relationships and the confidentiality of any patient-related health information.

## PRACTICE PEARLS

- Nurses and other healthcare providers must be technologically savvy.
- Nurses and other healthcare providers need to know the law and policy about patient privacy and confidentiality.
- Social media should only be used to improve patient access to accurate and appropriate information.

---

## THE PACE OF CHANGE

One of the most memorable recurring dreams nurses have in common goes like this:

> The shift was very busy, and I spent the entire time running from room to room doing assessments, taking vital signs, giving medications, and doing minor procedures. I barely had time to take a break or finish my documentation before the shift was nearing its end. It was a tough day, with provider and family challenges. I really felt I had too many sick patients to adequately care for, but it was almost time for the end of the shift report to the oncoming nurse. Whew—I had survived! Then, at the end of the shift report, the oncoming nurse asked me about Patient X. I politely told her I was not assigned Patient X. She looked surprised, so we verified the daily assignments for each nurse per the assignment sheet. And there it was in plain black and white—Patient X was assigned to me. Oh, no! Would they still be alive since I had not seen them all shift? They had missed all their medications, assessments, and vital signs. How could nobody have known? Did the charge nurse not go in and check on the patient when rounding? Did the patient not have any clinical needs or diagnostic testing that required consultation with a nurse or any other care providers?

And then the dreaming nurse wakes up from the nightmare!

Nursing and healthcare are fast-paced. Nurses experience a great deal of stress and must continually adapt to change with grace. Nielsen and Munir (2009) posited that the ability to effectively adapt to change shows tenacity and courage. The industry needs courageous leaders at all levels, now more than ever, to lead the way to a better system of health promotion and to focus on well-being and care. Our lives as we continue to age may depend on it.

The speed of life and work has increased exponentially, as described by Kotter (2011), who questioned whether people are really able to keep up with the new pace. The norm is no longer status quo; change comes at a rapid and unrelenting speed. Keeping up with the new pace of information, life, and change is difficult.

The COVID-19 pandemic showed us how fast things could really change—nearly in an instant. Most likely there will be even more change in the future that could be damaging to our health. Technology continues to drive the pace of change as improvements promise to enhance productivity, allowing nurses to do more with less or in the same amount of time. Could technology be another source of nurse and healthcare provider stress? Many practicing clinicians think so. Is the digital age really making people more productive? Not necessarily. And is better productivity making anyone providing the care healthier or more satisfied with their work?

Since 2020, there have been five generations of people in the workforce. Each generation brings its own set of expectations for their personal and professional lives (Putre, 2013). This diversity can provide a number of organizational challenges to current work process and business operations. Unintentional interpersonal conflict can result due to different styles of communication, work expectations, team values, and frames of reference.

In general, younger generations are more familiar with technology and are used to a faster pace of life. This is all they have known, and it is their "normal." For those who are older, human contact has always been valued; they are learning new technology and being introduced to the importance of work-life balance. Understanding the vast differences in preferences and expectations of each generation will be crucial for healthcare organizations of the future, where one size won't fit all for both recruitment and retention of key talent.

In addition, the aging of the US population has tremendous implications for the healthcare industry, both as employers of an aging workforce and as providers of services to a growing number of older patients (Harrington & Heidcamp, 2009). Who will fill the workforce vacancies as the population keeps aging and demand for services goes up? We know younger workers do not want or expect the same things from their work. Will they be able to fill the void as older workers retire? Will older workers feel compelled to stay in the workforce? If the Great Resignation during 2020–2022 from the COVID-19 pandemic was any indication of the future, we should all be worried.

The World Health Organization estimates the world population of those age 65 or over to be 1.5 billion by 2050, nearly triple the number in 2010 (Aetna, 2017). In addition, it is well-known that older individuals often experience more health conditions requiring medical treatment. This continued trajectory on a path where the demand for medical services (as highlighted by the pandemic) exceeds the supply of available resources (caregivers, supply, and space) is like a car careening toward a cliff. In addition, many have delayed care due to the implications of the COVID-19 pandemic. This has resulted in an inadvertent rise of the acuity of illness, and hospitals have increased lengths of stay—both due to sicker patients and being unduly burdened with those unable to transition to the next phase of care (Daly, 2020; Moore, 2020).

Is stress actually potentiating illness? Could we change our lifestyles to make an impact in acute care? Do we have time before we begin to suffer health consequences ourselves? Time is finite; more time cannot be created. Thus, we have to think intentionally about how time should be spent and what we are doing to care for ourselves and promote our own health. Could we decrease stress by spending less time in stress-invoking environments, or could the environments be made less stress-invoking? Both might be true. Because healthcare providers seemingly cannot change the pace, they must be willing to change themselves and the existing systems to build healthier places of work.

## PRACTICE PEARLS

- Understand what you can and cannot control in your environment to alleviate stress.
- Thoughts, feelings, and actions are connected. Be mindful about how you think and feel.
- You need to care for yourself first to be the best caregiver for others.
- Be resourceful, innovative, and creative in changing your workplace for the better.

---

## THE EFFECTS OF STRESS

Numerous studies, both in and outside of healthcare, have analyzed the effects of stress. In addition to reduced job satisfaction, stressed or fatigued workers may suffer health consequences, are more apt to make mistakes, are often unable to sleep and rest effectively, are absent from work more often, and experience a host of psychosocial distress, as described by Waddill-Goad in 2013. The new corporate business model of healthcare has fueled a dilemma for many nurses and other healthcare workers. Contemporary business practices and politics in healthcare have led to commercial value systems being instilled into professions that have been traditionally considered moral practice involving care and compassion (Roberts et al., 2012). The strain has produced more stress for caregivers in an already stress-laden environment. And the COVID-19 pandemic exposed political-laden turmoil, resulting in controversial decision-making about how public health emergencies should be handled.

A multitude of studies have shown that nurses and other caregivers have a propensity for burnout. The very nature of caring for others, sometimes without the ability to set limits (of time, compassion, etc.), potentiates the possibility for burnout. Articles found in the scholarly literature cite up to a prevalence of 40% of people feeling stressed and having the potential to become burned out in the workforce on any given day. Because burnout is known to result in physical, mental, and social consequences, why is it not more commonly discussed and addressed, and why aren't actions taken to prevent it? Is it an ignored phenomenon? At what cost?

Not only does burnout have personal consequences, but there are also organizational concerns that all relate to the bottom line, such as retention and turnover, employee satisfaction, clinical outcomes, medical errors, and patient satisfaction. Burnout is not a solely individual problem, as we know it stems from the social environment.

The US Bureau of Labor Statistics ranked nurses higher than average for musculoskeletal injuries from overexertion and bodily reaction in addition to other workplace injuries differing by age (US Bureau of Labor Statistics, 2018). And when a provider is absent, another is necessary to care for patients already in the queue or system. We also know mental health is just as important as physical health. On your very best day, it's possible to make a tragic mistake with disastrous consequences.

Because stress, fatigue, and burnout have serious penalties for both individuals and organizations, the healthcare industry must take note. Effective awareness and reduction approaches must be considered and implemented in the healthcare work environment. The potential for violence and incivility on the part of patients, visitors, and healthcare workers is escalating and must not be tolerated. Recognizing job stress and implementing other health and safety interventions targeted to the needs of nurses and healthcare providers in their work settings will facilitate the overarching goal of improving health and safety (Roberts et al., 2012). In turn, this will lead to safer and better patient care.

## PRACTICE PEARLS

- Recognize stress and its consequences.
- Attempt early intervention to mitigate stress.
- Adopt healthy coping strategies for stress tolerance.

# REFERENCES


Aetna International. (2017). *The ticking time bomb: Ageing population.* http://mark-ray.com/samples/AI--Ageing.pdf

American Holistic Nurses Association. (2015). *Holistic stress management for nurses.* http://www.ahna.org/Resources/Stress-Management

American Nurses Association. (2011). *2011 ANA health & safety survey: Hazards of the RN work environment.* https://www.nursingworld.org/~48dd70/globalassets/docs/ana/health-safetysurvey_mediabackgrounder_2011.pdf

American Sociological Association. (2014, August 19). Nurses driven mainly by a desire to help others are more likely to burn out. *Science Daily.* www.sciencedaily.com/releases/2014/08/140819082918.htm

ANA Enterprise. (2021, October 26). *New survey data: Thousands of nurses are still stressed, frustrated, and overwhelmed almost 2 years into the pandemic.* https://www.nursingworld.org/news/news-releases/2021/new-survey-data-thousands-of-nurses-are-still-stressed-frustrated-and-overwhelmed-almost-2-years-into-the-pandemic/

Centers for Medicare & Medicaid Services. (2014, October 6). *2014 definition stage 1 of meaningful use.* https://www.healthit.gov/providers-professionals/meaningful-use-definition-objectives

Daly, R. (2020, November 30). *Healthcare organizations prepare for sicker patients in 2021 due to deferred care.* Healthcare Financial Management Association. https://www.hfma.org/topics/hfm/2020/december/healthcare-organizations-prepare-sicker-patients-2021-deferred-care.html

Gupta, S. (2015, September 14). *Why America's nurses are burning out.* Everyday Health Media, LLC. http://www.everydayhealth.com/news/why-americas-nurses-are-burning-out/

Harrington, L., & Heidcamp, M. (2013, March). *The aging workforce: Challenges for the healthcare industry workforce.* The NTAR Leadership Center. https://heldrich.rutgers.edu/sites/default/files/2020-10/NTAR_Issue_Brief_Aging_Workforce_Health_Care_Final.pdf

Kelley, T. F., Brandon, D. H., & Docherty, S. L. (2011). Electronic nursing documentation as a strategy to improve quality of patient care [Abstract]. *Journal of Nursing Scholarship, 43*(2), 154–162.

Kotter, J. (2011, July 19). Can you handle an exponential rate of change? *Forbes*. http://www.forbes.com/sites/johnkotter/2011/07/19/can-you-handle-an-exponential-rate-of-change

Moore, D. (2020, May 19). Covid-19 patients are recovering, but with nowhere to go. *Boston Globe*. https://www.bostonglobe.com/2020/05/19/nation/covid-19-patients-are-recovering-with-nowhere-go/

National Council of State Boards of Nursing. (2018, November). *A nurse's guide to the use of social media*. https://www.ncsbn.org/brochures-and-posters/nurses-guide-to-the-use-of-social-media

Nielsen, K., & Munir, F. (2009). How do transformational leaders influence followers' affective well-being? Exploring the mediating role of self-efficacy. *Work & Stress, 23*(4), 313–329.

Putre, L. (2013). Generations in the workplace. *Hospital & Health Networks, 87*(1), 26–31.

Riffkin, R. (2014, December 18). Americans rate nurses highest on honesty, ethical standards. *Gallup*. http://www.gallup.com/poll/180260/americans-rate-nurses-highest-honesty-ethical-standards.aspx

Roberts, R., Grubb, P. L., & Grosch, J. W. (2012, June 25). Alleviating job stress in nurses. *Medscape*. http://www.medscape.com/viewarticle/765974

Slight, S. P., Berner, E. S., Galanter, W., Huff, S., Lambert, B. L., Lannon, C. L ., Lehmann, C. U., McCourt, B. J., McNamara, M., Menachemi, N., Payne, T. H., Spooner, S. A., Schiff, G. D., Wang, T. Y., Akincigil, A., Crystal, S., Fortmann, S. P., Vandermeer, M. L., & Bates, D. W. (2015). Meaningful use of electronic health records: Experiences from the field and future opportunities. *JMIR Medical Informatics, 3*(3), e30. https://www.ncbi.nlm.nih.gov/pmc/articles/PMC4704893/

Stimpfel, A. W., Sloane, D. M., & Aiken, L. H. (2012). The longer the shifts for hospital nurses, the higher the levels of burnout and dissatisfaction. *Health Affairs, 31*(11), 2501–2509.

US Bureau of Labor Statistics. (2018). *Occupational illnesses and injuries among registered nurses*. https://www.bls.gov/opub/mlr/2018/article/occupational-injuries-and-illnesses-among-registered-nurses.htm

US Bureau of Labor Statistics. (2020). *Occupational outlook handbook: Registered nurses*. https://www.bls.gov/ooh/healthcare/registered-nurses.htm

Waddill-Goad, S. (2013). *The development of a leadership fatigue questionnaire* [Doctoral dissertation, American Sentinel University].

# 1

# THE EFFECTS OF INHERENT STRESS

## OBJECTIVES

- Explore the stress-fatigue-burnout connection.
- Understand organizational stress.
- Understand the risks related to burnout.
- Define the health concerns resulting from stress, fatigue, and burnout.
- Define the practice considerations of managing stress.

Healthcare is an inherently stressful profession. Situations that providers of any healthcare service encounter on a regular basis are unimaginable to most people: life, death, and just about everything in between can be a "day in the life." Only recently have some of the experiences of nurses and other healthcare providers been profiled or highlighted by the news media, television, and social media—mostly due to the effects of the global COVID-19 pandemic. And most of it hasn't been good news. Although these venues do not always provide the most factual information, they have certainly raised public awareness—both about the impact to population health as a result of poor health choices and the realities of choosing nursing or healthcare as a profession.

## THE REALITY OF HEALTHCARE PROFESSIONAL STRESS

Stress at work is usually due to a number of intertwined issues. Ali et al. (2022) described the challenges for frontline nurses as the stress of taking care of patients, workload and assignments, communicating with colleagues, the nurse's or other healthcare worker's personal life, environment factors, emotional or physical stress, supervisory reports, community support, and problem solving, to name a few. Healthcare is a people business.

Where there are people, there will be clashes in thinking, values, and beliefs. In particular, nurses work with a variety of diverse types of people: different ethnic cultures, frames of reference, ages, faiths, educational levels, and more. The neutrality nurses and other healthcare workers must exhibit is sometimes in itself stress-producing when conflict arises and is contrary to their own feelings or beliefs. And nurses regularly play the role of peacemaker between many parties in an ambiguous industry filled with extreme chaos and change.

Dr. Hans Seyle (1956) has been credited as the first scientist to identify stress as a concept. His work, which spanned several decades beginning in the 1930s, identified stress as a difficult-to-define and subjective phenomenon.

Nevertheless, it is well-known and generally understood by most people that excessive stress leads to negative physical and emotional effects on the body and mind. A number of other researchers have since studied the effects of stress on the human body, the resulting adaption or maladaptation, and the ensuing consequences of each type of stress (positive, negative, and neutral stress—called *eustress*). Nurses and other healthcare providers often feel stress secondary to the work environment, whether it is real or perceived.

Waddill-Goad (2013) noted previous research over a decade, including work by Wells (2011), who cited Harvey et al. (2009), as well as Mimura and Griffiths (2003), suggesting that healthcare workers experience significantly more stress in the workplace than the wider working population. Thus, they must learn to tolerate a certain level of inherent stress that will always exist to some degree in healthcare settings, where there is a great degree of uncertainty and unpredictability. However, this is not generally taught in most formal education programs for the healthcare professions.

In addition, the healthcare environment has become quite complex and increasingly chaotic due to regulatory mandates, external influences, and excessive industry change. All healthcare providers must learn healthy skills to adapt to, effectively cope with, and adequately deflect and defuse day-to-day stress in order to survive. By becoming successful at stress-proofing and survival, healthcare providers can enhance their own practice and satisfaction at work. It is essential to recognize stress and the subsequent stressors early before you progress to fatigue and burnout.

Unfortunately, stress has a way of "sneaking up" on you in an insidious fashion. Sometimes before you know it, it is too late. It tends to come and go in irregular cycles or patterns, depending on life circumstances. Examples affecting the perception of stress include physical illness, injuries, mental exhaustion, fatigue, and attitudinal and/or behavior changes. Often, others recognize the warning signs before they become apparent to you. Loved ones and coworkers may recognize the signs before you do.

Before one reaches chronic fatigue (from stress) and realizes there might be a problem, burnout may be just around the corner. Nurses and other healthcare providers are especially at risk because they are experts in "carrying on" despite challenging conditions. For example, in the emergency department, a nurse will have several patients assigned for them to care for during their shift. One might be a patient with a lower acuity strain or sprain of a muscle or joint, a pediatric patient with a fever, a patient with unknown abdominal pain, and then in the adjacent room a patient might be complaining of back pain that turns into a major illness, such as a cardiac arrest from an abdominal aneurysm. In this type of stress-laden environment, care and tasks are constantly prioritized and reprioritized to get through the shift.

There is little time to process emotional or physical reactions predicated by stress. Stressful events, in any type of acute clinical environment, occur with some regularity. The inability or time to process the information leaves stress unchecked; that type of unresolved stress can layer upon previous experiences and progress over time from an acute issue to chronic fatigue and eventually lead to burnout.

## PRACTICE PEARLS

- Recognize that the healthcare environment is chaotic, fraught with unpredictability, and can be inherently stressful.
- Limit the effects of uncontrollable environmental influences that may cause stress by self-identifying early warning signals: feeling overwhelmed, experiencing mental and/or physical fatigue, and a change in thinking (positive to negative). These can all be remedied by taking a break.
- Learn to be emotionally aware. Emotional intelligence and practicing self-control are key strategies to overcome the effects of stress.

# THE PERSONAL STRESS–FATIGUE CONNECTION

In the 1940s, Forbes began writing about the symptoms of *fatigue*. He described it as strain from hurrying and worrying, emotional stress, and working to one's maximum capacity (Forbes, 1943). Fatigue produces nearly universal symptoms—people experience a similar feeling of "tiredness"—but the precipitating factors differ. The current dictionary definition of *fatigue* is "a state of mental or emotional strain or tension resulting from adverse or very demanding circumstances" (Dictionary.com, n.d.-a).

While some people experience fatigue from an extreme or serious illness, others experience it due to normal activities of daily life. A number of populations have been studied in relation to fatigue via a variety of research experiences: those with a multitude of illness types, industry- or job-specific occupational classes, as well as the public at large. Occupational health researchers estimate that 10% to 40% of the general population experiences fatigue on a regular basis (Waddill-Goad, 2013).

In 2020, the American Psychological Association's (APA) annual survey Stress in America found that year's survey results to be quite different from times past; they also noted the data has been collected annually since 2007 (APA, 2022). The 2020 survey revealed that most Americans have been profoundly affected by the global COVID-19 pandemic and have many concerns about the future. The unprecedented uncertainty is exacerbating symptoms for those who may have already had both diagnosed and undiagnosed anxiety, depression, and other mental health conditions (APA, 2022).

The entire population has experienced something none of us ever thought we would. It is believed by many that the disruption with school, jobs, the economy, supply chains, public health, and more will affect us for years to come. The World Health Organization (WHO) now estimates the worldwide excess death toll at nearly 15 million during 2020 and 2021 (WHO, 2022).

This estimate is many more deaths than a number of historic wars America has experienced—combined. It really is hard to fathom that level of death and destruction.

Nearly 8 in 10 people now say the global COVID-19 pandemic is a significant source of stress in their life (APA, 2022). The consequences of this stress were noted to be behavioral changes such as mood swings, angry outbursts, and physical body tension (APA, 2022). The same APA survey found that younger generations are suffering more mental and physical consequences from the level of uncertainty than older generations. For those of us who are older, we have life experience and lived through many changes in the country's overall direction, politics, economics, health, etc. in our lifetimes, giving us some hardiness for stress-producing events.

It is also well documented in the literature how the effects of stress and fatigue affect performance, skill, relationships, and health. Much of the research has been conducted outside of healthcare by the military, aviation, and nuclear industries; however, all of these industries, including healthcare, are considered to be high risk. Have we critically assessed nursing and other health professions and categorized them as high-risk careers? Is the risk of stress and its consequences taught in formal educational settings for healthcare professions? Is the risk well-known and understood by the practicing population of healthcare workers? The answer to all of these questions is not necessarily.

The North American Nursing Diagnosis Association (n.d.) defines *fatigue* as an overwhelming, sustained sense of exhaustion and decreased capacity for physical and mental work at the usual level. Fatigue is also described as acute or chronic, depending on the time frame it lasts and whether it succumbs to relieving factors. *Acute fatigue* is reversible and relieved by compensatory mechanisms; *chronic fatigue* is irreversible and impervious to compensation mechanisms (Beurskens et al., 2000). The difference between these two definitions is especially concerning with the length of time the global COVID-19 pandemic has persisted. What if too many healthcare workers suffer *irreversible* stress to the point of chronic fatigue?

Much of what has been studied and written about fatigue intertwines the two types—physical and mental fatigue, which may be difficult to separate, and one might potentiate the other. Which comes first? Could stress be leading to fatigue, thus causing unsafe conditions in the workplace? Or is fatigue leading to stress, thus causing unsafe conditions in the workplace? Is mental fatigue primary or secondary to physical fatigue? Can they both directly affect brain function? These are important and daunting questions that need to be addressed. Stress has the ability to change your brain (Mindful staff, 2016). You can read more here: https://www.mindful.org/what-stress-does-to-your-brain/.

A great deal of research exists relative to nurses and stress or fatigue for those working at the bedside. The occupational health industry has been concerned with fatigue as an unsafe malady in the workplace, and many think it is a risk that can be managed (Lerman et al., 2012). What about the bevy of other healthcare workers? What about healthcare leaders? Are the leaders aware of the consequences for themselves and the workforce they lead? Do leaders experience the same or similar symptoms? If so, what are the consequences to their leadership practice and decision-making?

Frings's (2011) study investigated inflexible thinking by those who are fatigued in rapidly changing work surroundings. Healthcare is a rapidly changing work environment. If inflexible thinking occurs in a chaotic environment, it could hypothetically be dangerous or even lethal. Early signs of stress and fatigue could signal performance danger when quick thinking is required.

## INEXTRICABLY LINKED: PERSONAL CHARACTERISTICS, RELATIONSHIPS, AND THE WORK ENVIRONMENT

Where we work and who we work with, in addition to our individual personality traits, is intertwined with work-related stress and the potential for burnout. Understanding these three drivers of stress and burnout are paramount to work fulfillment.

A nurse's or other healthcare provider's personality traits can be linked to the potential for burnout and the perception of work stress. Researchers have clearly demonstrated stress and burnout are not solely a result of working conditions. Not every employee has the same work experiences, is exposed to the same work conditions, develops work burnout, or has the same perception of stress. Two interesting relationships are, first, the neuroticism personality trait and the link to an individual's perception of exhaustion (Jennings, 2008). The second is the degree of a person's locus of control—or how much they believe they have control over their life—which has a relationship to stress and burnout.

Assessments for anxiety found a strong relationship to stress and work burnout (Jennings, 2008). Anxiety has two components—state anxiety, which is temporary and found when a person believes there is a threatening element of danger or harm, and trait anxiety, the more stable component that is considered a personality characteristic. In a separate study, a high degree of trait anxiety was a precursor to an individual's psychological stress (Jennings, 2008).

Further, the linkage a person has to other nurses and physicians they work with, direct management, and other departments they interface with had a direct impact on stress. Researchers also studied the link between interpersonal relationships with burnout and stress. Problematic interpersonal relationships with coworkers have the ability to increase the propensity for burnout, while positive experiences with coworkers positively impacted stress and burnout.

> To derive a better understanding of stress and burnout in the workplace, solid conceptualizations are needed that bring together the various pieces of the stress puzzle. At present, research is often conducted absent a solid theoretical and conceptual base. A more comprehensive blueprint of nurse stress and burnout in the work place needs to be developed. Empirical studies could then be conducted to investigate these very complex relationships, prospectively, over time. Once work stress is examined from a more solid theoretical and conceptual basis, then intervention studies can be initiated to assess the most useful ways to mitigate work stress. (Jennings, 2008, para. 30)

Conflict with physicians causes higher amounts of stress for nurses than poor interpersonal relationships with other nurses (Jennings, 2008). Specifically, the nurses' perception of verbal abuse involving physicians has more of an impact on stress and burnout. When looking at the frequency of verbal abuse at work, verbal abuse from another nurse was first, from patients was second, and from physicians was third (Jennings, 2008).

Having the right job in a supportive environment is key to any healthcare provider's work-related stress and the potential for burnout (Stone et al., 2008). For those searching for jobs, researching online hospital reviews (by current and past employees or patients), asking other peers their perception of the hospital, and researching public data for the hospital's publicly reported information can offer insight into the culture and priorities of the organization. During the interview process, it's important to ask about the culture of the unit for teamwork, conflict resolution, and management's actions when a nurse or physician exhibits inappropriate or abusive behaviors.

## PRACTICE PEARLS

- Recognize the connection between stress and fatigue.
- When you're feeling the effects of either stress or fatigue, choose to break the cycle.
- Address the cause of your stress and fatigue early on to prevent progression.
- Speak up about the effects of stress in your work environment.
- Ask your leaders what they are doing to combat stress and its effects in your work environment.

---

# ORGANIZATIONAL STRESS

The connections between stress, people, and organizations have been studied for decades. Most empirical studies of the connection between organizational stress and people blame discrepancies between human behavior and the organizational environment as the cause of stress (Edwards, 1992). Edwards (1992) suggested that this kind of stress stems from individuals' weaknesses in response to organizational stressors. Earlier, Lazarus and Folkman (1984) characterized stress as a process-based relationship, identifying three types of stress: positive, *eustress* (neutral) or *distress* (negative).

Lazarus and Folkman's transactional theory of stress and coping applies specifically to the nursing profession because nursing is a process. These researchers characterized stress between a person and their work environment as a changing process. They also heavily emphasized coping as a key strategy for adaption and optimal health. Nurses and other healthcare workers are immersed in a changing environment and must learn adequate coping mechanisms due to continual exposure to a plethora of adverse experiences. The ability to recognize stress—in real time—and its impact in the work environment is key to optimal performance in thinking and subsequent action. The healthy or positive experiences aren't usually the ones that leave a lasting impression. It is the negative experiences of grief, pain, and loss that all manage to take a toll and are frequently hard to forget.

Thus, effective coping is affected by *perception* (adequate or inadequate), *assessment* of the stressor (accurate or inaccurate), and *controllability* of the stressor (able or unable). What we think about becomes reality. Perception influences beliefs and behavior. If your ability to accurately perceive a situation or inadequately assess stressors is compromised, your response to the stressor may be insufficient. I know when I feel tired it makes a difference in how I respond to stress, and I bet it's the same for you, too. Stress, fatigue, and burnout all negatively influence your ability to precisely perceive, assess, and respond to internal and external stressors.

## PRACTICE PEARLS

- Work is only a small portion of your life. Treat it as such.
- Change the way you think to change your life.
- Think about what you need to do your best work or live your best life.
- All encounters, whether positive or negative, can be optimally reframed (with a shift in mindset) as a growth experience.

---

# THE RISK OF BURNOUT

Burnout first emerged as a social problem, not a scholarly construct. The concept was shaped by pragmatic practice rather than by academic concerns (Schaufeli et al., 1993). The study of burnout began in the 1970s as a result of a combination of personal and professional circumstances. Freudenberger (1974) coined the term "burnout," and measuring it has been a controversial issue ever since (Schaufeli & Van Dierendonck, 1993). Nearly simultaneously in the 1970s, those in research and practice began to study burnout. Researchers have since found that studying it is somewhat difficult because fatigue leading to other symptoms and eventually to burnout can have vague and variable descriptions. As study progressed over two decades into the 1990s, the scholarly literature reported more than 100 physical and mental symptoms describing the phenomenon or concept of burnout.

The most widely used definition for *burnout* to date is from Maslach and Jackson (1981), who describe it as a syndrome of emotional exhaustion, depersonalization, and reduced personal accomplishment. More contemporary definitions (after over 50 years of study) now found in the literature include new wording relative to an erosion of engagement. *Engagement* is newer nomenclature relative to satisfaction and has been measured by surveys in healthcare for patients, providers, and employees in recent times. Unfortunately, burnout has been associated with working conditions in the nursing profession for quite some time (O'Mahony, 2011).

O'Mahony (2011) summarized the consequences of burnout (based on previous decades of research) as low morale, increased absenteeism from sickness, decreased effectiveness and productivity, poorer job performance and patient care, and higher staff turnover. In 2015, another impending nursing shortage was on the horizon and an increased need for health services looming due to the aging population. At the time we professed that nursing could not afford to lose well-educated and trained nurses. Unfortunately, the global COVID-19 pandemic fueled many of the problems known in healthcare and compelled many healthcare workers (including nurses) to exit their workplaces, and some chose to leave the profession altogether.

Nursing and healthcare must be willing to change the culture of accepted stress, subsequent behavioral responses, and stress-producing work environments. The risk of nurses and others working in healthcare burning out is just too high in the current systems for practice. The aging of the population and the increased demand for healthcare services on the horizon signal a critical need for passionate and healthy providers.

Little information exists relative to the consequences of burnout in the nursing leadership population. It is suspected that when nurse leaders reach the point of burnout in their chosen career path, they suddenly do one of the following: take a break, change specialties by returning to clinical practice, or even quit nursing altogether. Numerous studies suggest nurse leaders are generally older than the average nurse due to the experience and expertise required by these roles (Waddill-Goad, 2013). In addition, nurse leaders may be more susceptible to fatigue secondary to stress-producing role demands. They often have high levels of responsibility, their role requires 24/7 availability, and there are few limitations regarding the amount of time they spend doing work-related tasks. Each of these factors increases the risk of burnout.

A recent study, using an emergency nurse sample, cited support from one's nurse manager as one of the most influential drivers for nursing burnout (Hunsaker et al., 2015). It is also well-known that most people leave their supervisors, not necessarily their position, when moving jobs. In addition, a correlation between burnout and turnover for intensive care unit (ICU) nurses was established (Shoorideh et al., 2015). Thus, burned out nurses and other healthcare workers will look for a change; both studies highlight the importance of nursing and other leaders knowing the symptoms of burnout, having a positive relationship with other team members, and especially forging a healthy bond between leaders and their direct reports.

Henry (2014) described six areas prone to increase the potential for burnout particularly in nurses; she adapted her conclusion of precursors to burnout from a previous study performed nearly a decade before by Maslach and Leiter in 2005:

- **Workload:** The amount of work to complete in a day and the frequency of surprising or unexpected events
- **Control:** Participation in decisions that affect the work environment and quality of leadership in upper management
- **Reward:** Recognition for achievement and opportunities for bonuses or raises
- **Community:** Frequency of supportive work interactions and close personal friendships at work

- **Fairness:** Management's dedication to giving everyone equal consideration; clear and open procedures for allocating rewards or promotion
- **Values:** Potential to contribute to the larger community and confidence that the organizational mission is meaningful

Each of Henry's (2014) described elements could easily be applied to others in healthcare. These precursors drive people to work excessively; skip meals and breaks; feel unappreciated, unrecognized, and unsupported by management; and experience cultures opposite to transparency, truth, and fairness. All these examples may lead nurses in any professional role or setting and other healthcare providers to experience burnout.

### PRACTICE PEARLS

- Learn to recognize the early symptoms that may lead to burnout.
- Find a work culture that fits your professional and personal values.
- Learn to value taking time to care for yourself.
- Know your mental, emotional, physical, and spiritual triggers before you hit your limit!

---

## HOW IS BURNOUT DIFFERENT FROM POST-TRAUMATIC STRESS DISORDER (PTSD)?

Emergency workers in Pisa, Italy, were studied in order to investigate the relationship between PTSD and burnout, as well as lifetime mood disorders, namely depression. These workers were selected because of their high exposure to traumatic and stressful work environments. More than half of the workers had at least one PTSD symptom in the *Diagnostic and Statistical Manual of Mental Disorders* (DSM-5) diagnostic criteria. Almost 16% reported all PTSD symptoms, and a significant correlation between PTSD and mood disorders, namely depression, was found. Using the compassion fatigue subscale, significant associations were identified with burnout and depression. This led to a link between PTSD, burnout, and lifetime mood disorders, particularly depression (Carmassi et al., 2020).

The stress of emotionally charged decision-making, heavy workloads, and extended work hours in emergency departments all contribute to burnout (Lall et al., 2019). Burnout can affect physical and mental health, cause sleep pattern changes, fatigue, difficulty concentrating, and irritability (Halbesleben et al., 2008). Burnout also impacts quality of care, patient outcomes, and absenteeism of staff (Halbesleben et al., 2008).

Depression, PTSD, and burnout have negative impacts on employees, patients, and organizations. Carmassi et al. (2020) suggested identifying at-risk individuals through screening tools or self-awareness and implementing prevention strategies to decrease the number of healthcare workers impacted. In addition to the categorized risk factors in Table 1.1, being young, female, having lower professional education, depressive psychological characteristics, and pre-existing mental health issues are contributing risk factors (Laposa et al., 2003; Mealer et al., 2009; Olashore et al., 2018).

Beyond screening employees for burnout/PTSD/depression, organizations can implement programs proven to improve resiliency against stressful and traumatic events. Employee reward systems, strategies to strengthen peer and manager relationships, and well-designed organizational structures are examples of programs found to help prevent employee burnout/PTSD (Schneider & Weigl, 2018). Employers should also support "protected" time for employees to seek professional help if needed (Schuster, 2021).

## PRACTICE PEARLS

- Find ways to gain control over tasks you are responsible for in the work environment.
- Invest in personal pursuits that bring joy and relieve work stress.
- Consider formal counseling if experiencing depressive symptoms.

---

Employees can self-intervene to reverse the trajectory of burnout. They may also be able to manage PTSD symptoms to prevent escalation to depression and negative outcomes. Suggestions include developing personal methods to achieve at least some control when work environments are chaotic, and investing in activities that bring relief from the burden of caring for others. When these interventions are not sufficient and additional support is needed, more formal mental health counseling should be considered. Healthcare workers should never perceive burnout as personal failure (Schuster, 2021).

The Mayo Clinic provides definitions and descriptions of both PTSD (https://www.mayoclinic.org/diseases-conditions/post-traumatic-stress-disorder/symptoms-causes/syc-20355967) and burnout (https://www.mayoclinic.org/healthy-lifestyle/adult-health/in-depth/burnout/art-20046642) on their educational webpage. The Mayo Clinic defines *PTSD* as "a mental health condition that's triggered by a terrifying event" with symptoms worsening or existing for months or years (2019, para. 1). Symptoms of PTSD can begin immediately after such an event or can start months to years after the event. The symptoms themselves come in four categories and can vary over time. The categories are:

- Intrusive memories
- Avoidance
- Negative changes in thinking and mood
- Changes in physical and emotional reactions

The Mayo Clinic (2021) defines *burnout* as a special type of work-related stress with physical and emotional exhaustion often related to a sense of reduced accomplishment and loss of personal identity.

A side-by-side risk factor, symptom, and complication list identified from our research of the literature is in Table 1.1. It identifies the similarities and differences in the disorders of PTSD and burnout.

Why do some people get PTSD or experience burnout and others don't? No one is really sure. The Mayo Clinic suggests one cause might be inherited mental health disorders. Many researchers associate a family history of mental health issues such as anxiety and depression to PTSD and to burnout.

**TABLE 1.1** COMPARISON BETWEEN PTSD AND BURNOUT

| | PTSD | Burnout |
|---|---|---|
| Risk Factors | Intense or long-lasting trauma<br>Jobs that increase trauma exposure<br>Mental health problems: depression/anxiety<br>Substance use/abuse<br>Lack of support system | Heavy workload and long hours or dysfunctional work dynamics<br>Being in a helping profession such as healthcare<br>Feeling that you have no control over your work/unclear expectations<br>Struggle with work/life balance<br>Lack of support system |
| Symptoms | Recurrent unwanted distressing memories or dreams of the event/reliving it<br>Severe emotional distress or physical reactions to reminders of the event<br>Avoiding thinking/talking about the event, avoiding reminders<br>Negative thoughts | Feeling as though you have to drag yourself to work/trouble getting started at work<br>Unexplained headaches/stomach or bowel problems<br>Little energy/productivity<br>Becoming cynical or critical at work<br>Feeling disillusioned about the job |

*continues*

**TABLE 1.1** COMPARISON BETWEEN PTSD AND BURNOUT (CONT.)

| | PTSD | Burnout |
|---|---|---|
| | Feelings of hopelessness/ detachment<br>Difficulty maintaining relationships<br>Loss of interest in things once enjoyed<br>Emotional numbness<br>Self-destructive behavior<br>Trouble sleeping/ concentrating<br>Easily startled, always on guard<br>Irritability, anger, aggressive outbursts<br>Overwhelming guilt/shame | Irritability/impatience with coworkers/customers<br>Difficulty concentrating<br>Little satisfaction from achievements<br>Using food/drugs/alcohol to feel or stop feeling<br>Changes in sleep habits |
| Complications | Depression/anxiety<br>Substance use/abuse<br>Eating disorders<br>Suicidal thoughts/actions | Excessive stress<br>Substance use/abuse<br>Type 2 diabetes/hypertension/ heart disease<br>Fatigue/insomnia<br>Sadness/irritability/anger<br>Vulnerability to illness<br>Depression leading to suicide |

# HEALTH CONCERNS RELATED TO STRESS AND WORKAHOLISM

Enlightened organizations have begun to take an interest in the abstract connections between mind, body, wellness, and health (Waddill-Goad, 2013).

A healthy organizational workforce makes for a healthy organizational bottom line: fewer costs for consumption of healthcare; less absenteeism; lower vacancy rates; lower turnover; improved employee satisfaction with the work environment; better customer experiences; higher quality metrics; better productivity; and satisfactory financial outcomes. Healthcare is a tough business requiring 24-hour-per-day and 7-day-per-week availability of adequate resources and highly trained personnel. The literature is rife with numerous examples citing health concerns relative to shift rotation and patterns of working off-shifts.

Nurses and other caregivers must begin to care for themselves, as they do others, by making their own good health and illness prevention a top priority. Not only will individuals benefit from the results, but their patients and associated organizations will as well. If nurses and other healthcare providers continue "business as usual" in their stress-laden work environments, their future individual health, career satisfaction, and success, as well as organizational outcomes, may all be at risk.

Nurses also have a strong tendency to become workaholics. Working fewer days with longer shifts allows nurses to take second jobs, work per diem, and pick up extra shifts in their primary place of employment. The definition of *workaholism* is to work compulsively at the expense of other pursuits (Dictionary.com, n.d.-b). Interestingly, the organization called Workaholics Anonymous was formally started by a *nurse* in the early 1980s in California. At nearly the same time, in various locations across the world, people began to notice a pathological aspect to work-related activity. They noticed that pathological activities, including work, were affecting them like other detrimental forms of addiction (Workaholics Anonymous, 2015).

Hospitals can fuel workaholic behavior for nurses and nurse leaders by providing less than optimal resources. Caring for patients and their caregivers is a common theme with nurses and workaholic behaviors. Too often the nurse or nurse leader is drawn into the pitfalls of being *needed* by the organization, their boss, or their peers to the detriment of themselves. These internal drivers or pressures are different than working an extra shift or just putting in long hours at the office. Nurses and leaders can be compelled by these internal pressures to keep working despite the negative consequences. Even when the person is not at work, they keep thinking about work. This sole focus on work is not healthy, as described by Clark in an article for the APA (2016).

Workaholism impacts overall work-life balance, which can blur the boundaries between a person's working life and personal life. Often, the balance is not evenly divided. There may be times when work increases more per workday than others. The problem comes when the time spent at work and the time at home thinking about work is routinely more than personal time off work.

This doesn't mean one should be sacrificed for the other. Rather, find a healthy balance where you can dedicate time to finding joy outside of work and not be consumed with thoughts about work. There can be a degree of homeostasis in work-life balance with good boundaries. Without limitations, the balance shifts and can have negative consequences on the other. The core of work-life balance is paying attention to the time spent for each—to ensure adequate mental well-being as well as physical well-being.

The symptoms of workaholism include higher work-related stress and job burnout rates, anger, depression, anxiety, and other psychosomatic symptoms (Osterweil, n.d.). Most workaholics are in denial about their behavior and their condition, and they often wonder why others do not work as hard as they do. The hallmark characteristics of workaholism as identified by Workaholics Anonymous (2015) are:

- A strong internal drive, in which work is a priority over other important things in life
- An inability to disengage or disconnect from work
- Working in excess of 40 hours per week on a routine basis
- Work negatively affecting relationships with family and friends due to obsession

- "Normal" practices are defined by routinely working while on vacation, while eating meals, on weekends, in bed, and while driving

While some of these characteristics may not be applicable to a clinical or bedside nurse's role, they certainly apply to a nursing leader or other healthcare leader's role. This definition and individual assessment should lead the industry to question if current work-related role expectations are healthy. Have we taken the consequences seriously? Are we promoting bad behavior with unrealistic expectations? Are healthcare workers really setting a good example for what good health and well-being looks like? Are healthcare leaders tuned in to being good role models for others?

## PRACTICE PEARLS

- Establish solid boundaries for hours of work, rest, and relaxation.
- Practice healthy habits: Engage in regular exercise, eat a balanced and healthy diet, get the recommended seven to nine hours of sleep per night, and take breaks when needed.
- Engage in positive coping strategies and change your current behavior. A few suggestions to decrease stress include talking about the stress, writing your thoughts and feelings in a journal, focusing on what you are grateful for, and taking regularly planned breaks from stressful conditions.
- Consider a planned "digital detox." Personal and professional technology advances and the resulting 24/7 availability can be an overwhelming source of stress and can lead to technology fatigue. Examples include limiting or eliminating access while on vacation, limitations on days off, and less access during non-work periods throughout the day. Ask yourself the following question, "Do I really need to be this available now?"

# PRACTICE CONSIDERATIONS

Theories, conceptual frameworks, and models are not discovered; they are created and invented based on facts, observable evidence, and the originator's ingenuity in pulling facts together and making sense of them (Polit & Beck, 2012). Nursing and other healthcare professions need a successful prescription to combat stress, fatigue, and burnout. Self-care is not selfish. In fact, taking better care of yourself allows you to be fully present in caring for others. Adaption and influence are known to affect performance (Waddill-Goad, 2013), and those working in healthcare need to learn how to compensate for stressful work environments.

An assessment—both individual and organizational—must be considered to identify the sources of stress. Individuals must take responsibility and learn to assess the predictors or precursors of stress, fatigue, and burnout. Organizations and individuals must share responsibility for the consequences of stress, fatigue, and burnout in the social environment. The responsibility for organizational stress lies solely within healthcare and other business entities. The leaders, particularly in healthcare, need to become adept at assessing their own organizations relative to the potential for stress, fatigue, and burnout for themselves and for their workforce. Leaders should be expected to initiate proactive steps to prevent the consequences of stress, fatigue, and burnout. This includes anyone in a leadership role.

Changes to current policy, practice, and procedure; role responsibilities; organizational design; and workload must be carefully planned and executed. Healthcare personnel are passionate and want to feel energized from their work. The norm of feeling overwhelmed should no longer be accepted or tolerated as "business as usual." A growing body of literature suggests that organizational leadership is closely associated with a variety of employee and organizational outcomes—the good and the bad (Kelloway & Barling, 2010).

Leaders at all levels in healthcare must take note of the current state of affairs and be willing to look in the mirror to see if their influence requires a change in course. For example, a supervisor must be willing to evaluate how their assigned shift runs: Do their coworkers get scheduled breaks? Are the patient assignments fair and equitable? Are they viewed by their peers as helpful and effective in the role? Leaders must have a level of introspection to assess their leadership style and its effect on their team. Organizations may benefit from "secret shopping" in the form of a survey for staff to evaluate the leader's performance in relation to reducing the stress on a given unit.

Nursing has traditionally promoted individuals who demonstrate independence, clinical competence, and enhanced productivity (Kerfoot, 2013). The same could be said for others in healthcare. In the future, traits such as a commitment to health and well-being should be equally considered. Commitment begins with the interview process and should be an integral component in the leader's annual job performance evaluation. We are in the business of health after all—and this should include promotion, prevention, and a back-to-basics philosophy. All leaders must adopt effective strategies for positively coping with their own stressors and then convey those abilities to influence the workforce they lead.

Richards (2013, p. 94) questioned whether a "scattered and splattered attention and drive-by focus" in the haste to get more done is hardwiring caregivers for disaster. The pace of nursing and healthcare continues to escalate in both speed and intensity. Richards (2013) calls *wellpower* a learned nursing ability for self-assessment, recognition of stress, and positive correction to adapt to stressful conditions. Adaption is believed to preserve wellpower.

Today's nurses and all others working in healthcare need wellpower. They must also embrace a questioning attitude, one of rational inquiry. Instead of focusing on, "How did things get to be this way?" (thinking in the past), a change in thinking such as, "What could be done to improve the current situation?" (thinking in the present) could be very beneficial. Participating in change may reduce stress from actual change.

Doing things the way we've always done them won't lead us to a better future. The global COVID-19 pandemic exposed many of the chinks in the armor in healthcare. In fact, it showed things could get a lot worse before they get better. The external changes in the healthcare industry are driving internal changes in practice (thankfully). Rather than resisting change, embracing it and being a part of improvement can be energizing. There are so many opportunities at present for system redesign: how we care for patients, expansion of telehealth, education and real corporate incentives for health promotion and illness prevention, etc.

Caring is the core business of healthcare (Williams et al., 2011), and nurses and other healthcare workers need to first care for themselves. We need to focus on health, wellness, and well-being. We must design and implement effective methods to prevent or decrease the effects of stress, fatigue, and burnout.

## CONCLUSION

This chapter introduced the timely topics of stress, fatigue, and burnout in nursing and healthcare. Highlights included a historical overview, relevant definitions, and real-life examples of how to decrease stress, the resulting fatigue, and the potential for burnout. While environmental stressors may seem impervious to change, we can change ourselves and our organizations one day at a time. We can change our response to stressors. However, this type of change won't be easy. It will require a deeper awareness of the negative effects of the present circumstances, clear recognition of the stressors and their impact, and thoughtful action to achieve a different response. The next chapter will explore and connect challenges in the healthcare business environment to what nurses and other healthcare providers feel in their practice.

# REFERENCES

Ali, H., Fatemi, Y., Ali, D., Hamasha, M., & Hamasha, S. (2022, May 25). Investigating frontline nurse stress: Perception of job demands, organizational support, and social support during the current COVID-19 pandemic. *Frontiers in Public Health.* https://doi.org/10.3389/fpubh.2022.839600

American Psychological Association. (2022). *Stress in America™ 2020: A national mental health crisis.* https://www.apa.org/news/press/releases/stress/2020/report-october#:~:text=More%20than%203%20in%204,history%20that%20they%20can%20remember

Beurskens A. J. H. M., Bültmann, U., Kant, I., Jan, H., Vercoulen, M. M., Bleijenberg, G., & Swaen, G. M. H. (2000). Fatigue among working people: Validity of a questionnaire measure. *Occupational Environmental Medicine, 57*(5), 353–357. https://doi.org/10.1136/oem.57.5.353

Carmassi, C., Bertelloni, C. A., Avella, M. T., Cremone, I., Massimetti, E., Corsi, M., & Dell'Osso, L. (2020). PTSD and burnout are related to lifetime mood spectrum in emergency healthcare operator. *Clinical Practice & Epidemiology in Mental Health, 16,* 165–173. https://doi.org/10.2174/1745017902016010165

Clark, M. A. (2016). *Workaholism: It's not just long hours on the job.* APA. https://www.apa.org/science/about/psa/2016/04/workaholism

Dictionary.com. (n.d.-a). *Fatigue.* https://www.dictionary.com/browse/fatigue

Dictionary.com. (n.d.-b). *Workaholic.* https://www.dictionary.com/browse/workaholic

Edwards, J. R. (1992). A cybernetic theory of stress, coping, and well-being in organizations. *Academy of Management Review, 17*(2), 238–274. https://doi.org/10.2307/258772

Forbes, W. (1943). Problems arising in the study of fatigue. *Psychosomatic Medicine, 5,* 155–157.

Freudenberger, H. (1974). Staff burn-out. *Journal of Social Sciences, 30*(1), 159–165. https://doi.org/10.1111/j.1540-4560.1974.tb00706.x

Frings, D. (2011, August 16). *Working together can help battle the effects of fatigue* [Press release]. APA. https://www.apa.org/news/press/releases/2011/08/fatigue-effects

Halbesleben, J. R. B., Wakefield, B. J., Wakefield, D. S., & Cooper, L. B. (2008). Nurse burnout and patient safety outcomes: Nurse safety perception versus reporting behavior. *Western Journal of Nursing Research, 30*(5), 560–577. http://dx.doi.org/10.1177/0193945907311322

Henry, B. J. (2014). Nursing burnout interventions: What is being done? *Clinical Journal of Oncology Nursing, 18*(2), 211–214. https://doi.org/10.1188/14.CJON.211-214

Hunsaker, S., Chen, H., Maughan, D., & Heaston, S. (2015). Factors that influence the development of compassion fatigue, burnout, and compassion satisfaction in emergency department nurses. *Journal of Nursing Scholarship, 47*(2), 186–194. https://doi.org/10.1111/jnu.12122

Jennings, B. M. (2008). Work stress and burnout among nurses: Role of the work environment and working conditions. *Patient safety and quality: An evidence-based handbook for nurses.* Agency for Healthcare Research and Quality.

Kelloway, E. K., & Barling, J. (2010). Leadership development as an intervention in occupational health psychology. *Work & Stress, 24*(3), 260–279. https://doi.org/10.1080/02678373.2010.518441

Kerfoot, K. M. (2013). Are you tired? Overcoming leadership styles that create leader fatigue. *Nursing Economics, 31*(3), 146, 147–151.

Lall, M. D., Gaeta, T. J., Chung, A. S., Dehon, E., Malcom, W., Ross, A., Way, D. P., Weichenthal, L., & Himelfarb, N. T. (2019). Assessment of physician well-being, part one: Burnout and other negative states. *Western Journal of Emergency Medicine, 20*(2), 278–290. http://dx.doi.org/10.5811/westjem.2019.1.39665

Laposa, J. M., Alden, L. E., & Fullerton, L. M. (2003). Work stress and posttraumatic stress disorder in ED nurses/personnel. *Journal of Emergency Nursing, 29*(1), 23–28. http://dx.doi.org/10.1067/men.2003.7

Lazarus, R. S., & Folkman, S. (1984). *Stress, appraisal, and coping.* Springer.

Lerman, S. E., Eskin, E., Flower, D. J., George, E. C., Gerson, B., Hartenbaum, N., Hursh, S. R., & Moore-Ede, M. (2012). Fatigue risk management in the workplace. *Journal of Occupational and Environmental Medicine, 54*(2), 231–258. https://doi.org/10.1097/JOM.0b013e318247a3b0

Maslach, C., & Jackson, S. E. (1981). The measurement of experienced burnout. *Journal of Organizational Behavior, 2*(2), 99–113. https://doi.org/10.1002/job.4030020205

Mayo Clinic Staff. (2019, July 6). *Post-traumatic stress disorder (PTSD).* https://www.mayoclinic.org/diseases-conditions/post-traumatic-stress-disorder/symptoms-causes/syc-20355967

Mayo Clinic Staff. (2021, June 5). *Job burnout: How to spot it and take action.* https://www.mayoclinic.org/healthy-lifestyle/adult-health/in-depth/burnout/art-20046642

Mealer, M., Burnham, E. L., Goode, C. J., Rothbaum, B., & Moss, M. (2009). The prevalence and impact of post-traumatic stress disorder and burnout syndrome in nurses. *Depression and Anxiety, 26*(12), 1118–1126. http://dx.doi.org/10.1002/da.20631

Mindful staff. (2016, February 3). What stress does to your brain. *Mindful.* https://www.mindful.org/what-stress-does-to-your-brain/

North American Nursing Diagnoses Association. (n.d.). *Nursing diagnoses for fatigue.* http://nandanursingdiagnoses.blogspot.com/2011/11/nursing-diagnoses-for-fatigue.html

Olashore, A. A., Akanni, O. O., Molebatsi, K., & Ogunjumo, J. A. (2018). Post-traumatic stress disorder among the staff of a mental health hospital: Prevalence and risk factors. *South African Journal of Psychiatry, 24,* 1222. http://dx.doi.org/10.4102/sajpsychiatry.v24i0.1222

O'Mahony, N. (2011). Nurse burnout and the working environment. *Emergency Nurse, 19*(5), 30–37. https://doi.org/10.7748/en2011.09.19.5.30.c8704

Osterweil, N. (n.d.). Are you a workaholic? *WebMD.* https://webmd.com/balance/features/are-you-a-workaholic

Polit, D. F., & Beck, C. T. (2012). *Nursing research: Generating and assessing evidence for nursing practice* (9th ed., Rev.). Wolters Kluwer; Lippincott, Williams & Wilkins.

Richards, K. (2013). Wellpower: The foundation of innovation. *Nursing Economics, 31*(2), 94–98.

Schaufeli, W. B., Maslach, C., & Marek, T. (Eds.) (1993). *Professional burnout: Recent developments in theory and research.* Taylor & Francis.

Schaufeli, W. B., & Van Dierendonck, D. (1993). The construct validity of two burnout measures. *Journal of Organizational Behavior, 14*(7), 631–647. https://doi.org/10.1002/job.4030140703

Schneider, A., & Weigl, M. (2018). Associations between psychosocial work factors and provider mental well-being in emergency departments: A systematic review. *PLoS One, 13*(6). http://dx.doi.org/10.1371/journal.pone.0197375

Schuster, B. L. (2021). Burnout, posttraumatic stress disorder, or both – listen carefully! *The American Journal of Medicine, 134*(6), 705–706. https://doi.org/10.1016/j.amjmed.2021.02.006

Seyle, H. (1956). *The stress of life* (1st ed.). McGraw-Hill.

Shoorideh, F. A., Ashktorab, T., Yaghmaei, F., & Majd, H. A. (2015). Relationship between ICU nurses' moral distress with burnout and anticipated turnover. *Nursing Ethics, 22*(1), 64–76. https://doi.org/10.1177/0969733014534874

Stone, P., Hughes, R., & Dailey, M. (2008). Creating a safe and high-quality health care environment. In *Patient safety and quality: An evidence-based handbook for nurses.* Agency for Healthcare Research and Quality.

Waddill-Goad, S. (2013). *The development of a leadership fatigue questionnaire* [Doctoral dissertation, American Sentinel University].

Williams, R. L., McDowell, J. B., & Kautz, D. (2011). A caring leadership model for nursing's future. *International Journal for Human Caring, 15*(1), 31–35. https://doi.org/10.20467/1091-5710.15.1.31

Workaholics Anonymous. (2015). *The history of Workaholics Anonymous*. https://workaholics-anonymous.org/contact-us/about-w-a

World Health Organization. (2022, May 5). *14.9 million excess deaths associated with the COVID-19 pandemic in 2020 and 2021.* [News release]. https://www.who.int/news/item/05-05-2022-14.9-million-excess-deaths-were-associated-with-the-covid-19-pandemic-in-2020-and-2021

# 2

# A SLICE OF REALITY

## OBJECTIVES

- Understand that healthcare is a business.
- Consider how organizational demands create stress.
- Explore how consumers affect the healthcare business.
- Explore how regulations and government affect healthcare business.
- Consider how transitioning to practice can help new graduates deal with stress.

When a person makes the decision to seek a career in nursing or healthcare, the most common reason is their innate desire to genuinely help people and care for them in times of need. The person must thrive on being challenged and enjoy the complexity of a difficult academic science curriculum. Many future nurses and other healthcare workers, were inspired by a person in the healthcare industry they met, who may have been a friend or a relative. They might also have been a patient or were involved with someone who was seriously ill. And they may have had the opportunity to admire the skill, dedication, and passion of the people who cared for their friend or family member.

The business side of healthcare is usually not one of the reasons why a person chooses healthcare as a profession. However, it is vitally important to remember healthcare is a business. The business of healthcare is complex and challenging; it will impact every healthcare worker's job in almost every specialty area they might encounter in their career. Every person in the United States and throughout the world feels the burden for access and the rising cost of healthcare. The cost of healthcare in the US specifically is unaffordable for many of its residents, as costs have continued to steadily escalate. By 2020, spending had reached nearly $4.1 trillion, with nearly one-third attributed to hospital care alone (Centers for Medicare & Medicaid Services [CMS], 2021d).

Healthcare is big business. Leaders in healthcare, including all members of the healthcare team, have the ability to influence much of what transpires in the industry. As an informed and responsible member of the healthcare team, we all need to perform at a higher level than ever before. We also need to be aware of the results of our decision-making. Stress, fatigue, and burnout can affect any person's ability to optimally perform their job. Not understanding how these factors influence patient outcomes and affect the cost of healthcare and can be extremely detrimental—both to the providers of care and their organizations.

# UNDERSTANDING THE BUSINESS OF HEALTHCARE

Healthcare is changing, and the days of "business as usual" are over. Many of healthcare's old systems simply do not work in the current environment. The global COVID-19 pandemic exposed much of the fragility in the systems. Healthcare in the US, in every aspect, is struggling with providing quality care in an economic environment where profit margins impact rising costs for labor, equipment, and supplies; building maintenance and capital improvements; as well as technology. Reduced reimbursement by both government and private insurance providers, and a continual push to improve the quality of care for well-informed consumers, is stretching the current system's limits.

For several years, both healthcare leaders and government policy-makers have used strategic tactics to reduce the cost of healthcare while attempting to improve the quality. The focus has been on improving patient safety by reducing errors, educating the public to be better healthcare consumers, forcing healthcare institutions to move to an electronic medical or health record, and increasing the investment in people whose sole focus is to identify and prevent medical fraud. In addition, the cost pressures presented by shortages of personnel are challenging even the best-managed organizations. Two studies, one in 2011 and one in 2018, refuted the claim that temporary nurses cost more than permanent nursing staff when *all* costs are taken into account: benefits, orientation, recruiting, administrative time, non-productive time (education), etc. (AMN Healthcare, 2018; Morgan Hunter HealthSearch, 2011). Has this changed since the COVID-19 pandemic? Do the *total* costs for temporary healthcare labor now really exceed a permanent hire?

I've always thought an interesting experiment might be to outsource an entire department of nurses to see the *true* impact on cost, productivity, patient satisfaction, quality, provider experience, etc. If we used all the of current metrics—we could truly see the difference. Temporary nurses are focused on providing a needed service, often on short notice. The best ones are readily able to assimilate into the staff milieu of a given area with little onboarding. Their incentives are equally aligned with the organization for providing an excellent outcome-focused service or product. And, should they not be up to the task or be as competent as expected, they can be nearly immediately replaced (by the next shift unless they are a danger to others).

There are other industries where the entire workforce is "temporary." Think about professional sports or any other contracted service. The engagement is time-limited and purely based on performance. If they don't perform, the arrangement is modified or terminated. I wonder if this would change the face of healthcare in a positive way by raising commitment and performance? I also wonder if providers of healthcare would feel differently if the arrangement could add more value for their contribution.

One area of healthcare where this type of thinking is more common is in the for-profit arena. Investments by private equity in healthcare have nearly tripled since 2015 (Medical News Today, 2022). As a result, approximately 25% of all hospitals in the US are now owned by private equity. Private equity is all about a return on investment or profit. What remains to be seen is the true impact on quality in healthcare.

In the past, healthcare has been a supply-driven system organized around how physicians practice (Porter & Lee, 2013). The movement toward a patient-centered system focused on the needs of patients is the path of the future. How does healthcare change a currently fragmented, physician-driven system to a value-based healthcare system? The patient-centered movement began with the 2006 book *Redefining Healthcare*, by Michael Porter and Elizabeth Teisberg.

The authors first introduced a value agenda. Porter and Teisberg set forth a "vision for the healthcare system where everything in the system is aligned around its fundamental purpose—patient health" (2006, p. 381). This unique vision painted a different picture of a future healthcare system. The key initiatives were integration strategies that increased value to the patient, rather than just increasing *volume* of the services provided.

To create this new healthcare system, these authors described how all healthcare clinical professionals, leaders, insurance companies, governmental leaders, technology developers, and pharmaceutical companies must look at what they are doing to improve value for the patient. In addition, they must be sure the service they provide is available to all patients equally (Porter & Teisberg, 2006). Today, now a decade and a half later, we know that is not the case.

The timing for envisioning a new healthcare paradigm couldn't be better after experiencing the multi-year global COVID-19 pandemic. Much has changed in the world of work and a true reset is in order. We must take our valuable lessons learned, adopt new best practices leveraging technology, focus on improving the nation's health (versus treating disease), and more.

### PRACTICE PEARLS

- Identify and eliminate process or system waste in your workplace.
- Be involved in staff councils or committees to affect clinical practice and operational decisions.
- Caring and compassion are the heart of nursing and healthcare; be a patient advocate and the communication link to other healthcare disciplines to deliver best-in-class care.
- Patients trust nurses; nurses are the best people to discuss their fears and concerns. Use this leverage to offer reasonable solutions to patient health and well-being challenges.

---

## ORGANIZATIONAL DEMANDS: PILLARS, METRICS, AND TARGETS

Healthcare is a very data-intensive business. In recent years, most organizations have adopted a cache of tools from general business models to track, trend, and compare outcomes, often referred to as dashboards. The generic example in Table 2.1 shows how a system of "pillars"—each a specific aspect of a business—can be displayed with measurable goals, targets, results, and action plans for course correction. It's important to understand how your organization views success. Do they measure against national, regional, or local benchmarks or prior year performance? Do they look at rates or raw numbers when evaluating goals and measuring improvement?

### TABLE 2.1 SYSTEM OF PILLARS WITH MEASURABLE GOALS AND TARGETS

| XYZ Valley Community Hospital, Departmental Strategic Plan Support | | | | | |
|---|---|---|---|---|---|
| Performance and Quality Improvement Measures | | | | | |
| 90-Day Action Plans | Target | June | July | August | Action Plan |
| **Service** | | | | | |
| **Finance** | | | | | |
| **People** | | | | | |
| **Quality** | | | | | |
| **Growth** | | | | | |

Healthcare organizations providing inpatient care, outpatient care, and ambulatory surgery have designated quality measures that must be reported to a national database and to CMS. Many organizations are also required to report quality measures to private insurance companies to meet contractual arrangements or for reimbursement purposes. The majority of the measures are focused on clinical care, and have financial incentives tied to the outcomes of the care. Healthcare systems provide this information to outside agencies in multiple ways. As the increased use of electronic medical or health records has expanded in hospitals and clinics, the electronic record must have the ability to retrieve data via reports from patient care documentation. If the reports cannot be retrieved from an electronic system, the data must be collected manually. It's now hard to believe that we used to do this on a regular basis as it was the only option.

The organization's leadership has a responsibility to designate staff who review and report the required patient-related data that is accurate and timely to the requesting entity. The importance of compliance with reporting of accurate quality metrics has been heightened. Reimbursement incentives are now connected to the results of the measurable quality metrics collected by healthcare organizations. Patient outcome data has become one of the top priorities in many healthcare organizations' agendas. Thus, patient-related documentation must be timely and as accurate as possible, as well as have sufficient details to validate clinical procedures and standards of care.

Reimbursement for Medicare patients has changed from a volume-based fee-for-service system to a value-based payment system. Participating hospitals are paid for inpatient acute care services based on the quality of care, not the quantity of care such as the number days the patient was hospitalized, supplies used for patient care, special equipment to perform procedures, and implantable devices. This is an extreme change in historical industry practice, affecting all aspects of healthcare: strategic planning for new and continued services offered to the community; hiring and retaining the best care providers; chasing patient satisfaction to add value; improving organizational performance; monitoring clinical outcomes; and, clinicians' practice patterns to yield the best financial results. Hence, it is imperative for all healthcare providers to understand how comprehensive, error-free, and up-to-date clinical documentation can impact a cascade of events in the overall organizational system.

The US Congress authorized the (inpatient) Hospital Value-Based Purchasing (VBP) as a part of the Patient Protection and Affordable Care Act which was signed into law in early 2010. The VBP system has been ongoing and is an effort to reward the best providers of healthcare. Each year, a percentage of the Diagnosis Related Group's payment-for-service model (for Medicare inpatient services) is withheld by Medicare. This percentage is held until the results of the quality metrics are reported and finalized. You can learn more about it here: https://www.cms.gov/Medicare/Quality-Initiatives-Patient-Assessment-Instruments/Value-Based-Programs/HVBP/Hospital-Value-Based-Purchasing

Correct coding of medical services in the patient's health record is imperative. These codes are substantiated by clinical documentation that identifies medical conditions such as major and minor diagnoses, complications, procedures, etc. that can be billed to insurers. Missing or adding a code can be quite costly, and it may be perceived as inadvertently fraudulent. There is a relatively short correction period allowed for errors; hence, the emphasis on accuracy.

Overall, hospitals whose results fall below the benchmark do not receive the withheld reimbursement percentage, and hospitals that exceed the benchmark receive a value-based bonus payment. The percentage of payment withheld has increased each year in order to push hospitals to continue improving the required set of quality measures, thus improving patient outcomes. As the VBP system has evolved, the percentage withheld was escalated each year to reach a maximum of 2% in 2017 and has remained at that level (CMS, 2021c). The withheld amounts are pooled, and it is now possible for a hospital to earn back a value-based incentive payment that may be less than, equal to, or more than the applicable withheld amount for that year (CMS, 2021b).

The governmental quality measures have been changing every year since the creation of the quality program. In the beginning, the metrics were related to the percentage of times a recognized evidence-based process guideline was implemented. In the first two years, the clinical process measures were valued at 70% and the patient experience measure was valued at 30%. As organizations performed better (rates reached 98%–100%), the bar was raised to no longer measure processes but instead to measure patient outcomes.

In 2015, the four quality domains measured were: 1) clinical process of care, 2) patient experience of care, 3) outcome, and 4) efficiency (CMS, 2014). For 2015, CMS cited the VBP metrics as follows:

- **Clinical process of care:** 13 measures with a value weight of 20%
- **Patient experience:** 8 measures with a value weight of 30%
- **Outcome:** 5 measures with a value of 30%
- **Efficiency:** 1 measure with a value of 20%

Since that time, the program has evolved and now includes measures aimed to (CMS, 2021a):

1. Reduce readmissions for certain health conditions and hospital-acquired condition reductions
2. Provide incentives for graduate medical education programs and indirect medical education
3. Enhance technological-based programs

You can learn about the quality program and the measurable compensatory metrics here: https://www.cms.gov/medicare/quality-initiatives-patient-assessment-instruments/hospitalqualityinits

As the years have passed since initial programmatic implementation, the process and patient outcomes for disease have hit the desired quality targets. Measures have been changed to other disease categories requiring improvement. The challenge for the healthcare industry is to push forward toward better patient outcomes across all disease states, while reducing cost and expanding patients' access to care. In addition to access, the system must begin to shift to one of prevention instead of being wholly encumbered by the treatment of illness. It seems like the majority of resources have been focused to measure the outcomes of poor health (landing one in a hospital) versus the prevention of illness in the first place.

## THE HEALTHCARE INDUSTRY'S MOST VALUABLE ASSET: THE PEOPLE

As the global COVID-19 pandemic has shown, without qualified healthcare personnel, patients cannot be adequately cared for—especially in a hospital setting. Nurses are responsible for the majority of patient care; they can influence and have the ability to improve a large percentage of clinical measures when given the appropriate environment and resources to do so. When searching for the most up-to-date listing of reportable measures in a hospital setting, the search returned 554 measures. You can learn more here: https://www.cms.gov/Medicare/Quality-Initiatives-Patient-Assessment-Instruments/QualityMeasures/CMS-Measures-Inventory. Shifting nursing resources to the front-end of the healthcare system (to prevent illness) could stem the shortage of personnel needed to care for sick individuals.

Nurses specifically have the ability to influence measures in clinical process, patient experience, and communication between and among the various disciplines of clinical care providers. In the area of patient outcomes, nurses make a significant difference through the use of critical communication in the event of a changing patient condition. They, along with other members of the healthcare team, are tasked with monitoring patient progress with nursing and medical interventions. Regarding efficiency, many organizations have undertaken initiatives related to process improvement and standardization in order to improve their operations and team member experiences in the workplace. Assessment and evaluation are two key areas about which healthcare providers must develop keen awareness.

Patients have much shorter stays or visits in their healthcare encounters than in times past. Nurses must determine if patients clearly understand their discharge instructions and what they need to do for an optimal recovery to prevent an adverse outcome or readmission. Read more about CMS's Quality

Measurement and Quality Improvement here: https://www.cms.gov/Medicare/Quality-Initiatives-Patient-Assessment-Instruments/MMS/Quality-Measure-and-Quality-Improvement-.

## PRACTICE PEARLS

- Nursing-sensitive indicators impact the quality of care.
    - Focus on the assessment and care of skin integrity to prevent hospital-acquired pressure ulcers.
    - Focus on the prevention of patient falls.
    - Always wash your hands to prevent the potential spread of infection.
    - Ambulate patients early and often; bed rest often delays recovery.
    - Remove urinary catheters as soon as possible.
    - Nurses have the ability to influence patient experience: Be a reliable communication conduit for the patient, family, and other members of the healthcare team.
    - Patient education is crucial for appropriate follow-up care. Use teach-back to assess whether patients understand their care plan.
- Consider shifting nursing resources to the front end of the healthcare continuum to prevent chronic conditions from progressing to require hospitalization.

---

A review by CMS of the results of 25 CMS quality-reporting programs from 2006 to 2013 showed significant progress in care improvement and cost reduction for Medicare patients. Of the 119 publicly reported performance rates, 95% showed progress, and 35% of the 119 measures exceeded the 90% metric of success (Earl, 2015). The CMS deputy administrator for innovation and quality/chief medical officer at the time, Patrick Conway, reported the nation has made clear progress in improving healthcare by achieving the three aims: 1) better care, 2) smarter spending, and 3) healthier people (Earl, 2015). This work continues today.

Positive improvements resulting from the push by governmental quality organizations and insurance companies for outstanding quality metrics will result in the continued refinement and expansion of the program. It is predicted that new quality metrics will continue to replace the old and be measured and reported in all areas of healthcare. It is essential for nurses and other healthcare clinicians to become familiar with these quality metrics and become comfortable with others viewing their documentation and measurable practice outcomes. For experienced nurses, this may be somewhat disconcerting and a source of stress. Nursing care is now under a spotlight and is being showcased—good, bad, or otherwise, whether we like it or not.

The intention of this government intervention is good. CMS is using the quality metrics as a lever to transform the delivery of healthcare. The focus has been with the Medicare population, but it is likely all Americans will receive a collateral benefit from this quality measurement program. Healthcare professionals have become immersed in system reform, engaged in clinical and outcome improvement, and they are striving for results to achieve better care in a better system. However, overall progress feels *slow*.

Patients rely on their medical providers to provide the most up-to-date information and best-in-class care. As a result, another shift is occurring as evidenced by the growth of integrative medical approaches, functional medicine, and intermixing Western medicine with other worldly methods. Since patients are now better informed, they are more educated about disease processes and are able to take more responsibility for their own health and well-being; sometimes this means avoiding traditional medical providers altogether or choosing what used to be labeled as "alternative" approaches for their care. Some examples include meditation, acupuncture, massage, herbal medicine, biofeedback, etc.

There also have been a number of changes in recent years in government norms recommended to the population. Since 1992, the US Department of Agriculture has provided a nutritional food pyramid outlining food intake.

However, it was changed in 2010 to "My Plate" as a new guideline for proper nutrition due to the increasing obesity epidemic in both adults and children and the growing challenges with food security (USDA National Agricultural Library, n.d.). The goal: Make smarter food choices. More information about the latest plan of Dietary Guidelines for Americans from 2020-2025 can be found here: https://www.dietaryguidelines.gov/sites/default/files/2021-03/Dietary_Guidelines_for_Americans-2020-2025.pdf.

## PRACTICE PEARLS

- Be mindful of what you put in and on your body.
- Consider the source of your food: made at home, from the grocery store, from local farms, or in restaurants.
- Consider the ingredients in the packaged food you eat: Can you pronounce the words and do you know what all of the ingredients are?
- Consider the choices you make with food: Is what you eat good for you?
- Consider if your lifestyle habits are affecting your health in a negative way.
- Consider learning more about nutrition and the implications for ill health and chronic disease.

# HOW U.S. POLICY-MAKING HAS AFFECTED HEALTHCARE TODAY

Over the last several decades, there have been a number of changes in food and agriculture policy, as well as, drug policies in the US. Genetic modification to organisms has shifted farmer growing practices to volume or shorter turnover in crops for higher overall yields and worldwide dietary patterns have been shifting due to the diversity of available food options (Kearney, 2010). Kearney (2010) posited accompanying the changes in overall food consumption have coincided with considerable health consequences. He cites urbanization, food industry marketing, and trade policies as being the major drivers linking the nutritional "transition" and increasing rates of obesity, as well as, chronic health conditions.

In addition, there are more packaged, prepared, and preserved foods on the market than ever before. Fast food has been well-adopted due to the increasing speed of life with myriad technological advances. However, to date few have taken note of the actual ingredients in these modified foods. One food activist has taken it upon herself to ask many tough questions of the largest food producers in North America. Vani Hari, also known as "the food babe," experienced her own health crisis spawning her interest in what was actually in her food after her dietary patterns landed her in a hospital (Food Babe, 2022). She has spent nearly every day since helping others take a different path toward health and well-being by understanding what is in your food, where it comes from, and learning that food truly is medicine. Her philosophy is that food is meant to heal, not harm.

Newly devised substances such as pesticides, herbicides and fungicides have peppered the media in recent years in relation to how they may have affected the food supply with subsequent litigation. And, with the changing dietary patterns around the world are the health consequences really known? Could our new dietary patterns and the foods we choose be damaging our health? Some think so.

As a counterbalance to these policy changes, a movement is underway to get to the root cause of illness and to raise awareness to be mindful of what we put in and on our bodies. The specialty of Functional Medicine is defined as "a systems biology-based approach that focuses on identifying and addressing the root cause of disease" by the Institute for Functional Medicine (2022) and is growing. They believe each symptom or medical diagnosis may contribute to one's overall health condition(s). And, their emphasis on lifestyle factors is aimed to improve one's health and well-being by making more informed daily choices to lessen the need for medical intervention at a later date.

Additionally, a shift in how drug research is done began several decades ago when research studies began moving from academic settings to commercial research run by private entities (Abramson, 2022). As described by Abramson (2022), this change brought new relationships with potential conflicts of interest, a change in the *pure* peer review process, added increased potential for bias, little to no government oversight, fueled a lack of drug efficacy testing before new releases, and more. These corporate giants have grown large and now have been responsible for many well-known healthcare related catastrophes exposed by the media such as: the number of harmful drugs released and then recalled, their contribution to the opioid crisis, price gouging, industry consolidation driving business monopolies, enhanced market influence, direct to consumer marketing, a lack of cost control, and more (Abramson, 2022; Ramaswamy, 2021). Not only is this a tragedy for medical professionals who rely on accurate and timely peer-reviewed data for best-practice decision-making, but the patients themselves.

## CONSUMER INFLUENCES IN HEALTHCARE

With increased access to the internet across the world, consumers of healthcare (patients) are better educated. They are able to stay better informed about happenings around the world, timely news, and healthcare's latest trends than at any previous time in history. Today's consumers are demanding healthcare systems and experiences that accommodate their busy schedules, provide useful information that can be obtained quickly and easily, and that allow them to be involved in decision-making. These consumers are different from those in the past because they also demand better access to care and better communication and a new level of participation with their healthcare providers. Plans of treatment are often devised jointly and executed via creative methods.

The growing availability and ease of access to the safety and quality outcomes of an organization and its providers is born from the advent of healthcare consumerism. Healthcare consumerism is the push by the public to make the access and delivery of healthcare services more efficient and cost-effective. This boils down to the goal of delivering the highest quality care at the lowest prices.

During his tenure, President Trump signed Executive Order 13877 to help increase healthcare transparency (2019). The executive order mandated that healthcare providers publish the cost of medical procedures before consumers receive them.

The Biden Administration has continued to push this effort and issued an interim final rule that allows for the following provisions (CMS, 2021e):

- Ban surprise billing for emergency services
- Ban high out-of-network cost-sharing for emergency and non-emergency services
- Ban out-of-network charges for ancillary care at an in-network facility in all circumstances
- Ban other out-of-network charges without advance notice.

Though slow moving, healthcare agencies, payers, tax and benefit professionals, and of course employers are starting to provide information on how patients can make more informed decisions about their healthcare, along with offering financial incentives.

These shifts may seem draconian to management teams steeped in the historical functions of healthcare, but the end results are intended to be optimized for patient care:

- Improved medical care
- Improved outcomes of that care
- Lower operating costs for healthcare organizations, physician groups, and independent providers
- Reduced costs of healthcare and healthcare insurance

More information on the development of price transparency can be found at: https://www.cms.gov/healthplan-price-transparency

In addition to healthcare, many other organizations have been affected by these industry changes; more of the cost of benefits has been passed along to employees, causing a new financial strain. A common cycle of stress is outlined here:

**Change ➔ Stress Perceived as Negative ➔ Adverse Consequences**

According to Gill (2022) in *Consumer Reports,* medical costs have risen 30.7% since 2011, and US healthcare spending is now in the low trillions, which is approximately 20%+ of the gross domestic product (GDP). It is also well-known that many patients have good intentions to be compliant with their treatment plans until they learn the cost. This often potentiates tough decisions related to what they can afford in addition to their usual household spending. Often, they choose to forego medical interventions, which may potentiate greater cost from more complicated care at a later date.

Healthcare providers who understand the nuances of demand consumerism and its influence on the marketplace will thrive. The impact of better quality and outcomes secondary to tuned-in healthcare providers and patients will facilitate the shift from an illness-based focus to a system of prevention. Healthcare costs will decrease and the population at large will be healthier.

It could be as simple as it's all in how you look at it (change). A new view of change producing stress is outlined here:

**Change → Positively Viewed Stress →
New Ideas for System Improvement**

A future challenge to healthcare organizations, as well as clinicians, will be to understand the interplay between internal and external customers. Those outside of healthcare are driving much of the industry change (especially, those who pay for it). They now expect higher quality at a more reasonable cost. It will be necessary to develop better ways of proactively working with suppliers of healthcare to accommodate changing demands of the modern consumer. Many of the systems in healthcare have been designed by and for the providers, not the payers or consumers. As this changes, the modern consumer will expect immediate access, accurate communication, and collegial collaboration between all types of team members in an expedient fashion.

Today's healthcare consumer is empowered to demand quality, safe, and easily accessible care. Per Press Ganey (2021), when healthcare consumers were polled, 54.4% believed the overall healthcare process is more arduous today than in 2019 (50.4%). The top barriers to consumers accessing healthcare are availability of appointments, finding physicians and hospitals in their insurance network, as well as the time it takes to manage this process. With over 65% of consumers using the internet for healthcare answers, this powerful method for accessing information can influence a patient's decision-making for healthcare choices. A few popular patient-facing websites are healthcare entities, WebMD (https://www.webmd.com/), Healthgrades (https://www.healthgrades.com/), Medicare.gov (https://www.medicare.gov/care-compare/?providerType=Hospital), and believe it or not—Facebook (https://www.facebook.com).

## Social Media

Social media cannot also be excluded from influencing patient decision-making. The weight of other consumers posting negative experiences about healthcare encounters with a particular institution or provider may be significant. Healthcare organizations or providers who fail to see that consumers and payors are taking the reins in the industry do so at their own peril.

According to Evan Kirstel from the Forbes Business Council, "Social media is now a driving force in the healthcare community for disseminating information, advocating for change, and connecting communities in the pursuit of better healthcare" (2022, para. 2).

Healthcare organizations have the opportunity to build passive confidence from the communities they serve by providing credible and easily accessible health education. This can include disease management, increasing awareness, and advocating for change that can impact the social determinants of health. In addition, it can serve to rapidly share new discoveries, research, and treatments with the public.

Organizations need to recognize that use of social media as a communication tool is no longer one medium, and the information must be credible and from a trusted source. It is a communication tool, and as such requires facilitation and closure of complete feedback loops, where the public can ask questions, get responses to the queries, and gain access to services that might benefit them.

Use of social media is not without risk. For the individual(s) in organizations who manage content, privacy needs to be held in the highest regard. Any post made on a company's website must exclude patient identifiers to comply with healthcare related privacy law (HIPAA, the Health Insurance Portability and Accountability Act). More information about HIPAA can be found here: https://www.hhs.gov/sites/default/files/privacysummary.pdf.

All content must be professional and not contain damaging information for the reputation of providers, individuals, or the institution.

## Telehealth Technology

A perfect example of utilizing available technology occurred during the global COVID-19 pandemic when many routine health needs were able to be taken care of via telehealth. Providers and government entities have been historically slow in adoption. People are busy in this fast-paced world and need efficient access to consultation and care. Not only did it improve access to care for patients during the pandemic (think, care anywhere), it has also improved efficiency for patients and some providers as well. Previously, telehealth had only been a gradually growing industry (Chakrabarti, 2019). For years, it has been a critical adjunct to provide specialty consultations and care in rural settings by linkage with larger facilities and their bevy of specialists. This allows patients who live in less populated areas to obtain better access to specialists for expert care despite their geographic locale. According to Press Ganey (2021), "Today, the patient experience encompasses every step of the healthcare journey, including navigating the web, scheduling, billing, insurance, and beyond."

## Consumer Expectations in 2022

Consumers expect the provider and healthcare entity to address and resolve their clinical condition (whether realistic or not).

Healthcare organizations and providers who fail to recognize that consumers are technologically savvy, more educated, and have set expectations for their care, may have difficulty sustaining business. COVID-19 shifted many industries to allow employees to work from home. Healthcare must also shift many long-standing practices and adjust its paradigm. For example, healthcare consumers now expect secure electronic patient portals to check their lab results, schedule online appointments, utilize technology to request their provider refill existing prescriptions, be able to communicate with their providers, and more.

## Healthcare Cost Shifting

One of the most controversial changes in healthcare is the continued shift in cost to the consumer. As companies who do provide health insurance for their employees constantly change the coverage and benefit plans, it requires a change in consumer behavior regarding knowledge, access, and consumption.

Many Americans view healthcare access and treatment as a right; however, it has become a costly privilege. This change has made consumers more conscientious about their healthcare decisions (Mangan, 2014), which may be good since we got a glimpse of the challenges the future holds during the COVID-19 pandemic.

Many of the traditional systems in healthcare have been designed by and for the providers, not the payers or consumers. In times past, patients usually followed their doctor's advice. Now, consumers are much more educated, wary of cost, and often tell their medical providers what they want or negotiate the outcome they desire. Ideally, this will lead to better health but may be a bit painful for current providers along the way (especially those used to a more paternalistic system).

Modern healthcare consumers also want to ask difficult questions about their care and treatment plans. They expect nearly immediate answers. And, sometimes it just doesn't work that way. The healthcare system's ability to satisfy consumer demand for convenience, access, and timely information will have a significant impact on where consumers take their business. Consumers will decide with whom and where to receive care, giving thought to quality, outcomes, and the entity's overall success in the delivery or approach to healthcare.

# THE SILVER TSUNAMI

The term "silver tsunami" originated in the 1980s, as discussions of the increase in the aging population began to occur (Barusch, 2013). The term can be found in economic and healthcare publications alike. Research about the silver tsunami in healthcare is moderate. A search in CINAHL with no restrictions reveals only 39 pieces of work. Some of those are focused on specialties in healthcare such as chiropractic care, audiology, and massage (Alexander, 2011; Foxworth, 2019; Veto, 2015). Others are focused on the need to educate leadership and initiate organizational change to manage the specific expectations of the baby boomer generation (Hannum, 2020). There is also a great deal of research about the mental health care needs of this population, which are likely to go unmet as mental health care professionals dwindle in numbers and cases of dementia increase (Bees, 2021; Canady, 2017; Schwartz, 2011). The silver tsunami is now impacting healthcare and will continue to do so, particularly in areas of workforce shortages such as nursing.

## CO-MORBIDITIES WITH AGING

Most people recognize that with additional years of life come additional ailments related to health. When these ailments are chronic conditions (diabetes, heart failure, renal disease, etc.) or create chronic illnesses (migraines related to a brain tumor), patients end up with lifelong struggles that can decrease their independence and increase their reliance on the healthcare system. Lenti et al. (2022) performed a study from November 2017 to November 2019 analyzing the co-morbidity status of elderly patients admitted to an internal medicine unit in Italy. Of the study participants, 96.2% had two or more comorbidities, 72.7% experienced poly-pharmacy (defined as five or more medications), hospital length of stay in this group was 14 days versus the hospital average stay of nine days, and the 30-day mortality rate was 12.9% versus 3.8% in the rest of the hospital population. It did not matter if the patient had a primary chronic condition with associated aliments or if they had multiple chronic conditions; the presence of these illnesses contributed significantly to the decline of the aged patient. Sheung-Tung in 2018 reported that each additional chronic illness is associated with an increase of 3.2 medical consultations per year and a 33% increase in medical costs.

## FALLS IN THE ELDERLY

A common surgical procedure in the active elderly is joint replacement. Non-active elderly tend to remain non-active either out of habit or because they feel that relaxation in retirement is a priority. Regardless of the reason, sarcopenia (a loss of muscle mass and strength) can result. In a two-year frailty and aging cohort study, Seo and Kim (2021) found associated falls in elderly women who experienced sarcopenia. Approximately 30% of the elderly experience at least one fall each year (Kwan et al., 2011). Falls are also the cause of approximately 95% of all hip fractures among the elderly; 20% of elderly adults suffering from hip fracture die within a year following the incident (Centers for Disease Control and Prevention [CDC], n.d.-b).

## CONFUSION IN THE ELDERLY

Confusion in the elderly is a common complication from a variety of issues including but not limited to cerebral vascular flow restriction; urinary tract infection; electrolyte imbalance or abnormal lab values; infection or fever; poly-pharmacy; the effects of analgesia, delirium, and dementia; or Alzheimer's disease. Implications of confusion in the elderly during hospitalization include an increased length of stay, either directly related to the confusion or because of an unexpected health complication resulting from the confusion resulting in increased medical care–related costs (Lin et al., 2015).

## THE IMPACT ON HEALTHCARE PROVIDERS

The increase in the elderly population has not gone unnoticed in healthcare. The impact on pre-hospital care alone is significant. Emergency Medical Services reports that patients 65 years and older utilize their services twice as often as younger populations, and patients 85 years and older utilize them three times as much. Elderly people account for one third of all traumatic deaths (Barishansky, 2016).

Chiropractic physicians are publishing about the unique perspectives of working on the elderly with more frail bodies (Foxworth, 2019). Orthopedic nurses report spending more time doing screenings; implementing preventive measures to avoid falls, wandering, and injuries; providing calming reassurance and education to both patients and families; and doing all of the ever-expanding work with fewer staff being scheduled (Rogers & Gibson, 2002). Schwartz (2011) suggested that more outpatient services should be offered to better support the growing geriatric population. However, expanding services will be challenging as fewer healthcare providers are available to fill current or new roles.

## WHAT CAN BE DONE?

The traditional business-focused medical centric healthcare delivery system, while supportive of organizational and clinic patient volumes, is no longer the safest way to manage elderly people with multiple co-morbidities (WWTW, 2015). Traditionally, clinicians schooled in large university medical centers have been required to attend training about how to address only a single problem at each patient encounter. If the patient had more than one issue, they were required to schedule another appointment.

This approach is inefficient and not patient-focused despite being promoted by current payor's billing practices. This is complicated for patients and providers alike, as well as very discouraging. It also negatively affects patient satisfaction, impacts patient throughput, and often does not address the deep concerns of patients. These interwoven complexities of co-morbid conditions require an all-inclusive look at each patient, not each individual symptom.

Geriatrics is thankfully already a focus for many clinical disciplines; for example, medicine and advanced practice nursing both have geriatric specialty certifications. These specialists are trained to manage patients individually. This includes addressing the inter-relation of co-morbid conditions and the patient environment (where and how the patient lives, family situation, finances, diet, physical activity, and more).

Utilizing a collaborative multidisciplinary approach to improving health (physician, nurse practitioner, nurse, dietician, physical therapist, social worker, etc.) can help ensure all components of a patient's care are addressed to the fullest extent, thus offering the best chance for a good quality of life. Wellness visits, while they may be extensive, are less expensive and traumatic than illness in elderly patients with co-morbidities. However, it has unfortunately been shown that there is no evidence to support wellness visits decreasing overall healthcare costs (Watkins et al., 2021).

Dementia and Alzheimer's are serious concerns in the elderly population. The Alzheimer's Association reports there are an estimated 6.5 million Americans age 65 and older living with Alzheimer's dementia in 2022. Seventy-three percent of those affected are 75 years of age and older (Alzheimer's Association, n.d.). Burnout, which is known to exist in healthcare, often expands its reach to home caregivers when patients develop dementia. It can be very stressful for all involved. The constant attention required quickly becomes exhausting for the care provider.

Kerry Jordan, at the University of Central Arkansas (UCA), knows this feeling all too well. Dr. Jordan teaches at the School of Nursing at UCA. When her parents began to exhibit signs of dementia, she and her husband, Kirk, sold their home and purchased one with an in-law suite so they could better oversee their care. As her parents aged and their dementia worsened, their physical health declined. Kerry found herself overwhelmed and in desperate need of help. Taking advantage of the opportunities that exist at UCA, Kerry developed an interprofessional clinic utilizing all healthcare professional student groups (Assaf, 2022). This is an excellent example of using innovation to solve an unmet healthcare need.

Patients and their families (should they choose to participate) now can experience group and individual therapies with all healthcare student groups including physical therapy, occupational therapy, speech therapy, nursing, and psychology. This has been a stepping stone for community awareness and health policy reform addressing caregiver support. Other universities have similar programs. These types of programs are great examples of interdisciplinary community resources that can support families and patients, as well as primary healthcare providers trying to manage a tsunami of patients with acute conditions as their health declines and dementia ensues. It is important for all healthcare organizations and providers to know existing community resources to support their practice, patient, and family needs. These programs also encourage future healthcare providers to consider geriatrics as a specialty.

## MINING SILVER

The advancement of DNA searches and companies providing genetic services such as Ancestry.com raised awareness to the origins of heritage. The 2020 global COVID-19 pandemic promulgated inquiry of family history, especially related to health, and the value of lessons learned through previous life experiences (e.g., the Spanish flu pandemic). This shows the necessity of collecting data from a comprehensive family history as part of the initial assessment for a patient. The history and physical examination, as well as past health, teaches us what to expect in the future. The impending silver tsunami will mostly likely not only be a wave of overwhelming volumes of patients that need care, but it is also a vast treasure of knowledge and experience from which we have an opportunity to learn. The baby boomer generation has deeply influenced American culture from war protests to civil rights advancements. They also hold the greatest wealth in the US population, provide a large group for aging studies, and have the potential to greatly impact the outcomes of future generational aging for healthy outcomes.

## PROVIDER RESPONSIBILITY

Hospice services and in-home care for the chronically ill are of great importance for the aging population. In addition, the health insurance industry has embraced annual wellness visits provided not only by the patient's selected primary care physician, but also by the insurance plan itself. Businesses such as Signify Health allow healthcare providers to perform home assessments for some health insurance payors. In this example, they also ensure patients have plans of care and understand their plan and how best to follow the plan appropriately for optimal health. Utilizing community resources and working together in interdisciplinary teams can optimize patient independence, provide families the support they need, and has the potential to keep the silver tsunami at bay, or at least facilitate a scaled-down version of the volume of people needing healthcare by diversifying care options and locations.

## THE INFLUENCE OF REGULATION

A large portion of the US population is covered by federal or state payor agencies in order to gain access to healthcare. It is unusual to find a healthcare provider or agency that does not accept patients covered by a government-sponsored program. Thus, the majority of all healthcare agencies must meet the regulatory standards and requirements of their respective state standards and the federal standards established by CMS. An online manual of regulations is regularly published to allow easy access for clientele. To ensure regulations are followed, most state agencies have been engaged in the monitoring process.

> In a 2020 report for National Healthcare Expenditures (NHE) from 2018 data, the largest shares of total health spending were sponsored by the US federal government (28.3 percent) and households (28.4 percent). The private business share of health spending accounted for 19.9 percent, state and local governments accounted for 16.5 percent, and other private revenues accounted for 6.9 percent. (CMS, 2020)

Regulatory surveyors may make announced or unannounced visits to healthcare sites. Visits may be prompted by consumer complaints related to care and treatment, access, or any other alleged violation in the regulations. Routine reviews of quality data are commonplace. Onsite reviews are required to determine if the quality of services meet professionally recognized standards of practice in healthcare. There are several independent organizations who also survey healthcare entities against their specified set of quality, operational, and work process related standards. More information about each can be found here:

- AAAHC: Accreditation Association for Ambulatory Health Care | https://www.aaahc.org/
- The Joint Commission Standards for Joint Commission Accreditation and Certification | https://www.jointcommission.org/standards/
- Det Norske Veritas: DNV Healthcare - Accreditation Organization for Hospitals and Healthcare Facilities - https://www.dnv.us/assurance/healthcare/ac.html
- The Foundation for the Malcolm Baldrige National Quality Award: https://baldrigefoundation.org/what-we-do/our-impact/health-care.html

Nursing is greatly affected by compliance with regulatory requirements and accreditation standards. Generally, staff nurses and other healthcare providers are somewhat unaware of the monumental amount of guidelines that must be followed. While this may seem like an administrative responsibility in some organizations, to comply with regulatory accreditation, there are standards that address clinical care and are specific to nursing and those who provide direct patient care. Nurses who work in an organization accredited by The Joint Commission or other quality survey body can have an unambiguous impact on the care delivered and adherence to the standards.

A number of references have been provided in this chapter for access and review of a multitude of healthcare entity requirements. Organizations are influenced by federal and state regulations, accrediting organizations such as The Joint Commission, DNV, Baldridge, AAAHC, and payers.

The decision to be surveyed by The Joint Commission is a voluntary choice by any organization. If the organization does choose to be surveyed by an accrediting organization such as The Joint Commission, the organization will have deemed status with CMS if they receive accreditation. If an organization chooses not to seek accreditation with an approved regulatory body, CMS will independently survey the organization approximately every three years. Read more about CMS and hospitals here: https://www.cms.gov/Medicare/Provider-Enrollment-and-certification/CertificationandComplianc/Hospitals.

The purpose of healthcare accrediting agencies is to collaborate with and evaluate healthcare entities against a set of recognized industry-specific standards to ensure quality and safety for the public. These activities help promote safe and effective care for patients. Approximately 70% to 80% of The Joint Commission standards are directly related to patient safety. In addition to the standards, The Joint Commission accreditation process includes health-related outcome measures. These measures are another way The Joint Commission holds healthcare organizations accountable for delivering safe and quality care (Wadhwa & Huynh, 2022). The certification the organization receives following their survey by The Joint Commission can be used as a report card for consumers to decide where they want their care to take place. You can read more about it here: https://www.jointcommission.org/what-we-offer/certification/. A 2017 comparison in Becker's Hospital Review of accrediting agencies can be found here: https://www.beckershospitalreview.com/hospital-management-administration/hospitals-and-health-systems-which-is-the-best-accrediting-source-for-your-organization.html.

Most organizations build compliance with regulations into their strategic plan executed via daily operations. Activities include safety checks, surveillance, and visual observation of work processes to confirm compliance. Surveys are becoming more frequent, and real-time readiness is crucial. Figure 2.1 illustrates one approach to reach successful organizational outcomes.

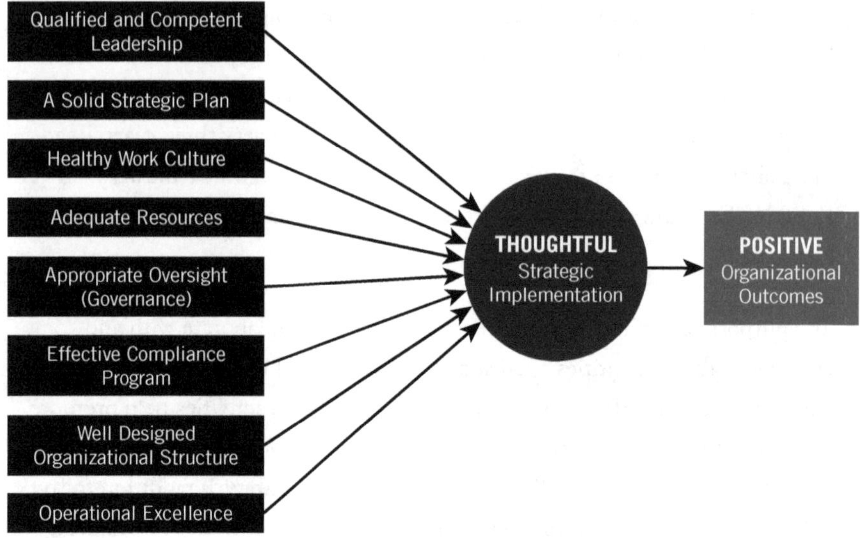


**FIGURE 2.1** Organizational model for success.

For example, the applicable standards for compliance with CMS are similar to The Joint Commission regulations. Nursing is a key participant in survey activity as they usually lead and coordinate the care of other ancillary disciplines. The majority of healthcare operations include areas of regulations focusing on patient care standards, infection control, medication administration, care coordination, patient safety, environment of care, and life safety. The process for The Joint Commission standard development occurs with input from healthcare professionals, providers, subject-matter experts, consumers, government agencies (including the Centers for Medicare & Medicaid Services), and employers. These agencies seek input from nursing when developing new or revised regulations and standards. Nursing's participation in development of the measures and standards is an example of how the profession advocates for safe and effective care (Wadhwa & Huynh, 2022). After the standards are proposed using scientific literature and expert consensus, they are reviewed by the board of commissioners. For a new standard to be added, it must meet certain criteria—it must be related to patient safety or quality of care, have a positive impact on health outcomes, meet or surpass law and/or regulation, and have the ability to be accurately and readily measured (The Joint Commission, 2022).

## THE IMPORTANCE OF TRANSITION-TO-PRACTICE PROGRAMS FOR NEW GRADUATES

> A determined effort to focus new nurses on the positive aspects of the nursing profession can successfully extinguish a great deal of the negativity that new graduates often feel, and can promote a smoother transition into practice. (Dyess & Sherman, 2009, p. 409)

In recent years, the National Council of State Boards of Nursing (NCSBN) has expressed concern about the training and retention of new graduate nurses. If the issue of retention of new graduates is not corrected, the results could have a major impact on the availability of nurses in the US to meet patient demands for nursing care.

Wolters Kluwer (2022) conducted a study, The New Nurse Readiness Survey, three times over a ten-year period (2012-2022) to look at the gap between theory and practice for new nurses. In this study it was determined that only 23% of new nurses had entry level competencies to practice. The NCSBN also looked at data as part of the survey, and determined that 50% of entry-level nurses are involved in practice errors and of these errors, 65% were related to poor clinical decision making. So why are new nurses so ill prepared to enter the workforce? The ongoing problem with access to clinical sites limits the experience that new nurses need. Frequently, during the COVID pandemic, nursing students were prohibited from entering the clinical setting and had to resort to online clinical experiences. The need for trained faculty, including clinical instructors remains a challenge for nursing programs.

Improving a novice nurses' ability to utilize critical thinking, which leads to clinical reasoning and clinical judgment, should be the focus of nursing education, not passing the NCLEX exam. This was pointed out in the Wolter Kluwer study (2022) in which nurse educators and practicing nurses were asked about their perception of education and practice. When posed the question regarding preparedness to practice today versus graduates of 5-10 years ago, educators felt 46% of grads were less prepared versus 66% of those in practice. These two groups were also asked about factors that made nurse graduates more prepared; educators felt that 54% of new nurses had better critical thinking and clinical judgment while only 26% of practicing nurses felt this to be true. Given this information, it becomes evident that a program to better prepare novice nurses is for employers to utilize a transition to practice format of orientation.

Table 2.2 was retrieved from the NCSBN website and demonstrates the need to create transition-to-practice programs for new graduates (NCSBN, 2015).

**TABLE 2.2** THE NEED TO CREATE TRANSITION-TO-PRACTICE PROGRAMS FOR NEW GRADUATES

| The Problem | The Impact |
|---|---|
| New nurses care for sicker patients in increasingly complex health settings. | New nurses report more negative safety practices and errors than experienced nurses. |
| New nurses feel increased stress levels. | Stress is a risk factor for patient safety and practice errors. |
| Approximately 25% of new nurses leave a position in their first year of practice. | Increased turnover negatively influences patient safety and healthcare outcomes. |

The first year of a new job in any profession is stressful. The transition from nursing student to registered nurse (RN) is one of the most difficult and stressful job transitions (Dyess & Sherman, 2009). The NCSBN has identified the critical elements in Figure 2.2 that can contribute to clinical errors and employee turnover (NCSBN, 2015).

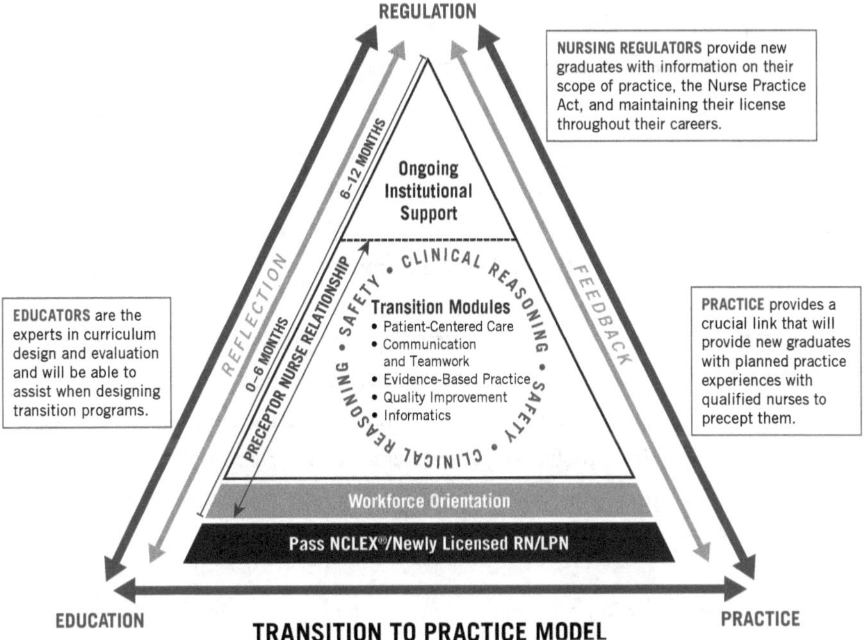


**FIGURE 2.2** Critical elements that contribute to clinical errors and employee turnover. *©NCSBN, 2015. Excerpted with permission from https://www.ncsbn.org/transition-to-practice.htm.*

Each new nurse must assimilate into a new work environment. In addition, learning confidence, the application of recently acquired skill, and clinical decision-making are more complex and develop over time. One of the leading nursing experts in transition-to-practice is Patricia Benner, who developed the "Novice to Expert" model of nursing skill development (Benner, 1984). Benner supports situational clinical coaching or guided clinical decision-making to help new graduates transition to practice. She believes coaching is not effective if it is delivered in a non-supportive organizational culture. The environment must welcome new graduates into the organization, be supportive of active learning, and be cognizant of the stress new nurses feel during the first year of nursing (O'Keeffe, 2013).

The NCSBN completed a multi-site study of transition-to-practice, including 105 hospitals in three states to study the impact of using a model for transition-to-practice. The program was created by the NCSBN and compared transition-to-practice with hospitals that established residency programs with nurses who had limited orientation (Spector et al., 2015). The study involved more than 1,000 newly hired nurses in their first year of work. Survey questions were completed online by participants in four intervals: 1) at baseline, 2) at 6 months, 3) at 9 months, and 4) at 12 months.

Post transition, the new registered nurses and the preceptors both completed an assessment of competence (Spector et al., 2015). The study findings concluded that specific outcomes such as self-reported errors, use of safety practices, work stress, job satisfaction; competence as reported by the new nurses and their linked preceptor; and hospital data on retention, were significantly better when transition programs had the following characteristics:

- A formalized program that is integrated into the institution, with support from higher administration
- A preceptorship, and the preceptor should be educated for the role
- A program that's 9-12 months in length
- Content that includes patient safety, clinical reasoning, communication and teamwork, patient-centered care, evidence-based practice, quality improvement, and informatics
- Time for new graduates to learn and apply the content and to obtain feedback and share their reflections
- Customization so the new graduates learn specialty content in the areas where they are working

In review of other transition-to-practice studies, the time for new graduate transition-to-practice occurs over an 18-month period (Halfer & Graf, 2006). The most critical time appears to be within the 3 to 12 month time frame. During this time, new nurses struggle with being overwhelmed and feeling that they have too much to do (Halfer & Graf, 2006). At the 12-month mark, nurses who felt satisfied with their job, satisfied with job competencies, experienced professional respect, had easy access to information, and had become part of the team were considered successful (Halfer & Graf, 2006).

The need for transition programs for new graduates has been discussed as early as the 1970s. Marlene Kramer (1974), in her book titled *Reality Shock,* described the transition from an educational setting to the service setting where there is a different set of priorities. Patricia Benner, in her study *From Novice to Expert,* focused on skill acquisition (Benner, 1984). The need for a transition-to-practice has been identified by many organizations, including The Joint Commission, The Carnegie Study of Nursing Education, and the Institute of Medicine. The increasing complexity of healthcare is another good reason for organizations to establish a transition-to-practice program (Spector et al., 2015).

In 2014, data collected in the Spector et al. study indicated that 33% to 48% of hospitals have comprehensive evidence-based nurse residency programs offered by employers. The programs are more often than not in hospitals with over 250 beds (Spector et al., 2015). In 2009, there were just slightly more than 5,000 hospitals in the US, according to hospital census data by the Centers for Disease Control. Seventy percent of the hospitals in this study operated fewer than 200 beds (CDC, 2017). Today, there are just over 6,000 hospitals in the US, and you can read more about them here: https://www.aha.org/statistics/fast-facts-us-hospitals.

Positive aspects of a residency program for new graduate nurses are the promotion of critical thinking, fostering peer networking and colleague discussions, and support for their professional role transition throughout the first year of practice (Halfer & Graf, 2006). The results from the NCSBN study indicate that a structured transition program improves patient safety by decreasing errors and negative safety practices in new graduate nurses. In addition, the nurses rated themselves as more competent, had less work-related stress and increased job satisfaction, and were less likely to leave their position during the first year (Spector et al., 2015).

As a profession, the support for transition-to-practice must come from nursing, as well as other top leadership. Nurses are the largest professional group in healthcare. To move the nursing profession to the next level, nurses need to support each other: preceptors and staff, staff with each other, staff and leaders, leaders and educators, and so on. As a new graduate, each nurse must decide how to apply learned practices. Standards are meant to guide appropriate behavior. Having a mentor is key, as these relationships and discussions have a positive influence on the new graduates as they transition into practice (Dyess & Sherman, 2009).

### PRACTICE PEARLS

- Nurses must be supportive of their peers.
- Expert nurses must mentor novice nurses.
- Nurses are lifelong learners who want to continue learning and apply their recently acquired skills in a supportive environment.
- All nurses want to feel that they are an important part of an effective team.
- Nurses should have opportunities and support for professional development.

## PREVENTING INCIVILITY, BULLYING, AND WORKPLACE VIOLENCE

Incivility, bullying, and violence in the healthcare setting also play a role in healthcare personnel shortages. The pending threat of emotional or physical abuse can affect both job satisfaction, as well as the ability for nurses and other healthcare personnel to provide the safest, highest quality care for patients.

The American Nurses Association (ANA, 2015) defines incivility and bullying as follows:

- *Incivility:* one or more rude, discourteous, or disrespectful actions that may or may not have a negative intent behind them
- *Bullying:* repeated, unwanted, harmful actions intended to humiliate, offend, and cause distress in the recipient

Both are acts of aggression that can be enacted verbally, or non-verbally through behaviors and physical acts. None of these behaviors are acceptable and should be confronted by the individual, group, and leaders as soon as possible to maintain a cohesive working environment.

*Workplace violence* is the act or threat of violence, ranging from verbal abuse to physical assaults directed toward persons at work or on duty. The impact of workplace violence can range from psychological issues to physical injury, or even death. The American Hospital Association (AHA) reports healthcare workers suffer more workplace injuries because of violence than any other profession (AHA, 2022). They asserted 44.4% of nurses reported an increase in physical violence since the global COVID-19 pandemic began, and 67.8% reported an increase in verbal abuse (Byon et al., 2021). The National Institute of Occupational Safety and Health (NIOSH) stated that the most common type of violence in healthcare settings is from patients, visitors, and other customers or clients. It can take the form of physical assault, non-verbal acts (threats, sexual harassment, verbal abuse, etc.), and acutely or chronically harm both the victim, witnesses, and even end in death (NIOSH, 2020). Unfortunately, we have seen these types of violence against healthcare workers play out in multiple incidents of stabbings, shootings and more at this writing in late 2022.

Beyond the immediate trauma, consequences for nurses and other healthcare providers include low morale, a potential loss of productivity resulting from lack of trust, dysfunctional team cohesiveness, and a sense that the work environment is hostile and dangerous. These types of events can fuel increased job stress, absenteeism, family turmoil, and worker turnover.

In response, the ANA published a position statement encouraging nurses, professional nursing organizations, healthcare system employers, and legislators to mitigate further occurrences of violence. Key points included (ANA, 2015):

- The nursing profession will not tolerate violence of any kind from any source.
- Nurses and employers must collaborate to create a culture of respect.
- The adoption of evidence-based strategies that prevent and mitigate incivility, bullying, and workplace violence must be a priority; the promotion of health, safety, wellness, and optimal outcomes in healthcare must be evident.
- The statement is relevant for all healthcare professionals and stakeholders, not exclusively to nurses.
- Stakeholders who have a relationship with the healthcare workplace also have a responsibility to address incivility, bullying, and workplace violence.

More recently, the ANA recognized that healthcare workers in inpatient facilities experienced workplace violence–related injuries requiring days off from work at a rate of at least 5 to 12 times higher than the rate of private-sector workers overall (ANA, 2019). In the brief, they encouraged promoting and instilling a culture of "zero tolerance" for violence in the workplace and called for policy and procedure to officially state the same. Additionally, the ANA published three levels of prevention to help focus on improving specific standards and competencies in the workplace (2019):

I. Primary Prevention: Stopping violence before it occurs by developing education and other strategies to identify risks, increase buffers, and reduce vulnerabilities in order to prevent workplace violence.

II. Secondary Prevention: Immediate and effective response to violence (including emergency care) with interventions intended to address emergent short-term consequences and reduce the negative impact of workplace violence.

III. Tertiary Prevention: Long-term responses to violence by implementing interventions intended to reduce the long-term negative and rehabilitation consequences of workplace violence.

Today, the healthcare industry is appealing to state and federal legislators to enact laws and regulations to protect healthcare workers from workplace violence. Here is an excerpt from the ANA that offers suggestions on how you can get involved:

> Tackling workplace violence will take a united effort. To that end, we have collated a series of promotional and educational resources that can help you and your colleagues reduce incidents in your workplace, and help create safe health care environments by advocating for change. (ANA, n.d.)

## PRACTICE PEARLS

- Take time to understand your organization's policies and procedures for managing difficult patients, workplace violence, and how to report concerns.
- Consider taking courses on managing difficult people, patients, and situations. The Crisis Prevention Institute courses are common in many healthcare organizations.
- Be alert to your surroundings and the environment; assess the insidious signs and symptoms of agitation from those around you. Quite often pain, a long wait, bad news, and even a change in clinical condition can be cause for a visitor, coworker, or patient to aggressively lash out.
- Get involved in your organization, community, or professional organizations to help make the "healing" workplace the safest it can be.

# CONCLUSION

Organizational change can't be rushed and always causes some degree of chaos. The healthcare industry is undergoing a wave of unprecedented change. While external forces are driving much of these changes, nurses and other healthcare providers of clinical care are central to the new system's success. Thus, this wave provides a positive opportunity for all providers to share their unique set of skills in bettering healthcare. Keeping the stressors in perspective will allow an open mind for improvement to evolve. Change takes time, talent, and skill for optimal execution. The next chapter explores nursing and healthcare as an art versus a science and explains how it is really a combination of both.

# REFERENCES

Alexander, S. (2019, August 1). Are you ready for the silver tsunami? *Massage Magazine* (279). https://www.massagemag.com/silver-tsunami-117096/

Alzheimer's Association. (n.d.). *2022 Alzheimer's disease facts and figures*. https://www.alz.org/media/Documents/alzheimers-facts-and-figures.pdf

American Hospital Association. (2022). *Fact sheet: Workplace violence and intimidation, and the need for a federal legislative response*. https://www.aha.org/system/files/media/file/2022/06/fact-sheet-workplace-violence-and-intimidation-and-the-need-for-a-federal-legislative-response.pdf

American Nurses Association. (n.d.). *Violence, incivility, & bullying*. https://www.nursingworld.org/practice-policy/work-environment/violence-incivility-bullying/

American Nurses Association. (2015, July 22). *Incivility, bullying, and workplace violence* [ANA position statement]. https://www.nursingworld.org/practice-policy/nursing-excellence/official-position-statements/id/incivility-bullying-and-workplace-violence/

American Nurses Association. (2019). *Reporting incidents of workplace violence* [Issue Brief]. https://www.nursingworld.org/~495349/globalassets/docs/ana/ethics/endabuse-issue-brief-final.pdf

AMN Healthcare. (2018, May 18). *Traveling nurses cost less than staff nurses: KPMG study*. [Blog post]. https://www.amnhealthcare.com/amn-insights/nursing/blog/traveling-nurses-cost-less-than-staff-nurses/

Assaf, C. (2022, April 15). *UCA program fills need for cognitive care workers service learning for students*. Fox 16. https://www.fox16.com/news/education/uca-program-fills-need-for-cognitive-care-workers-service-learning-for-students/

Barishansky, R. M. (2016, August). The silver tsunami: Are you ready? *EMS World*. http://www.cygnusinteractive.com/global/arc/main-ems.php?preview&id=64.

Barusch, A. S. (2013). The aging tsunami: Time for a new metaphor? *Journal of Gerontological Social Work, 56*(3), 181–184. https://doi.org/10.1080/01634372.2013.787348

Bees, J. (2021). The coming "silver tsunami" of dementia patients. *NEJM Catalyst, 2*(9). https://doi.org/10.1056/cat.21.0296

Benner, P. (1984). *From novice to expert: Excellence in clinical nursing practice*. Prentice Hall Health.

Byon, H. D., Sagherian, K., Kim, Y., Lipscomb, J., Crandall, M., & Steege, L. (2021). Nurses' experience with type II workplace violence and underreporting during the COVID-19 pandemic. *Workplace Health & Safety, 70*(9). https://doi.org/10.1177/21650799211031233

Canady, V. A. (2017). AMHCA fears 'silver tsunami' in wake of MH Workforce Crisis in rural areas. *Mental Health Weekly, 27*(31), 1–3. https://doi.org/10.1002/mhw.31143

Centers for Disease Control and Prevention. (n.d.). *Older adult fall prevention*. http://www.cdc.gov/HomeandRecreationalSafety/Falls/adultfalls.html

Centers for Disease Control and Prevention. (2017). *Table 89. Hospitals, beds, and occupancy rates, by type of ownership and size of hospital: United States, selected years 1975–2015*. https://www.cms.gov/Research-Statistics-Data-and-Systems/Statistics-Trends-and-Reports/NationalHealthExpendData/NHE-Fact-Sheet

Centers for Medicare & Medicaid Services. (2014, December 18). *Hospital value-based purchasing*. http://www.cms.gov/Medicare/Quality-Initiatives-Patient-Assessment-Instruments/hospital-value-based-purchasing/index.html

Centers for Medicare & Medicaid Services. (2015, March 2). *2015 National impact assessment of the Centers for Medicare & Medicaid Services (CMS) quality measures report*. http://www.cms.gov/Medicare/Quality-Initiatives-Patient-Assessment-Instruments/QualityMeasures/Downloads/2015-National-Impact-Assessment-Report.pdf

Centers for Medicare & Medicaid Services. (2020). *National health expenditure (NHE) fact sheet*. https://www.hhs.gov/guidance/document/national-health-expenditure-nhe-fact-sheet-0

Centers for Medicare & Medicaid Services. (2021a). *Acute Inpatient PPS*. https://www.cms.gov/Medicare/Medicare-Fee-for-Service-Payment/AcuteInpatientPPS

Centers for Medicare & Medicaid Services. (2021b). *Hospital value-based purchasing program*. https://www.cms.gov/Medicare/Quality-Initiatives-Patient-Assessment-Instruments/HospitalQualityInits/Hospital-Value-Based-Purchasing-

Centers for Medicare & Medicaid Services. (2021c). *The hospital value-based purchasing (VBP) program*. https://www.cms.gov/Medicare/Quality-Initiatives-Patient-Assessment-Instruments/Value-Based-Programs/HVBP/Hospital-Value-Based-Purchasing

Centers for Medicare & Medicaid Services. (2021d). *National health expenditures 2020 highlights*. https://www.cms.gov/files/document/highlights.pdf

Centers for Medicare and Medicaid Services. (2021e). *Press release HHS announces rule to protect consumers from surprise medical bills*. CMS Newsroom. https://www.cms.gov/newsroom/press-releases/hhs-announces-rule-protect-consumers-surprise-medical-bills

Chakrabarti, O. (2019). Telehealth: Emerging evidence on efficiency. *International Review of Economics & Finance, 60*, 257–264. https://doi.org/10.1016/j.iref.2018.10.021

Dyess, S. M., & Sherman, R. O. (2009). The first year of practice: New graduate nurses' transition and learning needs. *The Journal of Continuing Education in Nursing, 40*(9), 403–410. https://doi.org/10.3928/00220124-20090824-03

Earl, E. (2015, March 3). CMS indicates steadily improving quality measures. *Becker's Hospital Review*. http://www.beckershospitalreview.com/quality/cms-indicates-steadily-improving-quality-measures.html

Executive Office of the President. (2019). *The Federal Register*. Improving Price and Quality Transparency in American Healthcare To Put Patients First. https://www.federalregister.gov/documents/2019/06/27/2019-13945/improving-price-and-quality-transparency-in-american-healthcare-to-put-patients-first

Foxworth, R. (2019, November 5). The coming silver tsunami: An aging population and health care. *Chiropractic Economics*. https://www.chiroeco.com/aging-population-healthcare/

Gill, L. (2022, June). The remedy for big medical bills. *Consumer Reports*, 38–43.

Halfer, D., & Graf, E. (2006, March 24). Graduate nurse perceptions of the work experience. *Nursing Economics, 24*(3), 150–155.

Hannum, L. (2020). Change management communication—How it can prepare your organization for the silver tsunami. *Today's Geriatric Medicine, 13*(5), 6–8. https://www.todaysgeriatricmedicine.com/archive/SO20p6.shtml

The Joint Commission. (2022). *About our standards*. https://www.jointcommission.org/standards/about-our-standards/

Kirstel, E. (2022, January 24). Healthcare social media trends to watch in 2022. *Forbes*. https://www.forbes.com/sites/forbesbusinesscouncil/2022/01/24/healthcare-social-media-trends-to-watch-in-2022/?sh=51a86226434d

Kramer, M. (1974). *Reality shock: Why nurses leave nursing*. Mosby.

Kwan, M. M.-S., Close, J. C. T., Wong, A. K. W., & Lord, S. R. (2011). Falls incidence, risk factors, and consequences in Chinese older people: A systematic review. *Journal of the American Geriatrics Society, 59*(3), 536–543. https://doi.org/10.1111/j.1532-5415.2010.03286.x

Lenti, M. V., Klersy, C., Brera, A. S., Ballesio, A., Croce, G., Padovini, L., Ciccocioppo, R., Bertolino, G., Di Sabatino, A., & Corazza, G. R. (2022). Aging underlies heterogeneity between comorbidity and multimorbidity frameworks. *Internal and Emergency Medicine, 17*(4), 1033–1041. https://doi.org/10.1007/s11739-021-02899-2

Lin, W.-L., Chen, Y.-F., & Wang, J. (2015). Factors associated with the development of delirium in elderly patients in intensive care units. *Journal of Nursing Research, 23*(4), 322–329. https://doi.org/10.1097/jnr.0000000000000082

Mangan, D. (2014, January 6). *Health spending as share of GDP drops from first time since 1997*. CNBC. http://www.cnbc.com/id/101313516

Medical News Today. (2022). *What is private equity in healthcare?* https://www.medicalnewstoday.com/articles/private-equity-in-healthcare

Morgan Hunter HealthSearch. (2011, June 14). *Labor costs comparable for temporary and permanent nurses*. (mhhealthsearch.com)

National Council of State Boards of Nursing. (2015). *Transition to practice*. https://www.ncsbn.org/transition-to-practice.htm

The National Institute for Occupational Safety and Health. (2020). *Types of workplace violence*. Retrieved September 4, 2022, from https://wwwn.cdc.gov/WPVHC/Nurses/Course/Slide/Unit1_5

O'Keeffe, M. (2013, April 22). *Transition-to-practice programs may contribute to new grad success*. https://news.nurse.com/2013/04/22/transition-to-practice-programs-may-contribute-to-new-grad-success/#prettyPhoto

Porter, M. E., & Lee, T. H. (2013, October). The strategy that will fix health care. *Harvard Business Review*. https://hbr.org/2013/10/the-strategy-that-will-fix-health-care&cm_sp=Article

Porter, M. E., & Teisberg, E. (2006). *Redefining health care: Creating value-based competition on results*. Harvard Business School Press.

Press Ganey. (2021, December 1). *Consumer experience trends in healthcare 2021*. https://info.pressganey.com/e-books-research/press-ganey-consumer-trends-report-2021-1#main-content

Rogers, A. C., & Gibson, C. H. (2002). Experiences of orthopaedic nurses caring for elderly patients with acute confusion. *Journal of Orthopaedic Nursing, 6*(1), 9–17. https://doi.org/10.1054/joon.2001.0210

Schwartz, M. D. (2011). Health care reform and the primary care workforce bottleneck. *Journal of General Internal Medicine, 27*(4), 469–472. https://doi.org/10.1007/s11606-011-1921-4

Seo, K. cheon, & Kim, W. (2021). Association of different muscle mass indices, strength, and physical performance with falling in elderly: Results from the Korean frailty and aging cohort study. *Archives of Physical Medicine and Rehabilitation, 102*(10). https://doi.org/10.1016/j.apmr.2021.07.624

Sheung-Tung, H. (2018). Addressing the challenges of Silver Tsunami. *Journal of Orthopaedics, Trauma and Rehabilitation, 25*(1). https://doi.org/10.1016/j.jotr.2018.09.001

Spector, N., Blegen, M. A., Silvestre, J., Barnsteiner, J., Lynn, M. R., Ulrich, B., Fogg, L., & Alexander, M. (2015). Transition to practice study in hospital settings. *Journal of Nursing Regulation, 5*(4), 24–38. https://www.ncsbn.org/research-item/transition-to-practice-study-in-hospital-settings

USDA National Agriculture Library. (n.d.). *Dietary guidance*. https://www.nal.usda.gov/human-nutrition-and-food-safety/dietary-guidance

Veto, D. (2015). Silver tsunami: How to reach the wave of boomer patients. *Audiology Today, 27*(3), 26–33.

Wadhwa, R., & Huynh, A. P. (2022, March 9). *The Joint Commission*. StatPearls. https://www.ncbi.nlm.nih.gov/books/NBK557846/

Watkins, S., Astroth, K. S., Kim, M. J., & Dyck, M. J. (2021). Are Medicare wellness visits improving outcomes? *Journal of the American Association of Nurse Practitioners, 33*(8), 591–601. https://doi.org/10.1097/jxx.0000000000000411

WTTW. (2015, March 26). *What the 'silver tsunami' means for U.S. health care: An interview with Thomas Gill of the Yale Center on Aging.* Rx: The Quiet Revolution. https://rxfilm.org/problems/silver-tsunami-united-states-healthcare-thomas-gill-yale-center-on-aging-interview/

# 3

# NURSING AND HEALTHCARE PROFESSIONS: ART VS. SCIENCE

## OBJECTIVES

- Consider the characteristics that make nursing and other healthcare professions an art.
- Consider the characteristics that make nursing and other healthcare professions a science.
- Consider the characteristics that make nursing and other healthcare professions both an art and science and their relevance to stress, fatigue, and burnout.
- Learn about case studies showing professional stressors in action.

# INTRODUCTION

How often do you view a work of art and wonder what inspired the artist to create it? Do you ever wonder what question leads a scientist to pursue knowledge? As a nurse or other healthcare provider, what inspired you to make your career choice? What is/was the catalyst to pursue nursing or healthcare as a career?

Over the years, in personal conversation with friends and peers in the nursing profession, defining what nurses do is somewhat difficult to articulate. Nursing is the scientific basis for the care provided. Nurses can easily recite the normal range of a sodium level or the proper dose of acetaminophen for a 23-pound child. Yet, explaining why a nurse had "a feeling" to double check a patient because "their gut told them to" is much more difficult to quantify. Is it instinct? Is it intuition? Is it something that can be learned or was learned in training? Does it come from years of clinical practice?

Art combines two components of nursing practice: knowledge and skill. Comprehending evidence-based practice and the art of nursing supports the nurse in demonstrating technical competence, compassionate care, ethical decisions, and care that is individualized for each patient (Lima et al., 2022). While the art of nursing encompasses the nurse's technical skills, the art of compassion and caring are just as important. The nurse is a central figure in the patient's care and often sees the patient at their most vulnerable moments. The nurse's ability to incorporate the expertise of other clinical disciplines and identify and discuss patient fears, anxiety, or concerns at the time they are expressed is important (critical thinking and clinical judgment). Resolution must include working with other disciples as warranted. At times, there may be no solution. Compassion shown in the form of a caring hand to hold, a voice of support, and just being present in silence might be exactly what is needed. Supporting clinical disciplines offer expert knowledge in their areas of practice more on an intermittent or cyclical basis.

The science of nursing can be briefly described as the scientific discipline based on theory and research. The evidence is used to guide and improve nursing practice and the care nurses deliver. Sometimes referred to as *evidence-based practice,* scientific nursing concepts, constructs, and data are all used to identify and understand complexities of care. When art and science are merged, their elements of compassion, caring, intuition, evidence-based practice, and scientific constructs surface to produce the professional practice of nursing and the application to patient care. Most of the other clinical roles in healthcare also blend art with science: medicine, ancillary disciplines, etc. They also use evidence-based practice to guide their professions toward best practices.

There are many aspects to choosing a career in nursing or healthcare that create both intellectual and emotional issues for all providers. How often, when driving home, do you feel the need to call back and check in on a patient? How often can you not let go of the thought that you may have missed something or that there may be one more thing that you forgot to tell the oncoming nurse or other healthcare provider in a patient handoff? How often do you get easily sidetracked by work-related thoughts and they subsequently impact your life outside of work? For most nurses and other healthcare providers, these things occur on a daily basis. It is easy to find yourself feeling stressed until you get back to work and make sure the patient is or was OK.

These and other unresolved thoughts and associated feelings can lead nurses and other healthcare providers down the path to burnout. We often take on unnecessary responsibility for patients and others, when so much of it is out of our control. We blame ourselves if a patient's outcome is not favorable. We replay conflict-laden conversations in our heads. Why do we do this? What other profession besides those in healthcare takes on this type of burden?

Many of the other healthcare professions have much clearer or self-explanatory roles, such as a respiratory therapist, a laboratory technician, a medical doctor, a nurse's aide, a food service attendant or patient care assistant, and so on.

# DEFINING A NURSE AND WHAT THEY DO

A definition of nursing according to the American Nurses Association (ANA) follows:

> Nursing is the protection, promotion, and optimization of health and abilities, prevention of illness and injury, alleviation of suffering through the diagnosis and treatment of human response, and advocacy in the care of individuals, families, communities, and populations. (ANA, 2015b, para. 1)

More information can be found at this website: https://www.nursingworld.org/practice-policy/workforce/what-is-nursing.

The International Council of Nurses (2022, para. 1) defines nursing as:

> Nursing encompasses autonomous and collaborative care of individuals of all ages, families, groups and communities, sick or well and in all settings. Nursing includes the promotion of health, prevention of illness, and the care of ill, disabled and dying people. Advocacy, promotion of a safe environment, research, participation in shaping health policy and in patient and health systems management, and education are also key nursing roles.

More information can be found at this website: https://www.icn.ch/nursing-policy/nursing-definitions.

According to the National Council of State Boards of Nursing (2022, para. 1), a nurse is "an individual who has graduated from a state-approved school of nursing, passed the NCLEX-RN examination, and is licensed by a state board of nursing to provide patient care."

More information can be found at this website: https://www.ncsbn.org/resources/nursing-terms.page.

Given the multiple and differing definitions of nursing, it is not difficult to understand why nurses have problems describing exactly what they do and why they do it. A question often asked, that further adds to the confusion by both those in and out of the profession, is, "What is nursing: an art or science?"

## PRACTICE PEARLS

- Trust your "gut" or intuition.
- If something doesn't "feel" right, it probably isn't.
- Use the available scientific evidence—it can make or break your practice.

# NURSING AS AN ART

Chinn (1994) described art as not something that stands in opposition to science, but it is a part of all human experience. Art can express a feeling or what words usually fail to express. Art can bring a comprehensive experience to human consciousness if people are aware.

Artistic characteristics of nursing include:

- Creativity
- Intuition
- Insight
- Passion
- Collaboration

Lindeman (1999), in an editorial, summarized previous work by researchers Dock and Stewart from the 1920s about the art of nursing. Lindeman described how nursing would be lost, and possibly dangerous, without being guided by science. However, no amount of knowledge will ever make up for the lack of skills that constitute the art of nursing, and it is not something that can be formalized. As with any form of art, it reflects perceptions from the viewer and the art or artist who is performing.

Florence Nightingale stated:

> Nursing is an art; and if it is made to be an art, it requires as exclusive a devotion, as hard a preparation, as any painter's or sculptor's work; for what is having to do with dead canvas or cold marble, compared with having to do with the living body—the temple of God's spirit? It is one of the fine arts; I had almost said the finest of fine arts. (Dossey, 1999, p. 7; finestquotes.com, n.d.)

Finfgeld-Connett (2008) in her concept synthesis of the art of nursing, referenced relationship-centered practice and the artistic characteristics present in nursing. The artistic characteristics include kindness, compassion, healing touch, humor, and thoughtful doing. For nurses and other healthcare providers to provide this type of approach to patient care, they must be at their best. Developing a calm demeanor, a sense of a confidence with a peaceful spirit, and high regard for what they do is essential. This type of practice leaves little room for those who are stressed, fatigued, and burned out.

## EXPERIENCING THE ART OF NURSING THROUGH CASE STUDIES

How can we explain the "art of nursing"? Johnson (1994) reviewed all of the available literature relevant to the art of nursing and identified five distinct themes:

- Embracing the meaning in patient encounters
- Establishing a meaningful connection with the patient
- Skillfully performing (nursing) activities

- Developing an individualized course of action to care for patients
- Conducting your own practice of nursing) morally

The art of developing any type of clinical healthcare practice encircles the organic composition of knowledge, philosophy, spiritual beliefs, personal life experience, and professional experience to become a unique composition of *you.* It's how you individually practice your craft. This may be a completely different way to think of yourself as a healthcare professional and the novel contribution you make to society as a whole.

Patient interaction encompasses all of the characteristics stated by Johnson (1994) and can be best explained (or *shown*) through clinical practice examples. A series of examples, listed as cases, are presented throughout this chapter to illustrate nursing art versus science. (Each of these concepts could also aptly be applied to the other healthcare professions by inserting their professional role in the brackets.)

In each of the cases, consider if what is described was learned behavior for the nurses to act as they did. Or was it simple human kindness? Does it explain the "art" of practice?

***Case 1***

A 2-year-old had been a frequent patient in the intensive care unit. She had undergone multiple shunt revisions for hydrocephalus. The multiple revisions left a great deal of scar tissue along with a complication during the last revision. Both left her gravely ill and on a ventilator to assist her breathing; she was unresponsive to stimuli. One of the night-shift nurses who worked in the unit read to her every night and made sure that she had her own pajamas and her favorite stuffed animal with her. A bond had formed between the nurse and child. All of the staff knew the child would not survive. The night that she died, the nurse was on duty. She refused to let the child be taken to the morgue on the morgue cart. She wrapped her in her favorite blanket and carried her down the back steps to the morgue.

### *Case 2*

A young woman was in an auto accident, sustaining a severe head injury. She spent several weeks in the intensive care unit (ICU). A request was made to her family to bring in familiar items that she enjoyed, along with music. Her husband was a youth pastor and had a beautiful voice. Each day, he would come to her room and sing to her. Several of the staff, if time permitted, would join him and sing all of her favorite hymns. Often, other patients' family members would stand outside the door to hear the music. Other patients in the ICU would comment on how much they enjoyed the music. The patient went to rehabilitation for her injuries and made a marvelous recovery. After her discharge home, she commented to her husband that she remembers hearing choir music almost every day she was in the hospital.

### *Case 3*

A patient with Guillain-Barre syndrome spent several weeks in the hospital. He was an avid football fan and loved to watch the games on Sunday. Several nurses cared for him over the time he was hospitalized. On one of the Sundays, he thought the staff should all be involved in a football pool on the games for the day. The nurses who were on duty that day gladly granted his request. After his recovery was complete, he sent a thank you note to the staff commenting on how that day made him feel "normal" again.

### *Case 4*

On a busy night in the emergency department (ED), a radio call went out for a multiple fatality motor vehicle collision. One of the emergency medical services (EMS) crew members who responded to the scene came into the ED on a separate call later in the evening and was found in the utility room crying about the earlier call. Two little boys, brothers, had been killed in the accident. A beautiful baby girl was in the department with colic. She had settled down and was "a happy baby" waiting for discharge. One of the nurses talked with her parents and asked to "borrow" her for a few minutes. The nurse took the baby, walked over to the EMS crew member in the utility room, and placed the baby in his arms. She smiled and cooed at him. The nurse looked at the EMS crew member and made a simple statement, "Life goes on."

***Case 5***

A nurse was passing medications late in the evening. She entered a patient room to give the medications. The patient was in pain due to a kidney stone and had recently received a pain medication dosage to attempt to alleviate some of the pain. The nurse was busy and running behind. The patient made a simple request. "Can you please just sit and talk with me for a minute?" The nurse began to think of all she had to do before the end of her shift. However, she made the decision to sit with the patient. They had a wonderful conversation. During that time, the patient relaxed, and before the nurse left the room, he dozed off.

Each of these cases describes how a nurse's thoughts and subsequent behaviors were able to immensely comfort and influence others in a time of need. Being mindful, present, and not distracted—taking the time to notice another's distress—made all the difference to each of these patients by making a human connection. This "presence" requires nurses to skillfully cultivate a positive relationship with both stressors and stress.

Much of the recent adoption of science and technology in healthcare has challenged the ability to deeply connect with others. Many patients feel this has compounded the difficulty in truly connecting with their providers of healthcare.

### MEASURABLE ARTISTRY: SURGICAL PROCEDURES AND THE FIELD OF AESTHETICS

There is also a more literal artistic element to nursing and some healthcare specialties, such as aesthetics, wound care, intravenous insertion and surgery. Many providers have advanced degrees or certifications that elevate their practice to specialty niches where their artistic abilities are showcased. For example, the operating room nurse assistant, certified in wound closure, has the power to determine the appearance of the scar(s) left behind from a surgery. Scars continually remind a patient and their loved ones of what they've been through. Beautifully crafted suturing skills can leave minimal scarring and gentle reminders of life-saving surgeries, while large jagged scars may be a painful memory if they show Frankenstein-like suture tracks. Advanced practice nurses and others who practice the art of injectable wrinkle reducers and cosmetic fillers have artistic skills that mean the difference between beautifully lifted eyebrows and natural looking lip or cheek plumpness versus asymmetrical facial horrors.

## WHEN THINGS DON'T TURN OUT EXACTLY AS ENVISIONED

While art can be fun and relaxing, and the beauty created is powerful and satisfying, it can also be very stressful when there are high stakes in being artistic with a person's body and physical appearance. Just as there are high stakes in investing in people emotionally, artistic creativity can be risky for fear of both reputation and litigation. When one person responds negatively to a kind act or turns a nurse's or other healthcare provider's gentle words into something other than what was intended, fear can set in. When fear sets in, anxiety about all future encounters may follow. With anxiety and all of its emotional and physical components comes the cycle of stress, fatigue, and the potential for burnout.

***Case 6***

> A 42-year-old nurse executive is called to the medical-surgical floor to help with an unhappy patient. The 72-year-old woman is admitted for a thyroid imbalance that has led to some confusion. She is volatile with the staff and is refusing her medications and care. The nurse executive greets her warmly and tries to engage her in conversation. Soon they realize that they have a mutual connection. The patient's grandson and the nurse executive's son are in Taekwondo together. The patient remarks that her grandson is rambunctious, and the nurse executive laughs and says, "They are boys after all." The patient took her medication and was better to the staff with some encouragement from the nurse executive. That evening, the daughter of the patient calls the nurse executive at home and yells at her for talking about her son to her mother, saying, "How dare you criticize my child's behavior!"

Sometimes it feels as though no good deed goes unpunished. It did not take long for the nurse executive to feel the effects of burnout. Several sleepless nights ensued. People with good intentions hurt the most when they feel they have hurt other people. Good people are rewarded the most when they feel they have helped other people. Nurses and other healthcare providers who are making a positive impact are rewarded daily from those actions alone.

When the helpful nature is rejected, misunderstood, or received negatively, the damage to the provider may be severe. A little piece of the person's spirit is diminished, their artistic flame shines less brightly, and their willingness to give freely is impaired. This kind of entrapment creates a mental resistance that is physically demanding and emotionally draining; burnout ensues. Building hardiness helps to combat these feelings by strengthening responses to commitment (know you have done your best), control (understanding what you can and cannot control), and challenge (developing resilience to resist others negativity in your response).

## PRACTICE PEARLS

- Listen to your patients.
- Listen to the patient's parents or caregivers.
- Consider taking the time you need to encompass the art of nursing into your daily work representing the science of nursing. It will improve your practice.
- Think about how your stress impacts your work and the patients or others you care for in your work environment.
- When you're feeling stressed, take a moment to think about the experience you are having and the experience you would like to be having. How big is the gap?

---

## THE ROLE OF INTUITION IN NURSING AND HEALTHCARE

Finfgeld-Connett (2008), referenced the terms *empirical* and *metaphysical* knowledge in relation to the art of nursing. *Metaphysical* addresses characteristics that are not always apparent yet are intuitive to nursing practice. It is an important portion of nursing, and it relies on the nurse being in tune to their patient, peers, and most importantly, being in tune with themself. Buetow and Mintoft (2011) cited Haynes, Devereaux, and Guyatt's work in 2002 related to medical practice where evidence-based medicine also recognizes that clinical expertise, including intuition, is needed to integrate the clinical state and circumstances, research evidence, and patient preferences and actions. Both of these studies show the importance across clinical disciplines for the use of intuition in practice.

No one patient is the same as the next. Two patients' diagnoses may be the same, yet every other clinical and behavioral characteristic they exhibit are different. This generally produces a wide variety of outcomes. Nurses and other healthcare providers need to be able to recognize and acknowledge these differences to better care for each patient as an individual. Through the acknowledgement of these differences, providers are better able to help patients achieve their optimal levels of health. Caring for each patient individually requires careful thought and calculated risk-taking to address each of the differences to meet the patient's needs. An example is presented in the following case study.

***Case 7***

> A new graduate nurse was working on a surgical floor. Due to the fact that she was the newest nurse in the department, she was assigned a patient that the rest of the staff on her shift felt was "difficult" and did not want to care for. The new nurse entered the patient's room and immediately encountered a very angry woman experiencing mental health distress who suddenly began to cry. The nurse sat with her and asked her why she was angry. The patient shared with the nurse that she was the first one to acknowledge that she was angry and began to share the story of her illness along with her fears. The nurse and the patient developed a bond that lasted through each of her admissions and, subsequently, her death.
>
> The nurse in this case was in tune with her own feelings and chose not to enter the patient's room with a preconceived idea or bias secondary to her peers' perceptions of the situation. She took a risk by asking the patient a difficult question. The patient could have chosen not to share her feelings with the nurse and taken her anger (mental health distress) out on the new nurse. But by taking this risk, the new nurse helped to care for this patient by acknowledging her anger and removing it as a barrier. She was then able to proceed with the scientific elements of her physical care for the patient's clinical benefit.

## ARTISTIC KNOWLEDGE

Blondeau (2002) looked at nursing as a practical art and emphasized the concept of artistic knowledge in nursing through Adler's (1978) definition. Adler defined *artistic knowledge* as "making anything" and mentions that productive ideas are not enough to create an end product. Making things requires the knowledge and skill to take raw materials and create something more. If there is no end product then there is no realization of the idea, and it cannot be expressed.

Adler's (1978) definition of artistic knowledge can be applied to the practice of nursing and other health professions. The definition can best be described by applying it to a patient interaction:

> A patient presents with a set of symptoms they have developed. The patient is otherwise healthy and takes no medication. A nurse performs an initial assessment of the patient and relays the information to the medical provider. The medical provider assesses the symptoms (raw materials), orders testing and based on the findings (raw materials), prescribes a course of treatment (raw materials). The nurse carries out the orders and educates (something created from raw materials) the patient on the prescribed course of treatment. The patient acknowledges the treatment plan and schedules a follow-up appointment. Upon return for the follow-up appointment, the patient's symptoms have been alleviated and he has returned to a state of health (something created).

### PRACTICE PEARLS

- Every patient has a story to tell—listen.
- Be creative in your practice.
- To be at your best, take time for the "three R's": rest, recover, and refuel.

# NURSING AS A SCIENCE

To define the science of nursing, differences must be examined within science itself. In 1966, Hemple distinguished between natural and social sciences. Natural sciences include physics, chemistry, and biology and incorporate other areas such as anatomy and physiology. The social sciences, according to Hemple (1966) include sociology, political science, anthropology, and economics. Hemple (1966) went on to discuss that science is empirical and non-empirical. Empirical science attempts to describe, explain, and predict what occurs in the world we live in; where non-empirical science is not comparable and doesn't rely on data like a theory, faith or values (this or that, good or bad, etc.).

Scientific characteristics of nursing include:

- Deduction
- Fact finding
- Observation
- Testing and proving/disproving theories
- Collaborating

Nurses and medical providers similarly build a practice from the empirical science, as it provides the basis for the individualized care each patient receives. However, much of what is done in nursing and many of the other healthcare professions is non-empirical and falls under the category of social science (focusing on the human condition) as evidenced in the case studies in this chapter.

Manhart-Barrett (2002) defined nursing as a basic science; it is the application of the scientific art of using knowledge to practice nursing. Others define science in a slightly different way as being a collective body of knowledge composed of applied research along with testing theories. Research findings and the development of theories can be applied to generally any industry; and, certainly to a specific discipline such as nursing.

Parse et al. (2000) developed a definition of nursing science that is continually evolving. They define nursing science as a basic science. It encompasses substantive knowledge of the human-universe-health process while being discipline-based. Medicine is much of the same: continually evolving, based upon a specific body of science, etc.

These definitions lead to a question of significance. Cody (as cited in Daly et al., 1997) put forth a warning—the difficulty that nursing has as a profession with articulating what it does and its unique nature within healthcare has placed nursing at risk. Similarly, Nagle (1999) stated that nursing can be a matter of distinction or extinction. These views, albeit close and now over two decades old, bear a great deal of truth in nursing today. In addition, ancillary disciplines have evolved into specialty practice and removed some of the previous basic practice elements of nursing: ambulation, respiratory therapy, blood drawing, etc.

For experienced nurses, the ability to articulate the nursing process is defined by distinct steps. It begins with the assessment of a patient. The findings based on the assessment lead a nurse to plan interventions for the patient, with the patient. Those interventions are then implemented. After the interventions are implemented, at defined intervals, nurses reassess the effectiveness of the interventions. If the interventions are effective, the same course is followed. If the interventions are not effective, the entire process begins again—assessment of the patient, creating a care plan, implementation of clinical and non-clinical interventions, and evaluation of the process. Many of the other clinical disciplines follow a similar process to move the patient toward an improved health condition.

In recent times, this process has been expanded to include other elements such as nursing diagnosis and outcomes (ANA, 2015a). Nursing diagnosis weaves the nurse's clinical judgment with the client or patient's current condition; this facilitates a path forward for care planning. The addition of outcomes with planning focuses the care plan on measurable goals. This process of thinking and documentation of the overall care plan is shared with and among other clinical disciplines for care integration. More information about the nursing process and how it works can be found here: https://www.nursingworld.org/practice-policy/workforce/what-is-nursing/the-nursing-process.

There are some nurses in the profession who may question if this portion of the science of nursing has been replaced with clinical pathways and prompts in the electronic health or medical record that only require the click of a radio button. Or what about smart pumps that do not require a nurse to calculate the correct drip rate of a medication? Listening to a patient's apical pulse to count a heart rate is often done via a cardiac monitor. The cardiac monitor may not even be in the same room as the patient. The individual trained to surveil the monitor(s) is generally not a nurse. Automatic blood pressure cuffs are relied upon to take an accurate blood pressure. Pulse oximeters measure oxygen saturation and other technologic advances measure key vital signs; today's nurse just has to look at the readout on a machine.

However, interpretation—which takes into account all that a nurse sees with the patient—cannot be accomplished by machinery. *There is no substitute for a physical nursing assessment.* A great deal of information can be gained by what is seen, not seen and with the use of adjunctive technology. Does this advancement of technology take away from the science in nursing practice? Are today's nurses too dependent on equipment when they used to be dually dependent on assessment skills and knowledge? Each of these plays a crucial role in today's practice of nursing: physical and mental health assessment skills; environmental and situational awareness; the use of technology to gather data; and, assimilation via critical thinking and clinical judgment.

### *Case 8*

Not long ago, an anecdotal example of this issue occurred when an ED physician responded to an in-house incident in which a patient's condition was rapidly declining. The physician requested a current blood pressure on the patient and then watched as the nursing staff

> repeatedly pushed the button on the automatic blood pressure cuff in the attempt to get a blood pressure. The physician, in a moment of frustration, asked if anyone knew how to take a manual blood pressure.

A recent article written by Feliciano (2014) referenced a statement made by Dr. Rosalind Picard, a Massachusetts Institute of Technology professor who feels that robots should be made available to physicians and nurses to enhance the delivery of care. Feliciano (2014) noted efforts currently underway that could potentially lead to robots replacing nurses. Is that even possible? Have nurses become so dependent on technology that they could be replaced? Have nurses drifted away from the science that is the foundation for nursing practice? We don't think so.

Manhart-Barrett (2002) referenced previous work by other researchers in the 1990s who defined the science of nursing as a scholarly discipline, overlapping with other disciplines, all the while encompassing all that nurses do. Nursing is more than just providing care. Nursing science is theory- and research-based, as it requires specialized knowledge and utilizes methods other than those that are solely based in nursing science. However, nursing science is the core or essence of the discipline.

Idczak (2007) posited the science of nursing finds its base in the acquisition of skills and knowledge that occur throughout the nursing curriculum. The concept of *relatedness backward* describes how the skills are acquired in nursing. In this concept, the nurse acquires knowledge through looking back at a process and methodically scrutinizing the process to determine two things: what could have been done better and what worked well for the patient. An example, which is extreme yet defines it well, is presented in the following case.

***Case 9***

> A patient is to be transferred from the emergency department to the critical care unit (CCU) following the application of an external pacemaker for a heart block. Cardiac rhythm capture has been main-

> tained and the patient is delivered to the CCU. During the admission process, the patient is switched to the equipment that is present in the CCU. Cardiac rhythm capture was lost during the exchange and the patient did not survive. A root cause analysis (RCA) was conducted to determine the cause of the incident. All staff involved in the case were brought together in an attempt to gather information and understand what went wrong. This RCA process was meant to ensure this type of incident did not occur again. The nurses involved painstakingly reviewed every aspect of the case, including their care from the nursing perspective, and made recommendations to prevent any future occurrences.

In any root cause analysis process, all participants learn from the incident. And, most likely they will remember the mistakes that caused the extreme circumstances and it forever affects their clinical practice. To learn more about a root cause analysis and how it is conducted, see: https://psnet.ahrq.gov/primer/root-cause-analysis. To learn more about the importance of situational awareness and patient safety in healthcare, see: https://psnet.ahrq.gov/web-mm/situational-awareness-and-patient-safety.

# HOW ARE ART AND SCIENCE INTERTWINED?

Chinn (1994) declared the art of nursing as the art/act of the experience in the moment. It is the direct apprehension of a situation, the intuitive and embodied knowing that arises from the practice/praxis of nursing. Through this definition, the science of nursing can be interpreted to coincide with the art. Other healthcare professions may also have similar connection between art and science. What makes a nurse return to a room to check on a patient they just left? Many would say they just knew they needed to or had a gut feeling. How does a nurse know what to do in a crisis with a patient they have never met? Experience and embodied knowing; they both provide a solid foundation to appropriately respond in a crisis. When a disaster strikes, why is it the nurse who is relied on to handle the situation? Expert problem solving using the learned nursing process: assessment, diagnosis, outcomes/planning, implementation, and evaluation!

# CONCLUSION

Are healthcare disciplines art or science? There is no right or wrong answer to this question. Every provider of healthcare, regardless of where they are in their career path, what degree or degrees they hold, what department or setting they work in, could provide a definition and multiple examples to support art and science, or both.

Nurses and other healthcare providers must be mindful about what it takes to be at their best in caring for others. Mind "stress" only exists in what has happened in the past (such as PTSD) and what might come in the future (feelings of anxiety) not generally in the present. Emergent circumstances may dictate stress and appropriate action in the present. Thus, nurses and other healthcare providers need to be "mentally fit" as well as physically able to perform the job.

As technology continues to become standard practice in healthcare, pieces of both the art and science will be replaced. Yet, as nursing and healthcare research continues to evolve, clinical guidelines become standard, and evidence-based practices are implemented, new science will become prevalent. Science can never replace the art that fills an amazingly diverse profession. If one were to ask any patient who has been afraid before a procedure and comforted by a healthcare provider, they will tell you just the how special the provider was. If one were to talk to a family who tragically lost a loved one, most likely they would be able to describe how compassionate the healthcare worker was who helped them through the paperwork as an expert guide. Gather a group of nurses, and sometimes other healthcare providers, and they will share how a peer comforted them after a terrible shift.

If one were to ask a group of nurses specifically to describe how they knew to recheck a patient, they will respond, "I just knew." The same group of nurses could also describe many times they called back to check on a patient after the shift ended. It might even be in the middle of the night. When asked if there is another profession most nurses would choose, nurses emphatically state that there is nothing that they would rather do.

To be a dedicated artist requires commitment, sacrifice, talent, and a desire to create something beautiful, often out of something others would never see as beautiful. Artists make many sacrifices. Healthcare workers must work odd hours, off shifts, and holidays. They frequently miss family gatherings and milestones in their children's or other family members lives. They can sleep through a concert because they have been up for 36 hours. Christmas is often moved to another day on the calendar because it is their holiday to work. Healthcare providers often leave their shift hungry, exhausted, and barely able to think about what has to be done at home or in other aspects of their lives.

Nurses and some other healthcare workers witness more horror in a single day than most other professions in a lifetime. This has been especially true during the recent global COVID-19 pandemic. A distraught mother hands a nurse their lifeless child and expects the nurse to save her. A husband loses his wife of 60 years and cries on the nurse's shoulder; all the while, the nurse understands that it won't be long before he joins her. The indelible memories nurses and other healthcare workers now have from comforting critically ill patients unable to see or connect with family during COVID-19 has been heartbreaking. And, it has truly taken an emotional toll.

Nurses and those who choose the healthcare profession are like a piece of marble and the experiences are the hammer and chisel in the hands of the sculptor. Each patient cared for, each interaction with peers, each life experience slowly chips away, revealing more and more of the beauty beneath the surface. That beauty comes through in the way the healthcare provider interacts with patients, peers, family, friends, and complete strangers. It is the beauty that shines in the darkest moments.

The moments might include a nurse sitting with a family that tragically lost their 17-year-old son in an auto accident or the 88-year-old man whose wife passed away after 70 years of marriage. It is there when a physician delivers difficult news to a patient and the nurse is left at the bedside to "pick up the pieces" and help a patient and family comprehend what they have just been told. The beauty also shines through when a provider sees a patient walk for the first time after a major injury or hands a baby to a new parent.

Can nursing be quantified? Is it the same for other healthcare professions? Is it possible based on the components of each profession that are easy to define? And others that are fleeting? Is it art or a science? It might just be for each individual to decide.

In the next chapter, you will learn about nursing and healthcare leadership. Leadership is a specialty in itself and is often intertwined with diverse stressors. Nurses and other healthcare leaders regularly navigate among a multitude of stressful conditions in their daily work by balancing the needs of the organization, patients, providers, families, payors, and others. These complex conditions often produce immense stress, leading to fatigue and burnout.

# REFERENCES

Adler, M. (1978). *Art and prudence.* Arno Press.

American Nurses Association. (2015a). *The nursing process.* https://www.nursingworld.org/practice-policy/workforce/what-is-nursing/the-nursing-process/

American Nurses Association. (2015b). *What is nursing?* http://www.nursingworld.org/EspeciallyForYou/What-is-Nursing

Blondeau, D. (2002). Nursing art as a practical art: The necessary relationship between nursing art and nursing ethics. *Nursing Philosophy, 3*(3), 252–259. https://doi.org/10.1046/j.1466-769X.2002.00095.x

Buetow, S. A., & Mintoft, B. (2011, April 26). When should patient intuition be taken seriously? *Journal of General Internal Medicine, 26*(4), 433–436. https://doi.org/ 10.1007/s11606-010-1576-6

Chinn, P. (1994). Arts and esthetics in nursing. *Advances in Nursing Science, 17*(1), viii. https://doi.org/10.1097/00012272-199409000-00002

Daly, J., Mitchell, G., Toikkanen, T., Millar, B., Zanotti, R., Takahashi T., Willman, A., Barrett, W., & Cody, W. (1997). What is nursing science? An international dialogue. *Nursing Science Quarterly, 10,* 10–13. https://doi.org/10.1177/089431849701000105

Dossey, B. (1999). A Nightingale legacy: The art of nursing. *Creative Nursing, 5*(3), 7–9.

Feliciano, C. (2014, February 14). Robot replacing nurses: Is it really that far-fetched? *Nursetogether.com.* http://www.nursetogether.com/robot-replacing-nurses-is-it-really-that-f

Finestquotes.com. (n.d.). *Florence Nightingale quotes.* http://www.finestquotes.com/author_quotes-author-florence%20nightingale-page-0.htm

Finfgeld-Connett, D. (2008). Concept synthesis of the art of nursing. *Journal of Advanced Nursing, 62*(3), 381–388. https://doi.org/10.1111/j.1365-2648.2008.04601.x

Hemple, C. (1966). *Philosophy of natural science.* Prentice-Hall.

Idczak, S. E. (2007). I am a nurse: Nursing students learn the art and science of nursing. *Nursing Education Perspectives, 28*(2), 66–71.

International Council of Nurses. (2022). *Nursing definitions.* https://www.icn.ch/nursing-policy/nursing-definitions

Johnson, J. (1994). A dialectical examination of nursing art. *Advances in Nursing Science, 17*(1), 1–14. https://doi.org/10.1097/00012272-199409000-00003

Lima, J. J., Miranda K. C. L., Cestari, V. R. F., Pessoa, V. L. M. P. (2022, February). Art in evidence-based nursing practice from the perspective of Florence Nightingale. *Rev Bras Enferm, 75*(4), e20210664. English, Portuguese. https://doi.org/10.1590/0034-7167-2021-0664

Lindeman, C. (1999). From the guest editor: The art of nursing. *Creative Nursing, 5*(3), 3–4.

Manhart-Barrett, E. (2002). What is nursing science? *Nursing Science Quarterly, 15*(1), 51–60. https://doi.org/10.1177/089431840201500109

Nagle, L. M. (1999). A matter of extinction or distinction. *Western Journal of Nursing Research, 21*(1), 71–82. https://doi.org/10.1177/01939459922043712

National Council of State Boards of Nursing. (2022). *Definition of nursing terms.* https://www.ncsbn.org/resources/nursing-terms.page

Parse, R., Barrett, E., Bourgeois, M., Dee, V., Eagen, E., & Germain, C. (2000). Nursing theory guided practice: A definition. *Nursing Science Quarterly, 13*(2) 177. https://doi.org/10.1177/08943180022107474

# 4

# THE IMPACT OF LEADERSHIP IN NURSING AND HEALTHCARE

## OBJECTIVES

- Explore the idea of leadership.
- Consider the characteristics that make a good leader.
- Consider how good leadership mitigates stress.
- Learn techniques for lowering stress in a leadership position.

There is a great debate taking place in nearly every work setting about leadership. Are great leaders born or developed over time? Can leaders be shaped and created, or is leadership an instinct? Further discussion begs the question, is there a difference between leadership and management? How much influence does leadership have on operational outcomes?

What we do know is that leadership matters. It is perhaps the single most important element in any successful business enterprise (Mills, 2005). And leaders can lead from anywhere—not just in a formal leadership role. Good leaders are not afraid to take risks and are skilled at calculating the true cost of any change initiative.

However, not everyone who either chooses or ends up in a leadership role is meant to be a leader. The impact a leader can make—good or bad—is critical to the development of healthy workplace culture, the resulting work environment (policy and practice), and subsequent organizational performance (outcomes). The question needs to be posed: How are nurses and other healthcare providers trained for leadership positions? Is there formal training or are they put in the position to learn (like on-the-job training)? Are they provided a mentor? How are the new leaders supported? In addition, what ongoing training and support are provided to leaders as they grow in their leadership journey?

All nurses should be viewed as leaders due to their ability to influence others' decision-making: providers, patients, their peers, other clinicians, non-clinical team members, and formal leaders. Each level of either formal or informal leader also has a role. Informal leaders are crucial because they are often present, engaged, and influential. They have the ability to drive change among their peers. The informal leader can serve as a spokesperson for the unit, be the voice of reason, and have a stabilizing presence all while assisting the formal leadership in reaching their objectives.

## LEADERSHIP THROUGH LARGE-SCALE CHALLENGE

Never before, at least in recent years, has the importance of leadership been on display in healthcare for the world to see as it has during the global COVID-19 pandemic. The overwhelming, bone-deep fatigue and human suffering was unbearable to many. Now, turnover in nearly all positions is reaching new heights: At just 2% in 2019, turnover climbed to 18.6% in the Advisory Board's 2020 annual survey of over 200 health systems' nursing staff (Peng & Rewers, 2021). Vacancies are plaguing even the best-run institutions' and forcing unpopular decisions with service restrictions.

This presents quite a challenging dilemma when patients keep coming for services and there isn't anyone to care for them. The financial cost to an organization to replace a nurse in 2020 averaged $40,038 (NJSNA.org). This, along with the utilization of temporary staffing, may impact the cost and quality of care. A lack of trained personnel in all areas may cause delays in care, increase the opportunity for errors, and ultimately impact patient outcomes. The most difficult roles to fill are usually specialty areas which require more experience, specific education, and honed expertise; it doesn't look like this will be changing any time soon.

Peng and Rewers (2021) described how, while the recent increased rate of turnover is alarming, a more insidious problem has been at play with increasing turnover in *each* of the six years preceding the COVID-19 pandemic. They posited that leaders should be prepared for even more turnover in the future due to structural issues in the work environment (at the heart of nurse and other provider engagement) which remain unresolved, and compensatory motivation to leave for higher salaries and sign-on bonuses elsewhere. Here were their 2021 recommendations for how to combat these problems:

1. Embrace team-based care as a permanent solution to lessen staffing shortages and the associated challenges to providing quality care.

2. Implement entry-level worker competitive strategy.
3. Augment staffing and experience shortages with virtual care technology (i.e., e-intensive care units for critical care support).
4. Redesign RN total rewards to appeal to changing RN needs among the variable generations in the workforce.
5. Communicate the value proposition of working at the bedside.

In addition, leaders must not underestimate the impact of COVID-19 on the mental health of all healthcare workers. Burnout and stressful work environments are not new in healthcare—they were just exacerbated by the pandemic's complexities in an already chaotic system. And it doesn't seem like we have seen the worst of it. It has been extremely difficult both as a caregiver and a leader to feel helpless in a system overwhelmed with need. No amount of individual self-care can fix the work or social environment. That is up to the leadership to develop a culture where people want to work and be appropriately rewarded for it. The global COVID-19 pandemic has taken an undesirable toll on everyone in healthcare, and truly maybe every person on earth who experienced it.

## THE CONNECTION BETWEEN LEADERSHIP AND CULTURE

Leaders create structure through social interaction (Marion & Uhl-Bien, 2001). Social interaction can be simply described as the workplace culture built by relationships and encompassing how the work gets done. Cann (2016) diagnosed today's organizations as suffering from a recognition problem; they can't distinguish good leaders from bad ones.

He described weak leaders as follows (Cann, 2016):

- Their team routinely suffers from burnout.
- They lack emotional intelligence.

- They don't provide adequate direction.
- They find blame in everyone but themselves.
- They don't provide honest feedback. They are blind to the current situation.
- They are self-serving.

Unfortunately, Cann's description describes some leaders of today in nursing and healthcare. Their leadership behavior negatively influences the work environment and causes undue suffering by leading in a state of crisis management. Leadership is a specialty practice, evidenced by the number of advanced degree programs focusing specifically in leadership. These formal educational programs equip leaders with the skills to navigate the complexities of any leadership role (in various industries). The varied leadership programs offer insight to learners about emotional intelligence; how to delegate; how to give clear direction and follow up; engaging in clear communication; delivering performance reviews; becoming adept at business situational awareness; and common pitfalls. These assist leaders in avoiding the weak leader characteristics posited by Cann (2016).

Cohn (2012), after interviewing more than 60 Chief Executive Officers (CEOs) of very large global companies hiring leaders, surmised that they focus on the wrong things: candidate charm, academic credentials, and a stellar resume, when none of this has any bearing on leadership potential. In contrast to poor leadership, Cohn (2012) found that these seven fundamental leadership qualities are more effective at predicting future leadership success and are the hallmarks of great leaders:

- Integrity
- Passion
- Courage
- Vision

- Judgment
- Empathy
- Emotional intelligence

Stress, fatigue, and burnout among the workforce are all evident in negative work cultures. And now, leaders are more frequently than in past years being asked to do *even more* with less. When there is a leadership vacancy, it often goes unfilled, and another leader picks up the workload until a replacement can be found. This system is designed as a short-term fix. It's not a good fix to burden the leader with additional work in an area for which they may not have expertise. It is not unusual for the recruitment process to take several months to locate a candidate pool and determine the right fit to hire. When the temporary assignment is protracted, everyone suffers.

In areas where leaders are allowed to assist clinical staff (in some unionized environments this isn't possible), it can negatively affect the overall success of the unit. While patient care always comes first, the leadership functions cease as if they aren't important or valued. Leadership in healthcare must be viewed as its *own specialty.* It takes a learned and polished set of specific skills for recruiting, interviewing, and retaining staff; monitoring and improving quality measures while reducing risk for patient safety; building stakeholder relationships; preparing for and adjusting to budgetary constraints; evaluating patient and staff satisfaction; and constantly prioritizing and reprioritizing as necessary. Leadership cannot be overlooked nor unaddressed.

Leaders should not be saddled with their own crucial responsibilities, as well as expected to fill in (because they can) for all others under their areas of responsibility. When they do, the additional stress of working early and late to perform their own administrative duties takes a toll. It severely limits their ability for optimal health and well-being: time for self-care, meal breaks, spending quality time with family or friends, exercising, mental and physical downtime, etc. Combating stress, fatigue, and burnout is a shared responsibility in each organization, its leaders, and the employees who choose to work there.

### HOW POSITIVE LEADERSHIP PAYS OFF

A number of years ago, a training video depicting the culture of Southwest Airlines was developed to show the value of loyalty between a company and its employees; it described how to utilize trust to increase employee morale, develop superior customer service, and impact the company bottom line. Incidentally, Southwest Airlines has sustained positive financial performance in the difficult aviation industry where most all of their competitors have struggled. In January 2020, Southwest Airlines touted 47 consecutive years of profitability. However, during 2020 and 2021 the streak ended due to the dire effects of the global COVID-19 pandemic on the travel industry (Isidore, 2022).

A similar comparison can be made with healthcare leadership. It is so simple—the "golden rule" (treat others as you would like to be treated) goes a long way, and a servant leadership attitude should be a foundational element for leaders in healthcare, and especially in nursing. In addition, being nice and treating others with respect is just basic human kindness. Trust is also essential to develop an inclusive, healthy work environment where each member of the team feels valued.

## SERVANT LEADERSHIP

Robert K. Greenleaf coined the term *servant leadership* and first published his thoughts in an essay in the 1970s (Greenleaf Center for Servant Leadership, n.d.). Greenleaf described *servant leadership* as:

> The servant-leader is servant first… It begins with the natural feeling that one wants to serve, to serve first. Then conscious choice brings one to aspire to lead. That person is sharply different from one who is leader first, perhaps because of the need to assuage an unusual power drive or to acquire material possessions. (para. 2)

A servant-leader focuses primarily on the growth and well-being of people and the communities to which they belong. Healthcare deeply needs leaders now more than ever who have a clear sense of purpose, a passion for their work, and are laser-focused on health and well-being for both themselves and those they lead. The systems in healthcare also need radical transformation to be successful in the future by providing the best service and customer value.

## WHAT IS LEADERSHIP?

A single definition of leadership in the literature is elusive. Most descriptions of leaders are based on the context or the situation. A search of the nursing-specific literature revealed a multitude of examples offering differing singular definitions. Perhaps Cann's (2016) definition could be used in reverse to describe good leadership for any specialty. If so, Table 4.1 illustrates how they would compare.

**TABLE 4.1** COMPARING AN INEFFECTIVE LEADER AND AN IDEAL LEADER

| Cann's Ineffective Leader | Ideal Leader |
|---|---|
| Their team routinely suffers from burnout. | Their team is considered a dream team of leaders. |
| They lack emotional intelligence. | They exhibit emotional intelligence. |
| They don't provide adequate direction. | Their expectations are clear, and they are decisive when necessary. |
| They find blame in everyone but themselves. | They insist on a "no-blame culture." |
| They don't provide honest feedback. | They provide honest and candid feedback. |
| They are blind to the current situation. | They are aware of the current state of organizational affairs based on accurate data. |
| They are self-serving. | They exude an attitude of service. |

Working for an ideal leader sounds great, right? It also fits with what healthcare needs most to move forward in the whirlwind of current change.

A strong leader listens to others' concerns and provides follow-up with "circle" communication when issues are identified. Leaders also have a responsibility to create the support for a culture of safety throughout the organization—which includes employee responses to the social or work environment. A healthy work environment supports work-life balance.

A strong leader ensures that direct reports and other healthcare providers know what they value. This must include creating space for others to feel that they are heard and that the challenges they face in their work will be addressed (as best they can). Leaders' roles have become much more complex and important than in times past. They not only have responsibility for operational success, but must equally provide a supportive environment that promotes team success to deliver the safest and best patient outcomes. This is imperative for adequate recruitment and retention of talent. Talented individuals will no longer be subjected to poor leadership or poorly run organizations when they have a myriad of career choices.

## PRACTICE PEARL

"Do not follow where the path may lead. Go instead where there is no path and leave a trail."

–Anonymous

---

A memorable leader in history, Eleanor Roosevelt, was noted for her informal style. Her thoughts about leadership could be used today as guiding principles for nursing and healthcare:

- "You can often change your circumstances by changing your attitude; do one thing every day that scares you." This encourages leaders to reflect on their contribution and be willing to question the status quo and take risks.

- "Do what you feel in your heart to be right for you as you will be criticized anyway." This encourages leaders to follow their intuition and always do what is right no matter what the consequences.
- "To handle yourself, use your head; to handle others, use your heart." This encourages leaders to be thoughtful and caring when taking risks and driving change.

More pithy quotes from Eleanor Roosevelt can be found at https://www.goodreads.com/author/quotes/44566.Eleanor_Roosevelt.

Leadership can come from any position, and healthcare needs leadership at all levels. Nurses are in a unique position to offer leadership in all directions: with patients, with their peers, with other clinical colleagues, with those they supervise, and with their own supervisor. Each person can make a positive or negative difference from their contribution at work. Thoughtful and compassionate behavior results in honorable actions. Think about these nurses and their contribution: Florence Nightingale, Mother Teresa, Clara Barton, and Dorothea Dix (Nurseblogger, 2009). When you think about your role in healthcare, which type of leader are you? Are you a positive or a negative influence?

One of the greatest things a leader can do is be creative in their approach to problem solving. Much of what used to work in nursing and healthcare is no longer relevant for today's challenges. The global COVID-19 pandemic provided a platform for much creativity in the face of a crisis. Each day, those in healthcare devised novel solutions to unpredictable challenges. Most workers did not ever think we would see the day to reuse personal protective equipment, not be able to source the necessary supplies or their substitutes, be overrun with patients to the point that full capacity meant people were actually waiting *outside* the walls of healthcare facilities, creating alternative care environments in unconstructed spaces or in outdoor environments, and more.

Nikravan (2012) described exceptional leaders as those who help employees work through times of change by communicating extensively. Explaining the need for change and ensuring everyone understands the change increases the odds that the change will be successful. There was no shortage of opportunities during COVID-19, with rapid-fire changing directives from both external and internal sources. Leaders had to adapt and be agile in their actions and communications. The overwhelming amount of information was exhausting, and creative solutions had to materialize in real time.

Fear of the unknown peppered leaders' thoughts: what if they got sick, what if they brought the virus home to their families, what if too many of their staff got sick and could not provide care, what if the leaders got sick, where would we place all of the patients who needed care, what about staff member's children—where could they go and what about school; the list seemed never-ending. The leaders who were able to make it through the COVID-19 pandemic developed an immunity to the stress, fatigue, and burnout. But how did they do it? Read on.

## PRACTICE PEARLS

- Leadership can come from any organizational position (informal versus formal).
- Be a positive leadership influence on others—attitude and actions are everything.
- Nursing and healthcare are service professions—be a good example to others.

---

# THE LEADERSHIP-STRESS CONNECTION

Carlson (2009) described the chaos-filled healthcare environment as one with a dizzying pace of change with leaders showing weariness to continue, thus creating various degrees of satisfaction, too much positional turnover, health-related symptoms of stress, and a tendency to want to quit. Later, Waddill-Goad (2013) outlined stress as a concern in healthcare, specifically with executive nurses; the fine balance they must keep with multiple competing priorities served as a negatively contributing factor with strong organizational impact. Stress is known to lead to higher healthcare costs, inefficiency, staff turnover, increased sickness, and absenteeism in the workplace. These effects have been noted by the many diverse industries that have studied the effects of stress.

Shirey (2006) suggested stress is a negative factor in healthcare and nursing in a study over nearly *two decades.* This information is not new. Stress was shown to decrease the quality and the quantity of care, as well as job satisfaction. In a landmark leadership study, also over a 20-year period, Lieberson and O'Connor (1972) looked at the link between leadership, corporate, and environmental factors influencing organizational performance in 167 public companies. Their findings suggest that leaders are restricted in their ability to influence results due to the internal *structure* of an organization and its *culture* by blocked communication, factional conflict, and abortive bureaucracy. These results beg the question, "If there was more effective communication, less conflict, and less bureaucracy in the healthcare work environment, would nurses and other healthcare providers be less stressed, and would the organization achieve better results?" We believe the answer is yes!

During the global COVID-19 pandemic, there was not time for blocked communication, factional conflict, and the usual bureaucracy was seemingly shattered. This was one upside of the pandemic. Things got done with little interference. Could many of the new or revised processes now stick? Could an inventory of improvements in process be calculated to be used going forward?

The pandemic proved we could move fast and greatly simplify many of the complex work processes. Going forward the question is, can we stay with a solution-oriented approach, or will the industry revert back to a more comfortable approach of "command and control" that requires people to ask over and over again for the same problems to be solved? That depends a lot on how leadership responds.

# PRINCIPLES OF LEADERSHIP AND EXCELLENCE

Guyton (2012) identified a number of principles for successful nursing leadership, including:

- Share a commitment to excellence
- Measure what matters
- Build a culture around service
- Create a path for leadership succession

The first principle is a commitment to excellence. This aptly applies to all healthcare workers. Everything related to nursing and all of healthcare should meet a standard of excellence, and span of influence includes everything from caring for a patient to promoting the professions in a positive manner.

Another of Guyton's principles (2012) is to measure the things that are important. Currently, two of healthcare's most important regulatory metrics are patient experience and patient outcomes. But in the measurement of patient satisfaction or experience, the connection between nurse satisfaction and patient satisfaction is often overlooked. Nauert (n.d.) pointed out the direct correlation between customer satisfaction and employee satisfaction; the improvement is almost two-fold when employees have a high level of job satisfaction. In practice, this also seems to correlate. Happy employees lead to happier customers.

Here's a recent example tying patient experience and patient outcomes with a seemingly satisfied nursing staff. A friend described his recent hospital stay:

"The *entire* staff of nurses who cared for me were all temporary and did a fantastic job. They were caring, compassionate and did their job with precision and skill. I'll give them the highest score possible when I get my survey!"

The hospital and nurses' incentives were ideally aligned: provide excellent care and service with fair and equitable compensation. Was their excellent service because the nurses were completely engaged in their work and felt more valued? Whatever it was it showed and was different than previous hospitalizations. Was it because they knew they are only a day away from re-assignment (if they don't provide good care or service they are asked not to come back)? Is this a feasible and more cost-effective model to provide care in the future? Whoever the leader was, they were clearly building a culture around service.

In addition to the metrics of patient experience and outcomes, Guyton (2012) reminded leaders that growth and finance cannot be neglected. Each of these areas must be approached in a balanced fashion to create an optimal synergy of overall performance (customer service, people, finance, quality, growth, and so on). Nurses and other healthcare leaders need to be good role models with expert communication in planning growth and managing finance in the areas in which they are responsible. Information in the new age of healthcare needs to be shared, and organizations must be transparent. As previously described, employee engagement is necessary for the most successful outcomes in both business and service. Engaging healthcare employees in each of the balanced areas is perhaps more necessary now than ever before with cost pressures mounting from the fallout of the global COVID-19 pandemic. Difficult conversations in the future about lines of business, how work is done and by who will be unsettling for many in the workplace. However, in practice, when team members are informed about business challenges such as the cost of supplies and labor (engaged), they are able to make better choices in supply selection and the utilization of all available resources.

Guyton's (2012) principle, building a culture around service, is explained well by a servant leadership style. Nurse leaders particularly have an opportunity to serve many others by the decisions they make: medical care providers, patients, nurses and other healthcare team members. Their decisions can result in the design of improved systems; better patient and business outcomes; and a healthy work culture—or just the opposite. A culture in which customers and team members both feel valued is ideal and easily achievable in healthcare. In addition, one of the hallmark metrics of good leadership is low turnover; turnover is often solely caused from poor relationships between the involved parties.

Nothing causes more stress and frustration for leaders than vacancies with more work to be done than can be accomplished (where demand exceeds the available supply of resources). Why do most people change jobs? Research and experience suggest it is due to a less than optimal relationship with their direct supervisor. This also seems to be so simple; it is everyone's professional responsibility to create good relationships and a good work environment. Effective interpersonal relationships are paramount to a work environment that supports all healthcare providers and their practice. When successful, other problems often take care of themselves. Most measurable results in healthcare—employee, provider, and patient satisfaction or experiences, as well as financial and quality performance—are tightly intertwined with good relationship-building, efficient communication, and a healthy work environment. And, as brutally shown during the COVID-19 pandemic, it takes all members of the team being engaged to be successful.

Engagement can be a tricky thing. Several of the writers in this book have had the same or similar experience with nursing strikes: where the temporary nurses were onboarded the night before the unionized nurses left the facility. Without fail, the medical staff noticed a change during the strike in practice, attitude, and engagement with the "changing of the guard." Why? What was it that kept the permanent nurses from being highly engaged in their work, committed to providing excellent service, and being a fantastic team member? Did the leadership have some responsibility?

# BEING A GOOD LEADER

Building new leader programs or succession planning is vital for any organization, regardless of size. In smaller organizations, it is perhaps even more important. The fourth principle Guyton (2012) addressed was creating and developing leaders. A structured system of leadership succession is important for current and future leaders. Expectations are more clearly outlined, the desired characteristics and results are known, and organizations can create an effective leadership pipeline. Identifying internal and external talent is critical for optimal organizational skill planning. Frequently, internal informal leaders have a tremendous amount of influence and organizational knowledge. Commonly, what is needed is a formal system to hone their rudimentary leadership skills.

Guyton's (2012) additional and cited as vitally important principles are communication, accountability, reward, and recognition. Accountability begins with communicating clear expectations. Holding individuals accountable for their actions is a leadership skill that can be challenging to master; conversations about performance are often difficult and leaders must develop a tolerance for conflict. Many aspects of accountability are dependent on organizational policy and procedures. A single standard of leader communication, consistency, and follow-through is crucial.

Inconsistencies in communication cause confusion, which in turn cause stress and may affect morale. Take caution to prevent information overload. Consider multiple methods of communication to reach all intended parties. This includes written communications such as memos, email, etc. Other verbal communication channels such as huddles, informal hallway conversations, and short meetings can be used to reinforce written communiqués or for conversation or clarity. All communication strategies must embrace honesty and be timely and simple to reach and be understood by a diverse audience.

Success needs to be celebrated. Leaders and organizations who value employee contributions will reap the rewards. Giving credit where it's due and praising performance can go a long way. This is particularly important when individuals, groups, departments, and organizations are challenged. As leaders, it is easy to move on to the next thing or priority.

However, it is often the small things that make a difference in employee satisfaction. A simple hello, taking time to ask about how someone is doing, and being visible all yield positive rewards for leaders and staff. Reward and recognition are key strategies to make people feel valued. Taking the time to acknowledge employees for their professional contribution and personal accomplishments both carry a tremendous amount of weight. All too regularly, it is easy to focus on what is *not* going right versus what is. Nurses are trained to look for what is wrong. Decisions are made by a process of elimination. We make assessments and document by exception.

We need to consider changing our focus to looking for what is working and what can be improved in the work environment. This change in thinking or mindset might change the perception that "uncontrollable" external forces are causing stress, fatigue, and burnout. Control is an illusion and more often than not there are many factors in our environments we cannot control.

## PRACTICE PEARLS

- Strive for effective communication to build solid relationships. Only engage in healthy conflict and respectful debates. Less conflict means less stress.
- Pay attention to what is being measured in your work environment. What is your involvement and contribution?
- Learn about leadership and work to eliminate bureaucracy.
- Recognize a job well done and be accountable.

## THE FOUR T'S OF LEADERSHIP

Strategies to combat stress must be integrated into nursing and healthcare systems beginning with seminal education. Grossman and Valiga (2009) described four "T's" of leadership: truth, trust, teamwork, and training. Each is easy to implement into existing systems of leadership and communication.

- **Truth:** Leaders must be truthful even when the news is not good.
- **Trust:** Trust is built by being truthful and following through.
- **Teamwork:** Effective relationships require truth and trust.
- **Training:** It is essential to stay current with evidence-based industry practices.

According to teambuilding.com (2022), here are 10 important tips for building a high-performing team:

1. Think outside the box—this sets the tone for creativity and innovation.
2. Allow for professional development—use learning to strengthen team bonds.
3. Involve and engage all team members—be sure everyone participates to maximize team potential.
4. Highlight your team's strengths and interests—assign roles based on ability and expertise.
5. Use rewards and recognition—feeling valued at work links to well-being and performance.
6. Lead by example—model good behavior.
7. Respect your team's time and boundaries—be considerate and compassionate when scheduling activities.

8. Tend to conflicts before they happen—set clear goals and expectations to hold team members equally accountable.
9. Let team members weigh in—listening empowers others to feel valued and that their opinion matters.
10. Keep learning and improving—do your best to keep up-to-date and change course when necessary.

### PRACTICE PEARLS

- Team goals, roles, and guidelines must be clear.
- All team members must be invested in the outcome.
- Communication must flow freely and be truthful.

## STRUCTURE/PROCESS/OUTCOME IN SYSTEMS

The design of an organizational structure is critical, because it drives the subsequent work processes. Donabedian (1980) noted the structure/process/outcome connection in relation to quality. It also fittingly applies to business. Structure drives processes, which subsequently drive outcomes (good or bad) in a generally predictable fashion. The good largely drives good outcomes and the poor largely drives poor outcomes. Much of what transpires in the normal business of healthcare is not all that unpredictable.

There are patterns of predicting outcomes if you look at data. Healthcare has enormous amounts of data in current electronic systems. However, turning the data from often disparate systems into useful information has been historically challenging. Data-driven decision-making has also not been the consistent norm among many mid-level leaders. This is changing due to the number of required quality indicators, publicly reported data, growth in the acquisition of community hospitals by for-profit companies, and a strong focus on the clinical outcomes' connection to reimbursement or payment.

Design review can begin either at the top or at the base of an organizational structure. From the top, it might include analysis of the number of leadership roles, direct reports, span of control, and associated departmental fit with divisional responsibility. From the base, it may include analysis of skill mix, staffing patterns and plans, models of care delivery, and customer type and demand.

Each of the design elements drives work process. *Work process* consists of a number of steps that may be sequenced, dependent on previous results or independent of either. In recent years, a number of healthcare organizations have embarked on journeys to incorporate Lean or Six Sigma principles (more to come on these in later chapters) into their operations.

Both strategies have the ability to decrease variation, decrease defects, and improve overall cost and quality. Each begins with a standard approach to problem solving with a review of process steps and associated outcomes. Once the process (supported by data) is understood, changes can be recommended.

Healthcare is the most complex knowledge-driven industry in the world and represents one of the most important economic challenges in recent history (Glaser & Hess, 2011). Cox (2002) posited that you can transform something important into something urgent if you wait long enough. It has now been *two decades* since Cox made that statement. Healthcare seems to have been a "neglected" system, allowed to evolve on its own. And the evolution is not what it should be. It is a system based on illness and sick care versus one focused on population health and the prevention of illness. The current system is teetering on the verge of crisis, and making substantive change has become urgent. Hence, the number of outside sources driving investment in healthcare by those who desperately want to help fix it (Medical News Today, 2021).

Common nursing and other clinical procedures or business as usual has habitually layered new forms, electronic templates, techniques, and plans with little regard for past process analysis. Avoiding innovation by forward-thinking leadership and efficient system management has resulted in challenges of process, access, equity, and quality.

A sense of urgency now more than ever needs to become the new normal; inaction will be even more costly. Another upside of the global COVID-19 pandemic may be that is has spurred a great deal of change in a short period of time. If the momentum can remain high for overall system change, new ways of thinking may result in substantive changes for better health access, equity, and outcomes.

Nursing is constantly changing, so nurses cannot sit idly by and do nothing. They are the largest group of healthcare providers yet do not often use their collective voice. Nurse leaders need to be at decision-making tables and set the tone to embrace positive change. Nurses and all other healthcare providers need to embrace change for themselves and the public at large. Key traits for all of today's nurses and other healthcare providers should include competency in design, planning, explanation, and project or process implementation.

## PRACTICE PEARLS

- Does the organizational design support patient-care needs? Are the right people doing the right work?
- Does the department have efficient work processes?
- Does the work environment support good workflow (traffic patterns, location of equipment and supply, etc.)?
- Is leadership supportive of change related to improvement?
- Are the right people in the right leadership roles? Do they have demonstrated leadership expertise and competency?
- Are leaders trained for their positions?

## LEADERSHIP STRATEGIES TO MITIGATE STRESS

Interpersonal challenges can be one of the most concerning issues facing nurses, healthcare providers, and all leaders. Conflict causes a host of problems within organizations. Leaders must become stress tolerant to succeed in their assigned roles. They are often balancing priorities from a variety of sources: internal and external customer demands, financial pressures, labor shortages, as well as many others. Confidentiality is often required, and the inability to share information may potentiate feelings of stress. This requires leaders to balance professionalism with honesty and integrity.

Nurse leaders can suitably apply the nursing process method of problem solving to organizational maladies. Others can use it, too. Objectivity is key, and they must accurately assess the data in challenging situations as the first step. They must then analyze the available information, with the ability to ascertain additional material if necessary. They should only draw conclusions after careful assessment and analysis of the evidence and devise plans for a course of action, leaving time for appropriate pauses with evaluation. Timing might be everything. Rarely do others perceive organizational emergencies as true emergencies. Problems in general do not develop overnight and should not be solved in a thoughtless or reckless manner due to panic. Successful change takes time and thoughtful planning for precise execution and sustainability.

## APPROACH DECISION-MAKING MINDFULLY

Astute leaders make mindful decisions by considering the consequences. They take time for themselves and make time to be present for others. Sometimes taking time is the best strategy to decrease stress, fatigue, and the potential for burnout. Breaks can be invaluable whether they are a few minutes here and there for deep breathing, time for a walk, taking a *real* vacation, a planned break between jobs, or a formal sabbatical. The amount of time is relative depending on the intensity of the situation. It might be a short break, a long vacation, or extended time in between jobs.

A great deal of information is currently found in the literature about mindfulness. *Mindfulness* is simply defined as being aware and present. Awareness includes feelings, thoughts, and attention focused on the present moment. Rarely do we take time to stop "doing" and just "be." Learning to be is a key leadership trait; when you allow yourself space to be at your best, you are also better for others.

Future success should not be associated with busyness. Multitasking is a misnomer. When you are multitasking, you are not present in either or any task. Mindful individuals notice those who are not present. A lack of presence or not being in the moment and appearing disrespectful may signal trouble for leaders.

## INVITE IDEAS FROM THE TEAM

Engaged and empowered employees want to help. Let them! No person generally comes to work with adverse intentions. Positive leader and employee relationships can be developed. Providing opportunities for employees to share feelings, thoughts, and ideas can be powerful. However, leaders must listen and be present for others to feel heard.

### PRACTICE PEARLS

- Follow your instincts and trust yourself.
- Take the time to decrease stress and harness energy for positive outcomes.
- Empower others to assist in getting things done.
- Value yourself and those around you.

### PROVIDING A SAFE PRESSURE VALVE

A colleague shared a successful idea that she deployed in her work environment when employees presented an issue. The whiteboard in her office says the following:

- A "free &*$!@" in which the employee is allowed to come in and complain about something. With this option, they get what is bothering them off their chests and nothing more is said.
- The second option is to bring a problem forward for discussion along with possible solutions. The leader and employee work together to come up with a viable solution to the problem.
- The final option is the employee brings the problem to the leader, has no solution, and the leader takes over the problem. In this option, the employee supports the leader's decision for solution, regardless of whether they agree it was the right approach.

This problem-solving process has worked well and provides a sense of empowerment to employees because they know they have options and full leadership support.

## SET BOUNDARIES

Boundaries are one of the most challenging aspects of leadership. One must protect their time by managing their schedule utilizing the most pressing priorities, and be willing to change course with a moment's notice. This is often difficult when working with multiple stakeholders who have differing priorities and needs. The leader must be able to effectively communicate the current or changing priorities and clearly define their personal and professional boundaries to maintain their own mental and physical health. In addition, expectations for performance must be reasonable and objectively measurable. At times, workload and the priorities may need to be negotiated because there are only so many hours in a day and time is finite.

## USE MULTIPLE COMMUNICATION STRATEGIES

One of the most important tools that you can utilize to mitigate stress is communication. Leaders must communicate often and effectively. Some types of communication, such as delivering bad news, can be difficult but are essential for leadership success. Other communiqués, such as providing information via a short email or posting a notice, are simple. More complex communication may entail holding frequent staff meetings; this might be repetitive at different times and on different days, but the strategy is meant to ensure important messages are getting to each employee and being heard firsthand. Regardless of the type of communication, it is all essential. The well-informed and involved employee will be less stressed and develop trusting relationships with others and most importantly, with the leader. Trust what you believe in as a leader and value those around you to shape that vision.

### PRACTICE PEARLS

- Communication is key.
- Communicate often and in different formats.
- Communication needs to include everyone and is a two-way street.

---

## CONCLUSION

Being a leader takes courage, fortitude and hardiness. Learning about applying leadership in any healthcare role is essential and can be quite interesting. As described, there is no single definition of leadership but a collection of characteristics identifying excellence in leadership practice. All nurses and other healthcare providers should be viewed as having the opportunity to be leaders: in their specialty, with their peers, in their work unit, among their assigned patient group, and with friends and family. Taking ownership and feeling a sense of responsibility or control minimizes stress, subsequent fatigue, and the potential for burnout. The next chapter discusses professional integrity, associated dilemmas, and the nuances that facilitate connections between stress, fatigue, and burnout.

# REFERENCES

Cann, B. N. (2016, March 25). *Have you run into the (7) signs of weak leadership?* LinkedIn Pulse. https://www.linkedin.com/pulse/have-you-run-7-signs-weak-leadership-brent-n-cann/?articleId=6119050764343140352

Carlson, J. (2009). A retiring bunch. *Modern Healthcare, 39*(26), 6.

Cohn, J. (2012, February 14). *Why we pick bad leaders, and how to spot the good ones.* CNN. https://www.cnn.com/2012/02/14/opinion/cohn-pick-leaders/index.html

Cox, D. (2002). *Leadership when the heat is on.* McGraw-Hill.

Donabedian, A. (1980). *Explorations in quality assessment and monitoring: The definition of quality and approaches to assessment.* Health Administration Press.

Glaser, J., & Hess, R. (2011). Leveraging health care IT to improve operational performance. *Healthcare Financial Management, 65*(2), 82–85.

Greenleaf Center for Servant Leadership. (n.d.). *What is servant leadership?* https://greenleaf.org/what-is-servant-leadership

Grossman, S. C., & Valiga, T. M. (2009). *The new leadership challenge: Creating a future for nursing.* F. A. Davis.

Guyton, N. (2012). Nine principles of successful nursing leadership. *American Nurse Today, 7*(8). http://www.americannursetoday.com/nine-principles-of-successful-nursing-leadership

Isidore, C. (2022, January 27). *Southwest returns to profitability.* CNN Business. https://www.cnn.com/2022/01/27/business/southwest-earnings/index.html

Lieberson, S., & O'Connor, J. F. (1972). Leadership and organizational performance: A study of large corporations. *American Sociological Review, 37*(2), 117–130. https://doi.org/10.2307/2094020

Marion, R., & Uhl-Bien, M. (2001). *Leadership in complex organizations.* (Report 11). Management Department, Faculty Publications, University of Nebraska – Lincoln. http://digitalcommons.unl.edu/cgi/viewcontent.cgi?article=1012&context=managementfacpub

Medical News Today. (2021, November 10). *What is private equity in healthcare?* https://www.medicalnewstoday.com/articles/private-equity-in-healthcare

Mills, D. Q. (2005). The importance of leadership. In *Leadership: How to lead, how to live* (Chapter 1). MindEdge Press.

Nauert, R. (n.d.). *Employee satisfaction key for customer satisfaction.* PsychCentral. http://psychcentral.com/news/2011/06/02/employee-satisfaction-key-for-customer-satisfaction/26623.html

Nikravan, L. (2012). *Why creativity is the most important leadership quality.* Chief Learning Officer. https://www.chieflearningofficer.com/2012/05/30/why-creativity-is-the-most-important-leadership-quality/

NJSNA Nurses Weekly. (2020). *The cost of nurse turnover.* https://njsna.org/the-cost-of-nurse-turnover/

Nurseblogger. (2009, September 14). *25 most famous nurses in history.* http://onlinebsn.org/2009/25-most-famous-nurses-in-history/

Peng, J., & Rewers, L. (2021, October 6). *Why so many nurses are quitting (and what to do about it).* Advisory Board. https://www.advisory.com/daily-briefing/2021/10/06/nurse-turnover

Shirey, M. R. (2006). Stress and coping in nurse managers: Two decades of research. *Nursing Economics, 24*(4), 193–203, 211. http://www.medscape.com/viewarticle/543837

Teambuilding.com. (2022, October 9). *10 team building tips you must know in 2022.* https://teambuilding.com/blog/team-building-tips

Waddill-Goad, S. (2013). *The development of a Leadership Fatigue questionnaire* [Doctoral dissertation, American Sentinel University].

# 5

# PROFESSIONAL INTEGRITY

## OBJECTIVES

- Consider how nursing and healthcare is changing and how that affects the stress levels of all healthcare providers.
- Reflect how diversity (ethnic culture, tenure, age, and so on) in healthcare is positive for the entire profession of caregivers.
- Understand the level of preparation for new nurses or other healthcare providers and the impact on the profession(s).
- Consider what it means to be a "professional" nurse or other caregiver.
- Explore how different professional roles lead to different burn-out rates.
- Learn how to avoid boundary crossings.
- Consider how to manage stress while on the job.

Nursing along with others in clinical practice and integrity are synonymous with professionalism. To continue defining *best practice,* all healthcare providers must be truthful and transparent as they evaluate relevant research and innovative practice evidence.

The continuous evaluation of value in healthcare is the responsibility of each provider. This responsibility is central to supporting the integrity of nursing and medical practice for the individual and the professions. Evaluating and improving care proves the commitment to using evidence-based practice when providing care, treatment, and services to patients. Without constant evaluation of forthcoming evidence, the integrity of practice is lowered to a standard not reflective of excellence. Practicing in a healthcare role that does not merge the art and science of a caring profession may result in a less than meaningful practice.

Nurses are directly or indirectly involved in delivering the most care to patients. Thus, their participation in activities to improve care and reduce unsafe practices is paramount. And as nurses, we must redefine what the profession finds meaningful in relation to monitoring of safety, quality, and risk reduction activities associated with ideal nursing practice.

The evaluation of how nursing and other clinical practice adds value to the patient's care has three significant components: safety, quality, and risk. These major components are crucial to improving the daily methods, standards, and decisions that guide practice. The safety and quality components work to *proactively* protect the patient from harm while providing quality care. The risk component is a retrospective review of systems and processes that may have failed related to a patient safety error.

Engaging bedside clinicians to embrace and participate in designing their work to embed safety, quality, and risk reduction is essential to providing excellent care. However, this engagement does not come without challenges. Many providers may not fully understand their role in keeping professional integrity at the top of their mind. Integrity encompasses strong moral principles and honesty, which must be put into action by making continuous improvements in safety, quality, and risk reduction. In addition, the strong moral principles must guide their practice to be non-judgmental, caring, and compassionate for others. According to Coronado-Vasquez et al. (2017), "Patient safety and quality of care in a highly complex healthcare system depends not only on the actions of professionals at an individual level, but also on interaction with the environment."

When a care provider takes part in defining the measures to collect data, evaluate or find trends, and create actions to improve, they can have a direct impact on care in their area of practice. Nursing and other healthcare leaders need to foster and support staff participation in enhancing safety and quality while reducing the risk to patients. Who better to design the work than those doing it!

This includes open and transparent discussions of the three major components (safety, quality, and risk) and seeking feedback on how care can be improved. Other barriers may include an environment that is non-collaborative or not supportive for making improvement; providing care that is not patient-centered; or the leader's lack of support for open communication channels to collect feedback.

Nursing and other healthcare leaders can significantly influence the culture of an organization and ultimately the quality of patient care. Fostering an inclusive environment for key contributors provides valuable insight into how practice may be improved. Did you know nursing is the nation's largest healthcare profession  and is nearly three times the size of the physician profession (American Association of Colleges of Nursing [AACN], 2022)?

Just in the last seven years, the profession of nursing has now grown to nearly 4.2  million nurses with 84.1% employed in nursing according to the latest data from the AACN (2022). Compared to 2015, in a report from the Health Resources and Services Administration (HRSA), the US was estimated to have 2.6 million registered nurses, with 84.8% actively employed in nursing.

In addition, the majority of nurses, 58%, work in a hospital setting and deliver most of the nation's long-term care (AACN, 2022). The AACN (2022) projects a growth rate of 6% per year between 2021-2031 which is faster than the average of all other occupations.

As of 2020, most registered nurses enter the profession with a baccalaureate degree; and, 65.2% of nurses now hold a baccalaureate degree or higher. In 2020, the tally of advanced degrees for nurses showed only 14.9% of the nation's registered nurses held a master's degree and 2.2% a doctoral degree as their highest level of educational preparation. For advanced practice nurses, the need for advanced practice clinicians, leaders, researchers, and teachers far outstrips the supply (AACN, 2022).

## THE FUTURE OF NURSING

Nursing care is the core business in hospitals because people seldom are hospitalized unless they need nursing observation and clinical care. If healthcare continues to change as is being predicted, the percentage of nurses working in the inpatient hospital setting will decline over time as the nation begins to shift from an acute-care focus to prevention and better chronic-disease management. The only patients who will remain in the hospital will be complex patients and those patients who are no longer acute but do not have a safe place for transfer. This was showcased during the global COVID-19 pandemic, especially with acute care admissions. The elderly or immune-compromised residents of congregate living were not able to return to their previous living arrangement after their acute episode of care was complete in a hospital due to COVID-19 transmission worries.

As nurses are preparing for practice, consideration of the level of critical thinking and clinical judgment needs to take place. New nurses, entering practice post-pandemic, have been found to be lacking basic skills to practice. This is in part due to the lack of clinical practice experience as students.

Nursing and other healthcare students were not allowed in the clinical setting during the pandemic and were forced to mostly utilize virtual clinical practice and (if allowed) clinical simulations on campuses. According to a study by Kavanagh and Szweda (2017), only 23% of 5,000 graduate nurses who passed the national licensure exam (NCLEX) could demonstrate readiness to practice on entry-level assessments. These assessments were administered to determine the ability to critically think and utilize clinical reasoning. This same percentage was found to be unable to identify and manage a clinical change. Once a problem was identified, 54% of new graduates were not able to manage the problem effectively, and 23% lacked the urgency to do something about it (Kavanagh & Szweda, 2017). And this was *before* the global COVID-19 pandemic began.

In, 2021, Wolters Kluwer provided similar data in the report "Closing the Education-Practice Readiness Gap." The lack of nursing faculty along with clinical sites has impacted the ability to prepare new nurses to be able to critically think and make critical decisions in differing clinical settings. The lack of confidence to practice, based on the ability to think critically and utilize clinical judgment, adds to the stress that a new nurse experiences (Wolters Kluwer, 2021).

Read more about nurse readiness in the report here: https://www.wolterskluwer.com/en/expert-insights/survey-nursing-readiness

Nurses will continue to be desperately needed for those patients whose complex medical needs require hospitalization. The overall need for nurses is certainly not expected to decline due to a "graying of the population" and the rapid increase of patients with chronic disease. Effective transition to practice programs will be critical to allow those new to practice to safely transition.

The global COVID-19 pandemic has drastically changed the supply and demand economics. Approximately 194,500 registered nurse job openings are projected for each year over the next decade (US Bureau of Labor Statistics, 2022).

The education system as presently designed cannot meet the demand for new nurses given the continued problem with decreasing clinical sites and nursing faculty. This will continue to exacerbate the need for nurses when the supply is not able to match the demand. A continued focus on population health will expand the use of nurses in the ambulatory surgery center, outpatient, transitional, and home care settings. Many of the changes in healthcare to come are unknown and unpredictable; most likely this may produce anxiety and an underlying stress for nurses, as well as, other caregivers.

The Institute of Medicine (IOM), founded in 1970, underwent a name change in 2016 to the National Academy of Medicine. In 2010, they issued a report on the future of nursing describing the major roles and responsibilities of nurses in the following areas: direct patient care to teach and counsel patients; coordinate care and advocate for patients; and research and evaluate more effective ways of caring for patients (IOM, 2010). Even though one of the major responsibilities of nursing is direct patient care, nurses spend 80% of their time on documentation, medication administration, and communication with other providers. This leaves less than 20% of their time specifically for providing other types of direct care (IOM, 2010).

Read more about the IOM Report here: https://www.nursingworld.org/practice-policy/iom-future-of-nursing-report.

With implementation of the Affordable Care Act (ACA) in 2010, the United States had an opportunity to move to a higher-quality, safer, more affordable healthcare system by transforming the way healthcare was provided. While some headway has been made, there is still much work to be done. Incidentally, the ACA was the biggest change in healthcare since the creation of Medicare and Medicaid in 1965. Nursing, as well as, other healthcare professions have the potential to play a major role in changes by virtue of the number of nurses and medical providers, their adaptive capacity to change, and the versatility of their practice.

## PRACTICE PEARL

Now is a critical time for nursing to step forward to bridge the gap between coverage and access; to coordinate the complex care of patients with chronic illnesses; for advanced practice nurses to work to the full capability of their license potential as primary care providers; and finally, to see the value of nurses and enable their contribution across all practice settings and the healthcare continuum. (IOM, 2010)

---

Institute of Medicine (IOM). (2010). *The future of nursing: Leading change, advancing health.* https://www.nursingworld.org/practice-policy/iom-future-of-nursing-report/

Due to the close relationship of nurses with patients and their scientific knowledge of care processes across the continuum, nurses have an opportunity and ability to act as partners with all healthcare professionals and to lead the redesign of the healthcare environment (IOM, 2010). The challenge for nurses as well as other healthcare providers, will be to learn how best to balance the needs of patients without increasing their own stress and fatigue. Stress in nursing has been discussed since the 1950s; four main sources of anxiety remain among nurses: patient care, decision-making, taking responsibility, and change (Jennings, 2008).

Inherent stress in the role of a nurse and other healthcare providers is related to the physical labor of caring for others, working long hours (as well as rotating shifts), constantly dealing with human suffering, and complex interpersonal relationships with patients, families, and fellow healthcare staff (Jennings, 2008). With increasing pressure to focus on cost efficiencies, improved quality of care, the use of technology, and higher expectations by patient and families, nurses as well as other clinical providers of healthcare, will continue to feel the pressure to change the way they practice. Undoubtedly, this pressure will result in feelings of anxiety, stress, fatigue, and burnout for some nurses and other clinicians.

### PRACTICE PEARLS

- Be willing to ask for help when you need it.
- Develop supportive relationships with nursing peers, leaders, and other coworkers to reduce stress in your work environment.
- Help to develop a supportive team environment with other clinical colleagues.

---

## DIVERSITY IN NURSING AND OTHER HEALTH PROFESSIONS

The US Department of Health and Human Services, Health Resources and Services Administration (HRSA), is the department of the government whose primary mission is to improve health and achieve health equity through access to quality services, a skilled health workforce, and innovative programs (HRSA, 2017).

More about HRSA can be found here: https://www.hrsa.gov/about.

One of HRSA's primary roles is to evaluate the adequacy of the number of healthcare providers by category and the distribution across the nation to meet the demand for access to care (HRSA, 2017).

Key findings from their 2017 report were:

- Female workers represent the majority in 25 of the 30 US health occupations analyzed.
- There is considerable variation in racial and ethnic diversity by occupational groups.
- All minority groups, except Asians, are underrepresented in Health Diagnosis and Treating occupations.

- Hispanics, Asians, and Native Hawaiian/Pacific Islanders are underrepresented among Counselors and Social Workers (Community and Social Service occupation).
- Personal Care and Service Occupations is the most diverse occupational group, followed by occupations belonging to the Healthcare Support group.

The full report can be found here: https://bhw.hrsa.gov/sites/default/files/bureau-health-workforce/data-research/diversity-us-health-occupations.pdf.

Diversity in nursing and other healthcare professions is an especially important goal as our country is becoming more diverse; specifically, the nursing education community is working to ensure the nursing profession demographics match the needs of the population for accessible, affordable, and quality healthcare.

The same report published by HRSA in 2017 compared diversity in healthcare occupations (within the health workforce) to the diversity of the current US working-age population (16 years of age or older who are currently employed or seeking employment). With the exception of nursing being a predominantly female profession, the ethnic distribution was very similar to the current working population of the United States. This report shows continued progress by universities in their work to improve diversity in nursing and the other healthcare professions.

Table 5.1 shows a summarized table of percentages from the report, which highlights the diversity by sex and race of healthcare professions in comparison to the US working-age population (HRSA, 2017).

**TABLE 5.1** DIVERSITY: AN HRSA-BASED COMPARISON BETWEEN NURSING AND THE US WORKING POPULATION

| | Male | Female | Hispanic | White | Black | Asian | American Indian/ Alaska Native | Pacific Islander | Multiple/ Other Race Affiliation |
|---|---|---|---|---|---|---|---|---|---|
| US Working-Age Population (%) | 52.8 | 47.2 | 16.1 | 64.4 | 11.6 | 5.3 | 0.6 | 0.2 | 1.8 |
| Registered Nurses (%) | 9.6 | 90.4 | 5.7 | 73.5 | 10.4 | 8.4 | 0.4 | 0.1 | 1.5 |

The increase in diversity and a greater willingness to practice in underserved areas has resulted in improved access to care by healthcare providers who are culturally and linguistically skilled to provide appropriate services (National Advisory Council on Nurse Education and Practice, 2013). Most of the research on improving patient outcomes for minority populations has been done with independent providers. The role of nursing is especially important in diversity because of the personal relationship that occurs between a nurse and a patient. Properly matching patient and care providers relative to race and language creates what is referred to as *concordance*. By having race and language concordance, communication between the patient and care provider improves, resulting in better patient satisfaction and outcomes of care (National Research Council, 2004).

## DIVERSITY, EQUITY, INCLUSION, ACCEPTANCE, AND BELONGING

Diversity, equity, and inclusion (DEI) are representative of an inexhaustible list of terms that organizations are currently using when embracing and celebrating the many cultures our workforce and patient populations bring in 2023. People often think of diversity as differences in race and ethnicity. But diversity also applies to gender, gender identity, sexual orientation, size, language, religious and political beliefs, age, disability, education, and thought to name a few.

Diversity is an important consideration for any workplace. Specifically in nursing, a diverse workforce can be directly related to the quality of care, meaning that nurses who have traits, practices, beliefs, etc. in common with the patients they serve may be better equipped to care for and connect with the patients and populations. As such, many organizations have launched campaigns to promote understanding in the workforce hoping it translates to a healthier, more compassionate workforce with better-connected patient interactions. These efforts take many forms that may include Sexual Orientation and Gender Identity committees, Patient Family Advisory Councils (PFAC), advancement for inclusion on the Healthcare Equity Index (HEI) sponsored by the Human Rights Campaign, or more global council structures.

Since 2020, The Joint Commission has added queries about organizational processes that will lead to improved health equity. To date, surveyors have taken an inquisitive stance; however, they are scheduling special sessions to hear what organizations are doing to address health equity, and formal regulations are expected in the future. More information can be found on The Joint Commission's efforts related to health equity here: https://www.jointcommission.org/resources/patient-safety-topics/health-equity#t=_Tab_StandardsFAQs&sort=relevancy.

Creating an inclusive culture in healthcare is incredibly important in today's world. This begins by breaking down stereotypes and helping individuals recognize implicit or learned "feelings" about people, groups, etc. Subsequent behavior in response to those feelings is important for personal growth. Caregivers must exude compassion without judgment. Most people are doing their best given the circumstances in their life. Communicating everything as clearly as possible to others is crucial to promote diversity and inclusivity in your organization or workplace. People want to feel heard and be understood.

Here are two helpful websites to learn more about HEI and PFAC:

HEI: https://www.hrc.org/resources/healthcare-equality-index

PFAC: https://www.aha.org/patient-and-family-advisory-councils-podcasts-and-blueprint

## MULTIGENERATIONAL WORKFORCE

In 2022, there are five generations in the workforce (Jensen, 2022). Jensen (2022) described how this diversity of age, thought, experience, values, etc. may cause unnecessary tension and misunderstandings between and among the generations, potentiating conflict in the workforce. Those from the millennial generation are the largest component of the current workforce. They have grown up using technology, are used to moving at a fast pace, have different expectations of work, and have witnessed changing social values.

Jensen (2022) suggested three simple guidelines for a people-focused culture to follow:

1. Be curious: What can we learn from each other?
2. Incorporate best practices across generations and optimally mix teams of people.
3. Be patient: Allow time for a shared identity to develop across generations.

Age, experience, and the wisdom from challenges that come with it cannot be solely considered when looking at a population. The multitude of generations in the workforce and population at large present an exciting opportunity for us to maximize the knowledge and expertise of more tenured people while also bringing diversity of thought from younger generations. This mix of thinking is ideal for innovation and breakthroughs, especially in healthcare.

*"Change is not a criticism of the past; it just means tomorrow will be different."*

–Unknown source

Healthcare needs this diversity of thought, various experience, and insight to changing customer expectations now more than ever.

Consider the group of people you work with or interact with most: Every generation has been shaped by different experiences (recession and collapse of the housing market), defining world events (the Vietnam War, Desert Storm, and 9/11), the growth of technology (paper and pencil to handheld computers), the change from tethered phones to cellular devices, privacy or public sharing, and values (hard labor working toward an outcome versus digital age and social media influenced instant gratification). Each generation has been shaped by their experiences and what they've learned as a result. What can you learn from each other? Might your genuine curiosity open dialogue or improve the trust you share as you work together? Are there new ideas to be mutually shared and adopted?

The point is that we must gain an understanding of where each generation has come from in order to ensure we create an environment where each can thrive in the workplace and the world.

## GENERATIONAL BREAKDOWN

Baby boomers (1946-1961): This is a loyal and ambitious, goal-oriented generation that is motivated by promotions, professional development, and aspire to gain authority. They value hard work and have experienced many changes in their lifetimes. Their intellectual and organizational knowledge must be downloaded in short order, as many have already started retiring, taking their experiential wisdom and expertise with them.

Generation X (1961-1981): Born and raised during what may one day be known as "a technological renaissance," this group grew up as latch-key kids; they used the first microwaves, saw color televisions, began early game systems, used clunky home computers, and launched large cellphones—technology became mainstream. Though they prefer to work independently, they are known to be very collaborative, appreciate work-life balance, and prefer informal, rapid, and publicly communicated recognition.

Millennials (1981-1997): Millennials or Gen Y, are the first generation to be raised completely immersed in digital technology (with early access to the internet). Members of this generation are motivated by learning opportunities and professional development, mentoring from more senior work colleagues, feedback, and a positive workplace culture.

Gen Z (1997-2012): As the newest generation to enter the workforce, this generation appears to strive for meaningful work that is in alignment with their values. They want exciting projects they can be passionate about, complete quickly, and move onto other challenges. Incredibly tech savvy, and a product of constant technology stimulation, they excel at multitasking (if that's possible). One overt difference which appears to be surfacing, is that unlike their predecessors, they are very open with their knowledge and information sharing by seeking out public platforms. They know no privacy boundaries and have a preference for regular in-person public recognition.

## PRACTICE PEARLS

- Consider the generational makeup of your coworkers. Are there opportunities to build more collegiality and workplace satisfaction within the team?
- Celebrate individual and collective success. While this is generally welcome in open forums, younger generations prefer online platforms for appreciation where they can share their stories.
- Consider creating mentor programs between generations.

- Be aware that reverse mentorship programs are also popping up, where each employee is both a mentor and a mentee.
- Encourage feedback and group communication to identify mutual team goals.
- Ensure each generation is represented in team composition.
- Tailor coaching and motivational strategies to enhance performance to each individual.

Enhance employees' well-being by asking what is important to them. Wellness must be a part of performance management (as it is imperative to building a new workforce).

---

# DEFINITION OF PROFESSIONAL NURSING

Healthcare used to be defined by the care physicians provided when they diagnosed and treated a disease. This perspective caused confusion for nurses and other clinical professions who struggled to define their own professional role. Nurses have since demonstrated their differentiated skills and specialized knowledge, thus distinguishing their professional role from physicians and other clinical professions.

In the early development of an understanding or definition of nursing, Florence Nightingale, whose writings began in 1860, described nursing's activities as something that put patients in the best condition possible for nature to take its course (Nightingale, 1860). Over 100 years later, this landmark definition of nursing was contained in the statute of the New York State Practice Act of 1972, which has served as legal support for nurses' independent practice and has become a model for other states to use in their nurse practice acts. The definition enables nurses to claim a body of knowledge apart from medicine and to have authority over their own practice.

Here is the definition of registered nursing from the New York State Education Department (NYSED), Office of Health Professions:

> The practice of the profession of nursing, as a registered professional nurse, is defined as diagnosing and treating human responses to actual or potential health problems through such services as case finding, health teaching, health counseling, and provision of supportive care to or restorative of life and well-being, and executing medical regimens prescribed by a licensed physician, dentist, or other licensed healthcare provider legally authorized under this title and in accordance with the commissioner's regulations. A nursing regimen shall be consistent with and shall not vary any existing medical regimen. (NYSED, 2015, para. 1)

The New York State law began the movement in nursing to develop nursing diagnoses that describe a patient's response to health problems. In follow-up to this movement, the American Nurse Association (ANA) developed and published "Nursing: A Social Policy Statement," which describes nurses' responsibilities to patients and society; this further validates the advocacy role of nurses (ANA, 2010).

Here is the ANA's depiction of what nursing is from their website (ANA, n.d.):

> 21st Century nursing is the glue that holds a patient's health care journey together. Across the entire patient experience, and wherever there is someone in need of care, nurses work tirelessly to identify and protect the needs of the individual.
>
> Beyond the time-honored reputation for compassion and dedication lies a highly specialized profession, which is constantly evolving to address the needs of society. From ensuring the most accurate diagnoses to the ongoing education of the public about critical health issues; nurses are indispensable in safeguarding public health.
>
> Nursing can be described as both an art and a science; a heart and a mind. At its heart, lies a fundamental respect for human dignity and an intuition for a patient's needs. This is supported by the mind, in the form of rigorous core learning. Due to the vast range of specialisms

> and complex skills in the nursing profession, each nurse will have specific strengths, passions, and expertise.
>
> However, nursing has a unifying ethos: In assessing a patient, nurses do not just consider test results. Through the critical thinking exemplified in the nursing process, nurses use their judgment to integrate objective data with subjective experience of a patient's biological, physical and behavioral needs. This ensures that every patient, from city hospital to community health center; state prison to summer camp, receives the best possible care regardless of who they are, or where they may be.

In a discussion regarding the definition of nursing, Mason (2011) provided a summary of Patricia Benner's position relative to caring in nursing. Nurses must:

- Continue to demand an expert knowledge level
- Possess the ability to integrate physical, psychological, emotional, and social dimensions of health
- Demonstrate skill in administering supportive care
- Exude superb critical thinking and clinical judgment
- Hone their assessment skills
- Be proficient in coordinating care and advocacy

Incidentally, Benner continued to study various aspects of nursing practice from the time her landmark study was published in 1984 until she retired, and nursing practice has changed dramatically during the last five decades.

Currently, great challenges exist within nursing practice to appropriately delegate care to unlicensed personnel (if they are included in the care delivery model) and deliver care in challenging environments to far more complex patients. This can also be a source of stress, especially for nurses who want to "do it all." However, for the most cost-effective care and efficiency of care provision, care should be assigned based on education, skill, and licensure. And of course, there are some provisions that only a licensed registered nurse can perform. A joint statement on delegation (in a white paper) from the American Nurses Association (ANA) and the National Council of State Boards of Nursing (NCSBN) can be found at: https://www.ncsbn.org/public-files/NGND-PosPaper_06.pdf.

In addition, (in 2005) the National Council of State Boards of Nursing (NCSBN) published a position paper for guidance related to the responsibilities relative to nursing delegation titled, *Working with Others: A Position Paper,* which can be found here: https://ncsbn.org/public-files/Working_with_Others.pdf.

In the nursing profession, challenges occur not only with transition of novice nurses to competent practice but with the transition from competent to expert levels of practice. In addition, frequent job changes may also prevent nurses from reaching the expert level of practice in their specialty (Benner et al., 2009). Stress also increases for experienced nurses when there are few competent peers to serve as mentors or coaches for less experienced nurses.

The global COVID-19 pandemic exacerbated already known stressors for nurses and other healthcare professionals. Demand for care often exceeded the available caregivers in nearly every care environment, thus increasing the feelings of helplessness resulting in additional stress. And those caring for known COVID-19 patients also experienced greater stress due to fears about the disease itself or actually contracting the disease.

The pandemic created particularly damaging emotional injury for nurses and other care providers known as *moral distress* (Edmonson et al., 2022). Edmonson et al. (2022) described moral distress comes from knowing what the right things are to do but being unable to do them. In addition, the authors cited working in an environment where a caregiver's core values feel violated potentiates anger, frustration, guilt, anxiety, and self-blame; often, if left unchecked, these can lead to increased stress, fatigue, burnout, exhaustion, and more.

Over the past hundred years, the definition of nursing has been refined to reflect the development of a body of knowledge specific to nursing. Nursing has had a long and important legacy in healthcare. One of the most important roles is as an advocate for a better, safer, more humanistic healthcare system. It is important that nursing continue this legacy into the future with the highest standards of professional integrity and a focus of providing patient-centered healthcare.

## THE ADVANTAGES OF VARIOUS ROLES IN NURSING

With the aging of society and the increase in chronic health conditions in the population, healthcare systems are dealing with an increasing number of medically complex patients. Nursing is one of the major professions stepping forward to take on additional responsibilities. In the rapidly changing healthcare environment, nursing will continue to evolve as a profession with new and stimulating opportunities. Caring for higher-acuity patients will be more challenging for hospitals while organizations continue to receive smaller reimbursement. Nurses may be able to take on new or more responsibilities in hospitals, clinics, and care centers to help meet these new challenges.

One of the strengths of the nursing profession is the ability of nurses to work in multiple and different roles in healthcare. Feeling stressed in one area? Make a move to another area! Approximately 60% of nurses work in a hospital setting; however, many nurses have moved beyond the hospital to private practice, home health, hospice, long-term care, outpatient surgical centers, insurance companies, managed care companies, industry, nursing education, and more (HRSA, 2018). In the hospital setting, there are also many direct and indirect nursing roles such as critical care, emergency, surgical services (same day, sterile processing, operating room, post-anesthesia recovery, etc.), medical, surgical, pediatrics, mother and baby units, labor and delivery, care management, utilization review, leadership, risk management, quality or process improvement, education specialists, and more. On occasion, jobs are created by nurses who discover a problem and develop a solution that improves the delivery of care for patients.

When a nurse decides to pursue advanced nursing or non-nursing education or become certified in a specialty, they have the opportunity to become a leader in healthcare. The advanced practice nurse has an expanded scope of practice, which helps to fill a void relative to access and care for patients. The increased number of advanced practice nurses has opened another world for nursing to provide primary and preventive care. In many states, an advanced practice nurse's scope is expanded to the specialties of certified midwives, nurse anesthetists, family nurse practitioners, as well as nurse practitioners in cardiology, oncology, neonatal, and many other advanced clinical specialties. Professional nursing organizations have taken an active role state by state to increase the independence of the advanced practice role. In some states, nurses are allowed to practice rather independently, but in other states they must have a collaborative relationship with a sponsoring physician. In addition to advanced practice specialties in clinical areas, there are also opportunities in leadership, research, and education.

Registered nurses work collaboratively with all other healthcare professionals. Nursing has practice restrictions according to the scope of practice defined by each state's board of nursing. The practice rules are usually established by the state legislature delegating oversight by the state board of nursing. Nurses are generally not allowed to operate or practice independently. Nurses implement medical provider and other clinicians (licensed independent practitioners) orders so many times, people believe that nurses always operate under another provider's license. Each nurse is responsible for providing care under their own license. With more than three times as many nurses as physicians in the United States, nurses provide direct patient care utilizing provider orders for tasks such as medication administration, dressing changes, various treatments or therapies, and so on. There is opportunity for the nurse to master complex, multifaceted issues that affect our healthcare systems and the health problems in the population at large. The nursing role has expanded beyond the performance of tasks and procedures—nurses are effective collaborators in a multidisciplinary health team who help patients to navigate the complex health environment (Tiffin, 2013).

# NURSING INFORMATICS

> In attempting to arrive at the truth, I have applied everywhere for information, but in scarcely an instance have I been able to obtain hospital records fit for any purposes of comparison. If they could be obtained...they would show subscribers how their money was being spent, what amount of good was really being done with it, or whether the money was not doing mischief rather than good. (Nightingale, 1860).

These words, spoken by "the mother" of modern nursing over 150 years ago, hold just as true in today's healthcare system. Nightingale seems to have foreseen the need to track patient progress, aggregate data, and use the data to improve; all while illustrating the patient journey encompassing caring, value, and quality in care delivery.

Nursing informatics was recognized as a specialty by the ANA in 1992, earning its own unique scope and standards of practice. *Nursing informatics* is defined as "the specialty that transforms data into needed information and leverages technologies to improve health and health care equity, safety, quality, and outcomes" (ANA, 2022, p. 3).

The exponential growth of information, knowledge, and technology create a significant driver to optimize information technology (IT); especially when it comes to improving efficiency, quality, and safety of healthcare delivery. As practitioners, we know that the highest and most predictable care yielding safety and quality is rooted in standardization. While some healthcare entities have made considerable progress in system standardization, we have a long way to go before adopting a standard algorithm for human interaction. The nursing informaticist is the translator for turning data into information, information into knowledge, and knowledge into applicable nursing wisdom (ANA, 2022).

Working as a nursing informaticist can take many forms depending on the level of expertise a nurse acquires. This work may include enabling and improving clinical decision-making; managing information for knowledge integrity and security; and the ability to inform and influence top-level decision- and policy-making. The information collected creates a solid foundation and allows for sound clinical decision-making and formulating evidence-based practices.

Nurses interested in informatics might find themselves in the role of project manager, educator, researcher, policy influencer, entrepreneur, or executive leader. More information about the role can be found from these sources:

- American Nursing Informatics Association (https://www.ania.org/)
- Healthcare Information and Management Systems Society (https://www.himss.org/)
- American Telemedicine Association (https://www.americantelemed.org/)

# DEFINING PROFESSIONAL BOUNDARIES

Since 1999, when Gallup first included nurses in its survey on professional ethics and honesty, nurses have ranked the highest with over 89% of survey participants (DailyNurse, 2021); they have been ranked first every year with the exception of 2001, when firefighters were on top after the horrific terrorist attack on 9/11 (Riffkin, 2014). To date, that is 20 straight years of surveys (2002–2021)! The results of the survey reflect a special relationship or bond that is built between nurses and patients as well as with those who know them. Patients expect that a nurse will act in their best interest and will respect their dignity. Nurses have the privilege to care for patients when they are not at their best and often are the most vulnerable. Nurses' integrity and ethics must always stay at the highest level. And, the same applies to all other types of healthcare workers.

The National Council on State Boards of Nursing (NCSBN) now provides electronic downloads, hard copy booklets, videos, links to relevant articles, and an online course to learn more about professional boundaries. These references may be useful to other healthcare professionals as well. The references are found here: https://www.ncsbn.org/nursing-regulation/practice/professional-boundaries.page.

According to the NCSBN, nursing is defined via professional boundaries whose scope includes "the spaces between the nurse's power and the client's vulnerability. The power of the nurse comes from the nurse's professional position and access to sensitive personal information. The difference in personal information the nurse knows about the patient versus personal information the patient knows about the nurse creates an imbalance in the nurse-patient relationship" (NCSBN, 2014, p. 4). The NCSBN has published a pamphlet identifying professional standards to help nurses understand professional boundaries and work to establish and maintain those boundaries (NCSBN, 2014).

When a successful relationship develops between a nurse and patient, it is based on trust, compassion, and mutual respect. Such a positive relationship between a patient and nurse has been shown to improve patient outcomes (Duffy & Brewer, 2011). The goal is to develop a therapeutic relationship that "allows nurses to apply their professional knowledge, skills, abilities and experiences toward meeting the health needs of the patient" (NCSBN, 2014, p. 4). When this type of relationship occurs, the patient's dignity is protected, and it allows for the development of trust and respect between the nurse and the patient.

## BOUNDARIES AND THE CONTINUUM OF PROFESSIONAL BEHAVIOR

- It is your responsibility to delineate and maintain professional and personal boundaries.
- You should work with honesty and integrity within the therapeutic relationship.
- Examine any boundary crossing, be aware of its potential implications, and avoid repeated crossings.
- Variables such as care settings, community influences, patient needs, and the nature of therapy all affect the delineation of boundaries.
- Actions that overstep established boundaries to meet the needs of the nurse are *boundary violations.*
- Avoid situations in which you have a personal, professional or business relationship with the patient.
- Post-termination relationships are complex because the patient may need additional services. It may be difficult to determine when or where the nurse-patient relationship ends.

*National Council of State Boards of Nursing (NCSBN), 2014*

## PRACTICE PEARLS

- Think about what you need to do your *best* work and be willing to ask for it.
- Be honest and trustworthy.
- Learn about professional boundaries and the consequences of violations.
- Be on the safe side and never post work-related information on social media.

Environmental chaos, potentiated by a suboptimal work culture, can cause undue stress for nurses and other healthcare providers. Healthy work cultures may produce results that are just the opposite. The negative results of an unhealthy work culture may inhibit a team member's ability to focus on the very reasons they chose to work in healthcare: to create an effective provider-patient relationship and to feel as if their time is making a difference. All healthcare providers must learn to prioritize and remain objective and organized in their approach to care provision, leadership, or education to prevent undue stress, resulting fatigue, and the potential progression to burnout.

Behaviors considered inappropriate can be separated into three categories: boundary crossings, boundary violations, and sexual misconduct. Stress can unduly influence caregivers to act in unusual ways versus those behaviors occurring under normal working conditions.

## BOUNDARY CROSSING

The NCSBN defines a *boundary crossing* as a decision to deviate from an established boundary for a therapeutic purpose (NCSBN, 2014). Boundary crossing occurs when a nurse or other care provider goes beyond a therapeutic relationship. A boundary crossing is usually a brief excursion across a professional boundary that may be inadvertent, thoughtless, or even purposeful. It is usually justified by the person as meeting a therapeutic care need.

For example, a nurse could disclose personal information to reassure a patient. When this occurs, the nurse should consider this a cautionary flag and should closely consider whether this was the right thing to do. The following two cases describe situations where boundaries were crossed.

### *Case 1*

> A neonatal intensive care unit (NICU) nurse became especially attached to a premature infant. The family was from out of town. The parents had several other children, so they were not able to

come into town to see the infant very often. The nurse felt that she knew what the baby needed more than the parents since she was frequently at the hospital. When the baby was getting close to being discharged, the parents came to the hospital and stayed for a couple of days to learn the baby's post-discharge care needs. However, the nurse did not believe the parents were ready for the baby to be discharged, so she asked the physician to delay it for several days. She also got into an argument with one of the other nurses in the NICU because the other nurse believed the parents' knowledge was adequate for discharge. In this example, the nurse became too involved with the baby and should not have requested a delay (and potentially much more costly hospital stay) due to her feelings about the parents' ability to care for *their* child.

***Case 2***

A young adult male patient was admitted to a surgical floor after a somewhat complicated appendectomy. The nurse caring for the patient was very compassionate and provided good care. However, she spent more time with this patient than her others—he was a young, good-looking college student. The nurse was just slightly older than the student and she knew he was from another state and had no family in the area. She overstepped her boundaries in wanting to help him when she gave him her personal cellphone number and offered to give him a ride home when he was discharged. In addition, they began a texting relationship while he was still a patient in the hospital. The nurse should not have divulged her personal contact information or developed a texting relationship while the patient was still under hospital care.

## BOUNDARY VIOLATIONS

A *boundary violation* should be considered a danger signal or red flag. For example, if a nurse believes a pediatric patient's parents are not ready to safely care for the patient, the nurse must be sure objectivity reigns—if the nurse's relationship with the patient is "too close," their judgment may be clouded. The following case describes a situation where a nurse crossed a professional boundary.

### *Case 3*

A pediatric patient was admitted for a serious respiratory illness. The parents of the patient were young, and this was their first child. The nurse caring for the child had a number of years of experience as a nurse and three children of her own. During the course of the child's illness, the nurse witnessed a number of instances when she felt the parents were not attending to the child's needs (showing up late for meetings with the doctor, not responding appropriately when the child needed comforting, and so on). She wondered what would happen to the child when he was discharged from the hospital. Could or would the parents properly care for the sick child? In her haste to do "something" to remedy the situation, she called the state Child Protective Services agency on one of her days off to report the situation. Unfortunately, it did not meet the outlined criteria for reporting. However, the agency was obligated to investigate. Once the hospital was advised of the report (during the investigation), they felt education was necessary for staff. An educational program was provided for all staff to differentiate the licensing duty to report and the differences between the obligation and an emotional reaction to observations of parent-child interactions. In this case, the nurse overstepped her boundaries by not knowing the difference between what she was obligated to report and how she felt about the child's parents and their parenting skills. The nurse did not get into any trouble per se, but it did raise questions about her professional competency.

## SEXUAL MISCONDUCT

The last category, *sexual misconduct*, is the most serious violation. Nurses and other caregivers have the responsibility and duty to make sure this line is never crossed until the care provider/patient relationship has ended (Hanna & Suplee, 2012). It is the provider's responsibility to understand the laws and practice regulations that apply to boundary violations in their state of practice. The following case outlines an example of sexual misconduct.

***Case 4***

> An adult male patient was admitted for a major surgical procedure. While he was hospitalized, he was very overt about flirting with all of the nurses he encountered. For some nurses, it made them so uncomfortable they requested not to be assigned to his case. For others, they enjoyed the attention and flirted right back with the patient. However, one nurse took the flirting too far. When propositioned by the patient for sexual favors, she obliged. She thought she was doing nothing wrong and truly intended to help the patient in his recovery. Seemingly, she was unaware of her professional responsibilities and the boundaries outlined by law relative to the practice of nursing. The nurse should not have engaged in any sexual banter or subsequent contact with this patient. The hospital felt obligated to report the incident to their legal counsel and the board of nursing (BON). After investigation and a comprehensive review, her employment was terminated. The BON performed their own investigation and levied the appropriate consequences.

Clear sexual boundaries are crucial for patient safety (NCSBN, 2009). Violations of this type can have lasting repercussions for the care provider, the facility, and the patient. A comprehensive sexual misconduct guide was published to assist BONs in their education and case review by the NCSBN in 2009. The following information has been excerpted from the report:

> In the National Council of State Boards of Nursing's analysis of 10 years of Nursys® data (NCSBN, 2009), 53,361 nurses were disciplined; of those, 636, or 0.57 percent, were included in the following categories: sexual misconduct, sex with client, sexual abuse, sexual language or sexual boundaries. Therefore, sexual misconduct is not a common complaint to a Board of Nursing (BON). The actual prevalence, however, is not known. Indeed, 38 to 52 percent of health care professionals report knowing of colleagues who have been sexually involved with patients (Halter et al., 2007). (NCSBN, 2009, p. 2)

## MANAGING STRESS AND PERSONAL BEHAVIOR

Nurses learn about nursing boundaries when, as a student, they recite the "Nightingale Pledge" used in pinning ceremonies throughout the country. Some passages from the "Nightingale Pledge" that specifically address professional boundaries are, "I will abstain from whatever is deleterious and mischievous...maintain and elevate the standard of my profession...will hold confidence matters committed to my keeping...in the practice of my calling...and devote myself to the welfare of those committed to my care" (Gretter, 1893). The entire Nightingale Pledge (which has stood the test of time) can be found here: https://nursing.vanderbilt.edu/news/florence-nightingale-pledge.

These are important descriptions of the boundaries related to the responsibilities of a nurse. The pledge was created by Gretter and a committee for the Farrand Training School as a modified "Hippocratic Oath" for nurses as a token of esteem for the founder of modern nursing (Gretter, 1893). It has some similarities to the Hippocratic Oath adopted by medical professionals; the original Greek and revised version can be found here: https://doctors.practo.com/the-hippocratic-oath-the-original-and-revised-version. It is amazing to realize the intelligence and forethought, see the current relevance to today's practice, and note that the highest ethical standards have not changed in hundreds of years.

Due to the personal and intimate nature of caring in a nurse's professional role, nurses may be conflicted and may make moral judgments about a particular course of treatment for a patient (Cavaliere et al., 2010). This might cause the nurse to drift into inappropriate boundary decisions. It is not unusual for nurses to experience moral distress from situations surrounding end-of-life care decisions, institutional policy constraints, and situations which the nurse may believe affects their ability to provide quality care to their patients (Roberts et al., 2012). The situation that caused the moral distress (and the moral distress itself) may result in increased overall stress. This adds to already existing fatigue and leads to symptoms of burnout.

Stress often leads to unintended consequences, including inappropriate behavior. Although nurses learn about healthy behavior and ways to cope with stress in their formal academic programs, the realities of practice may be challenging. The appropriate use and misuse of prescription drugs in the US population is a grave public health concern and is reported in some fashion nearly every day by a variety of media sources. Unfortunately, healthcare providers are not immune; estimates of diversion and use among healthcare workers is suspected to be on the rise, but reliable statistics about prevalence are shrouded in clandestine secrecy (New, 2015).

Prescription drug abuse is on the rise among nurses (Brosher, 2014). Jason (2015) posited in her series of articles to better acquaint licensees with the Oregon Board of Nursing's requirements that there was a dearth of knowledge regarding impairment in the nursing population at large. Based on her research of the available data (including sources at the ANA), estimates were upward of 10% in 2015.

Today, new estimates say upward of 15% of healthcare workers now struggle with addiction or impairment according to an estimate by the NCSBN (Nyhus, 2021). These care providers using alcohol or drugs to an extent sufficient enough to impair performance could pose a risk to the public. These numbers do not include nurses or other healthcare providers who might be impaired due to mental health related issues.

Most healthcare organizations are aware of the potential for diversion of controlled substances and other pharmacologics; however, the degree to which they actively monitor healthcare workers varies. To learn more about diversion and its consequences, follow this link: https://www.ncsbn.org/public-files/Regulatory_Management_of_Substance_Use.pdf.

The greatest risk of nursing drug diversion is public safety: community or patient harm (Jason, 2015). Diversion in a healthcare setting is a criminal activity (New, 2015). Institutions have a duty to provide a safe care environment. A nurse on their very best day can make a mistake. Impairment or substance abuse exponentially raises the likelihood of an error. Due to the seriousness of the nature of diversion, some state agencies are considering formal programs requiring standardized organizational surveillance. In addition, regulatory agencies have taken note. Not only is there organizational regulatory liability and penalty potential, but the licensee faces a host of costly adverse consequences which could include civil penalties and negative publicity (New, 2015). Additionally, the professional healthcare worker may lose their license to practice their chosen profession.

One way to avoid crossing professional boundary lines is by increasing education of nurses and other healthcare professionals regarding violations. It is important to know how to identify early warning signs of professional boundary crossing and the resulting potential or real harm that may occur to patients, as well as the impact on other nursing and healthcare staff (Holder & Schenthal, 2007). Nurses have a professional responsibility to themselves, their peers, and their patients. Nurse practice acts in all states require nurses to mandatorily report unprofessional, illegal, and unsafe practices.

## RESOURCES FOR THOSE WHO NEED HELP

The NCSBN has a number of resources available for Substance Use Disorder in Nursing found here: https://www.ncsbn.org/nursing-regulation/practice/substance-use-disorder/substance-use-in-nursing.page.

Here are a few other resources:

- Help for the Healers: Resources for Impaired Healthcare Professionals | https://drugrehab.org/expert-area/help-for-the-healers-resources-for-impaired-healthcare-professionals/
- Alcohol & Substance Misuse | https://www.cdc.gov/workplacehealthpromotion/health-strategies/substance-misuse/index.html
- Drug diversion and impaired healthcare workers | The Joint Commission: https://www.jointcommission.org/resources/news-and-multimedia/newsletters/newsletters/quick-safety/quick-safety-48-drug-diversion-and-impaired-health-care-workers/#.Y1GHBHbMLIV
- Impaired healthcare professional - PubMed: https://pubmed.ncbi.nlm.nih.gov/17242598/
- Impaired Healthcare Workers Threaten Safety, but Also Need Support: https://www.reliasmedia.com/articles/148460-impaired-health-care-workers-threaten-safety-but-also-need-support

Alcohol use disorder is on the rise in the nursing profession, particularly during and following the global COVID-19 pandemic. In the 2022 Nurse Worklife and Wellness Study, which evaluated the use of numerous substances in 1,170 nurses, 354 reported the use of alcohol in the past year. Of that 354, 124 consumed alcohol only, while 231 consumed both alcohol and drugs and screened positive for substance abuse disorder (Rathburn, 2022). During the global COVID-19 pandemic, the added stress exacerbated the use of alcohol. Due to the stigma, potential loss of licensure and subsequent loss of income, many nurses and other licensed healthcare providers do not seek treatment for substance abuse.

Another barrier that exists related to treatment is the lack of coverage under most insurance plans and other third-party payers. Given these barriers, many nurses and other clinicians walk a thin line with their professional boundaries. Nurses, other healthcare providers, and employers need to be more aware of the consequences of stress and ensure that programs are available to assist nurses and other healthcare providers with this issue. Many treatment programs are noted as resiliency programs that support stress management with healthy coping techniques, group discussion of the trials and tribulations of a career in healthcare in a particular organization, and mutual support for positive decision-making and healthy choices.

Alcohol and other substances pose a serious problem not only to patients but those providing care to those patients. Estimations state that approximately 10% to 15% of all healthcare professionals will misuse some type of drug or alcohol at some point during their career (Baldisseri, 2022). Certain specialties within healthcare are at a much higher risk. Those that work in the psychiatric setting, anesthesia, and the emergency department fall into the higher risk group, as well as paramedics and emergency medical technicians due to the level of daily stressors in their work.

### *Case 5*

> An emergency department (ED) manager arrives in the department early in the morning. The night shift charge nurse meets her with the statement, "If I ever have to work like this again, I will quit and everyone will leave with me." After further conversation, it was determined that the ED physician was acutely intoxicated and had been rude to patients and staff. After questioning the charge nurse as to why she did not contact the manager or house supervisor, the charge nurse stated she did not want to get the ED physician in trouble. The medical director for the ED group was notified and the

ED physician was removed from duty and appropriately referred for rehabilitation.

This case points out the misguided loyalty peers exhibit for one another in healthcare. The concern over a friend's substance abuse or diversion is a struggle. Some peers may be single parents, attempting to further their education, etc., and no one wants to be responsible for the person losing their job. However, everyone makes choices, and our ultimate duty is to safely care for patients. This alone poses an ethical issue for those involved.

Many consider professional boundary crossing an occupational hazard in nursing and other healthcare professions. Human interactions put providers at risk if they do not have a clear understanding of their role and responsibility. For example, nurses are encouraged to develop caring relationships with patients, and patient satisfaction is often a direct measure of factors based on the relationship. Nurses and other medical professionals need to spend time to learn about professional boundary risks in formalized educational settings and in the work environment.

Incidents that come under public scrutiny in the media are generally stories of victim abuse or malpractice. These examples often result in mistrust and wariness between patients and nurses, or other healthcare providers, negatively affecting the provider-patient relationship. When an allegation surfaces or an actual violation occurs, the issues are generally referred to the state board of nursing or other healthcare profession for investigation. In particular, the state boards of nursing are the regulatory agencies responsible for protecting the public related to nursing practice. The protection is established by a set of statutes, rules, and regulations that make up each individual state's Nurse Practice Act. The Nurse Practice Act is the basis to determine appropriateness of a nurse's actions (Holder & Schenthal, 2007). Each licensed or certified healthcare professional has an established set of practice standards set by the issuing state.

A significant problem with alleged or actual boundary transgressions is they are often committed by well-educated professionals during a stressful situation. These transgressions are rarely deliberate exploitation, but a consequence of well-intentioned actions where a nurse or other healthcare provider rationalizes crossing professional boundaries for the benefit of the patient. Proactive consideration must be given to preventing boundary violations. Frequently, they begin with innocent boundary drift such as thoughts about what could be done to help a patient in a difficult situation. Boundary drift may progress to boundary crossing and even slip into a violation. Ideally, education to prevent boundary violation needs to occur before boundaries start to drift.

Managing appropriate professional boundaries is each healthcare professional's responsibility. The best prevention is the development of a strong awareness and education plan. This education must include definitions of professional boundaries, differentiation of boundary crossings, and examples of violations. Each professional has a "violation potential." Understanding how to assess and address your own and others' violation potential can help to prevent boundary crossings.

Violation potential is dynamic and can change over time in response to life events and personal vulnerabilities. Nurses must be aware of the risk for themselves and other healthcare professionals. Risk factors are adversely affected by unresolved trauma from childhood, experiencing family or close friends who have died, critical illness, and stress. Environmental elements include work setting, patient type, and a nurse's or another healthcare provider's experience. A person's violation potential can be increased by an unexpected stress catalyst such as a divorce, death, or career change. This may cause a well-intentioned nurse to cross the line that separates ethical from unethical behavior (Holder & Schenthal, 2007).

Support from nursing leaders, colleagues, and peers for strategies to address the inherent environmental chaos, stressful events, and subsequent feelings of stress must be a priority in the healthcare environment. Employee Assistance Programs (EAP) and human resource (HR) personnel can be excellent resources for those struggling with personal or professional stress.

## PRACTICE PEARLS

- Pay attention to the consequences of stress in the work environment.
- Use available organizational resources when necessary to assist with stress management (Employee Assistance Programs or human resources).
- Be supportive to others who are stressed.
- Employers need to provide resources related to substance abuse disorder.
- A reporting mechanism needs to be in place for individuals who have concerns regarding potential substance abuse in their peers.

---

# THE POWER OF CHOICE

We know from positive psychology literature that most people crave stability, like to have a feeling of being somewhat in control, and are generally safe with their basic needs met to live a reasonably productive life. However, the COVID-19 pandemic upended what we all knew as our "normal." The massive upheaval to daily life caused an immense amount of stress for most everyone.

Now, we must learn to strike a balance between the lessons learned over the last two+ years and the challenges which still exist today. It is imperative to make smart choices about what we feel is important for our lives and will also allow us to live with integrity. There is no time like the present to begin as we all have to "restart" somewhere.

Brower (2021) describes *choice* as the "goldilocks"—where we need just the right amount of alternatives. This can pertain to our work, our personal lives, or both. With just the right amount of alternatives, it balances choice with control. Brower suggests people need options for where they work, how they do the work, who they work with (the lifeblood of engagement), and leveraging technology. This helps each person live with intention for better balance of health and well-being.

Employee stress levels are at an all-time high and mental health issues are rife. The pandemic has caused a sea change in how we work and live—and one of the most difficult aspects is the loss of control we've endured. This is tough for all of us—and also for leaders and organizations. When people aren't at their best, well-being, happiness, and performance suffer and so do company outcomes (Brower, 2021).

Healthcare needs to take note and be creative and flexible in how work gets done to better outcomes. We must all become more human-centered—for both patients' and healthcare workers' optimal well-being.

# CONCLUSION

Healthcare professions have become increasingly diverse in the following areas: age, years of professional experience, gender, and ethnicity. This diversity should be viewed as positive for each profession as we more closely match the US population.

Diversity brings a wide variety of experiences, styles of thinking, and frames of reference. We know change is afoot, and new thinking is required to thrive in the healthcare systems of the future. Being a stellar professional in practice, educational preparation, and behavior is necessary for today's nurse and other healthcare professionals.

All healthcare workers must become creative in their work and tolerant of the chaos in healthcare as the system continues to evolve; a heightened awareness of environmental stressors leading to feelings of stress, the propensity for fatigue, and the potential for burnout must be paramount. Recognizing the signs of stress, fatigue and burnout is the first step in being able to take action to mitigate the consequences of intensely stress-laden work. The following chapter will explore the implications of existing silos in healthcare.

# REFERENCES

American Association of Colleges of Nursing. (2022). *Nursing fact sheet.* https://www.aacnnursing.org/News-Information/Fact-Sheets/Nursing-Fact-Sheet

American Nurses Association. (n.d.). *What is nursing?* https://www.nursingworld.org/practice-policy/workforce/what-is-nursing

American Nurses Association. (2010). *Nursing: A social policy statement.* Author.

American Nurses Association. (2022). *Nursing informatics: Scope and standards of practice* (3rd ed.). Author.

Baldisseri, M.. (2007). Impaired healthcare professional. *Critical Care Medicine, 35*, S106–S116. https://doi.org/10.1097/01.CCM.0000252918.87746.96

Benner, P. (1984). *From novice to expert: Excellence in clinical nursing practice.* Prentice Hall Health.

Benner, P., Tanner, C., & Chesla, C. (2009). *Expertise in nursing practice* (2nd ed.). Springer Publishing Company.

Brosher, B. (2014, August). Prescription drug abuse among nurses a growing problem. *Indiana public media news.* https://indianapublicmedia.org/news/prescription-drug-abuse-nurses-growing-problem.php

Brower, T. (2021, February 21). The power of choice and what matters most for the future of work. *Forbes.* https://www.forbes.com/sites/tracybrower/2021/02/21/the-power-of-choice-and-what-matters-most-for-the-future-of-work/?sh=692676e9c569

Cavaliere, T. A., Daly, B., Dowling, D., & Montgomery, K. (2010). Moral distress in neonatal intensive care units RNs. *Advanced Neonatal Care, 10*(3), 145–156. https://doi.org/10.1097/ANC.0b013e3181dd6c48

Coronado-Vázquez, V., García-López, A., López-Sauras, S., & Alcaine, J. M. T. (2017). Nursing involvement in risk and patient safety management in primary care. *Enfermeria Clinica, 27*(4), 246–250. https://doi.org/10.1016/j.enfcli.2017.04.009

Duffy, J. R., & Brewer, B. B. (2011). Feasibility of a multi-institutional collaborative to improve patient-nurse relationship quality. *Journal of Nursing Administration, 41*(2), 78–83. https://doi.org/10.1097/NNA.0b013e3182059463

Edmonson, C., Anest, P., & Gogek, J. (2022). A profession disrupted: Looking back to go forward. *Nurse Leader, 20*(3), 281–285. https://doi.org/10.1016/j.mnl.2022.02.010

Gretter, L. (1893). *Florence Nightingale Pledge.* https://nursing.vanderbilt.edu/news/florence-nightingale-pledge/

Hanna, A. F., & Suplee, P. D. (2012). Don't cross the line: Respecting professional boundaries. *Nursing, 42*(9), 40–47. https://doi.org/10.1097/01.NURSE.0000418612.68723.54

Health Resources and Services Administration. (2017, August). *Sex, race and ethnic diversity of U.S. healthcare occupations (2011-2015).* https://bhw.hrsa.gov/sites/default/files/bureau-health-workforce/data-research/diversity-us-health-occupations.pdf

Health Resources and Services Administration. (2018). *2018 national sample survey of registered nurses: Brief summary of results.* https://bhw.hrsa.gov/sites/default/files/bureau-health-workforce/data-research/nssrn-summary-report.pdf

Holder, K. V., & Schenthal, S. J. (2007). Watch your step: Nursing and professional boundaries. *Nursing Management, 38*(2), 24–29. https://doi.org/10.1097/00006247-200702000-00010

Institute of Medicine. (2010). *The future of nursing: Leading change, advancing health.* http://www.nursingworld.org/MainMenuCategories/ThePracticeofProfessionalNursing/workforce/IOM-Future-of-Nursing-Report-1

Jason, R. R. (2015). Monitoring the impaired provider. *Oregon State Board of Nursing Sentinel, 34*(1), 6–10. https://www.oregon.gov/osbn/pages/Impaired-Provider.aspx

Jennings, B. (2008). Work stress and burnout among nurses: Role of the work environment and working conditions. In R. G. Hughes (Ed.), *Patient safety and quality: An evidence-based handbook for nurses* (pp. 133–158). Agency for Healthcare Research and Quality.

Jensen, T. (2022, March 1). Multigeneration workforce—Not all employees are millenials. *Forbes.* https://www.forbes.com/sites/forbestechcouncil/2022/03/01/multigeneration-workforce---not-all-employees-are-millennials/?sh=22bb7eb76d14

Kavanaugh, J.M. & Szweda, C. (2017). The crisis in competency: The strategic and ethical imperative to assessing new graduate nurses' clinical reasoning. *Nursing Education Perspectives, 38*(2), 57-62.

Mason, D. (2011). *The nursing profession: Development, challenges and opportunities.* Jossey-Bass.

National Advisory Council on Nurse Education and Practice. (2013). *Achieving health equity through nursing workforce diversity.* http://www.hrsa.gov/advisorycommittees/bhwadvisory/nacnep/reports/eleventhreport.pdf

National Council of State Boards of Nursing. (2009). *Practical guidelines for boards of nursing on sexual misconduct cases.* https://www.ncsbn.org/books-journals/practical-guidelines-for-bons

National Council of State Boards of Nursing. (2014). *A nurses's guide to professional boundaries.* Author.

National Research Council. (2004). *In the nation's compelling interest: Ensuring diversity in the health professionals.* National Academies Press.

New, K. (2015). Preventing, detecting, and investigating drug diversion in health care facilities. *Continuing Education, 5*(1), 18–25. https://doi.org/10.1016/S2155-8256(15)30095-8

New York State Education Department. (2015). NYSOPnursing: Laws, rules & regulations: Article 139, section 6902. *New York State Office of Health Professions.* http://www.op.nysed.gov/prof/nurse/article139.htm

Nightingale, F. (1860). *Notes on nursing: What it is and what it is not.* D. Appleton and Company, reprinted by Dover Publications, 1969.

Nyhus, J. (2021, May). Drug diversion in healthcare: Prevention and detection for nurses. *American Nurse Journal, 15*(5), 26–30. https://www.myamericannurse.com/drug-diversion-in-healthcare/

Rathburn, J. (2022). Destigmatizing alcohol use disorder among nurses. *Nursing, 52*(7). 23–29. https://doi.org/10.1097/01.NURSE.0000832364.28141.12

Riffkin, R. (2014, December 18). Americans rate nurses highest on honesty, ethical standards. *Gallup.* http://www.gallup.com/poll/180260/americans-rate-nurses-highest-honesty-ethical-standards.aspx

Roberts, R., Grubb, P. L., & Grosch, J. W. (2012, June 25). Alleviating job stress in nurses. *MedScape.* http://www.medscape.com/viewarticle/765974

Tiffin, C. (2013, March 1). Beyond the bedside: The changing role of today's nurse. *Huffington Post.* https://www.huffpost.com/entry/nursing-school_b_1384285

US Bureau of Labor Statistics. (2022). *Occupational outlook handbook, registered nurses, job outlook.* https://www.bls.gov/ooh/healthcare/registered-nurses.htm#tab-6

Wolters Kluwer. (2021, January 20). *Closing the education-practice readiness gap.* https://www.wolterskluwer.com/en/expert-insights/survey-nursing-readiness

# 6

# THE INTERNAL STRAIN OF SILOS

## OBJECTIVES

- Understand the benefits and challenges of working as a team.
- Explore why the healthcare environment has become a mass of silos.
- Consider why the "silo" phenomenon is stress-inducing.
- Explore the different types of silos and how to combat them.
- Consider why competition for limited resources and personnel shortages lead to conflict among healthcare workers.

There is an infamous story about four people named Everybody, Somebody, Anybody, and Nobody. Although there doesn't seem be to a record of where the story originated, it resurfaces in the actual lives of healthcare professionals each day. The story goes like this:

> There was an important job to be done and Everybody was asked to do it. Everybody was sure Somebody would do it. Anybody could have done it, but Nobody did it. Somebody got angry about that because it was Everybody's job. Everybody thought Anybody could do it, but Nobody realized that Everybody wouldn't do it. It ended up that Everybody blamed Somebody when actually Nobody asked Anybody.

## THE CHALLENGES OF WORKING AS A TEAM

Healthcare is now a team "sport" where we must all work closely together; teamwork is critical. Interprofessional teaching and learning in healthcare has become more and more in demand with the objective of students entering the healthcare workforce already steeped in collaborative skills (Felgoise et al., 2019). While we will differentiate teamwork from collaboration, the mind-set of working together sets the stage for both concepts to work effectively. In 1965, Tuckman's groundbreaking research revealed four stages of team behavior: forming, storming, norming, and performing (Upwork, 2021). This process is commonly used when launching new team or improvement efforts:

- **Forming** begins with the team members getting to know one another.
- **Storming** occurs after team members become comfortable and begin to take risks by sharing contrarian views.
- **Norming** occurs when the team exhibits cohesion and is working toward a common goal.

- **Performing** is reserved for what Tuckman called "high-performing teams" who are able to function as a unified group and without conflict.

Later in 1977, Tuckman and Jensen added *adjourning* to the team process, whereby the team uncouples or dissolves the group dynamics in an attempt to move on. This step has also been called *deforming* and *mourning*, due to the feelings team members experience when this phase of their work comes to an end.

Teamwork in healthcare can have direct impacts on bedside care and processes that support patient care. Teams with synergy generate more creative ideas, find innovative solutions to problems, and implement strategic actions, which can be more effective than when a person works by themself (Mayo & Wooley, 2016). In cases where individuals aren't working with team synergy or social capital, the impact of effort lessens. You've heard the common phrase, "more heads are better than one." Strong consideration should be given to the addition of teaching ideal teamwork and team behavior in formal nursing, as well as other healthcare programs. Taking care of patients requires a multidisciplinary approach with a team of skilled individuals, each with their own area of expertise. While "everyone" is responsible for their own specialty, "everyone" also has to know how their work fits into the work of other disciplines.

Traditional organizational structures, especially in hospitals, have isolated clinical disciplines into silos. Nursing and ancillary clinical services have often been organized into their own service lines. Only recently have reorganizations integrated various clinical disciplines into more unified and inclusive reporting structures. This reorganization has allowed an opportunity for enhanced collaboration and improved teamwork among specialties. Examples include leaders working in dyads or triads to lead a specific clinical service or line of similar services.

Isn't it true that we sometimes find ourselves floundering through the day, wondering how we will ever get all of our work completed? A good analogy for being a nurse, leader, or other healthcare provider in today's complex healthcare environment is like standing in the middle of a tornado—where do you begin? Which task needs to be accomplished first? Most healthcare workers are good at prioritizing and can usually find the time to help a colleague in need. They can assist in task completion, make telephone calls to other disciplines, and provide patient care; however, when there are unplanned absences (such as a sick call) or when the daily plan does not unfold as expected, it can be quite challenging for the entire team to keep up with the required work.

Effective teamwork fosters the act of care providers asking other team members for help. Some team members may hesitate to ask their peer or peers for help for fear of being judged as less competent. The "tornado" of activity on any given shift can be lessened by leveraging the available resources. Asking for help should never be viewed as a weakness, but as a position of strength for the provider to offer safe, quality care for a patient.

In addition, team members must be willing to work collaboratively with the organization's leaders. An "us and them" culture is a breeding ground for trouble. Leaders unwilling to assist team members fail the team. Teams that are effective are inclusive and work well together to support coworkers by using efficient communication skills to promote quality and safe care.

Most nurses and other healthcare providers seek organizations who "walk the talk" by providing a work environment where people feel they are making a difference, are valued, can enjoy their job, and feel supported. When a nurse or other care provider believes they can speak honestly and openly about the daily challenges, their satisfaction with the work environment and team increases. This supportive milieu can lead to lower turnover rates, improved quality from effective care processes, and better customer satisfaction. In contrast, conflict occurs when any member of the team doesn't hold up their end of the bargain. At times, this may require leadership intervention.

It is important to differentiate between team or teamwork and collaboration. These terms do not have the same meaning. For example, *collaboration* can be the product of simple interactions between coworkers from the same or different departments. *Teamwork* is the process to reach an outcome when coworkers have clear, honest communication, a supportive culture, and are working toward a common goal or objective. Healthcare workers can foster better teamwork by learning how to effectively communicate or negotiate by becoming tolerant of listening to others with differing opinions and moving forward.

In an acute care setting, the work becomes much more difficult, because hospitalized patients can be quite ill. Bedside nurses and other care providers can sometimes team up and help each other out, but what they cannot do is complete each other's documentation. So even when teamed up for patient care activities, only part of the work can be done with a partner. Nurses and leaders in other roles, such as education or administration, can ask for help if they have teammates, but often they are solo acts left to their own resourcefulness to get way too much work done in one day's time. This makes the work more challenging and setting appropriate boundaries essential.

Learning to prioritize is a key strategy to achieve your goals and feel a sense of accomplishment. At the end of the day, there is often work left undone. Sometimes we are aware there is work left needing to be completed. Other times, we do not discover it until an audit is completed or a lawsuit is filed and there is nothing in the record to support the efforts of care that was provided. Learning to accurately prioritize begins in nursing and other academic healthcare programs and is continually improved throughout a career. By properly prioritizing, omissions and errors can be minimized.

# THE HEALTHCARE SILO PHENOMENON

Merriam-Webster's dictionary (2015) defines *silo* as "a tower or pit on a farm used to store grain." If you have ever visited a farm, you know that only one type of grain is stored in a silo at a time. If, for instance, a farm harvests both corn and beans, the corn is kept in one silo while the beans are kept in another. A second definition for silo is "an underground chamber in which a guided missile is kept ready for firing." In both instances, the purpose of the silo is to isolate the item for its protection. To be siloed is to be *isolated*. When silos occur in healthcare, roles become isolated, disciplines become isolated, departments become isolated, communication becomes isolated, and frustrations often arise. Being frustrated with the work environment, work processes, and work colleagues are the beginning stages of stress and fatigue and may lead eventually to burnout. Figure 6.1 shows some common silos found in the healthcare industry.

Healthcare has been known to have a number of inefficient work processes that have led to the creation of workarounds in the system. Workarounds are a prime offender for the establishment of silos and often violate established systems or policy. Silos result in difficulties with communication, teamwork, and effective collaboration. The person or persons who created the workaround are the only ones who know how it works. Communication, or the lack thereof, is a key contributing factor to errors in healthcare. Because healthcare is such a demanding field, providers who learn workarounds are often praised as being resourceful and efficient. While innovation in healthcare is sorely needed, new work processes must be communicated so that others are aware and can comply.

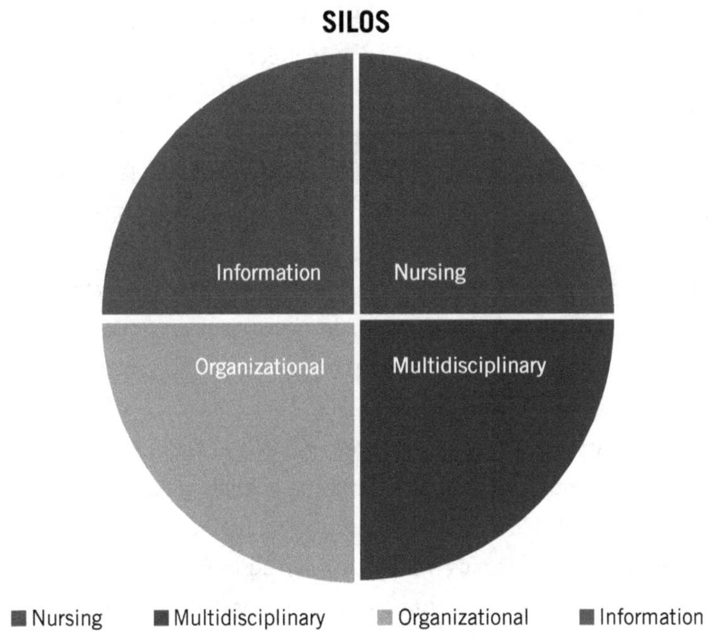


**FIGURE 6.1** Healthcare silos are often a result of difficulties with communication and effective collaboration.

One example of a workaround, likely to occur in a typical nurse's day, is related to securing enough intravenous medication pumps for post-operative patients. The post-operative unit might hoard and/or hide all the pumps they can find instead of following the hospital process of sending them back to the designated area for cleaning. This workaround is often a result of a day when the unit had a pump shortage. This approach might work for solving the unit's problem, but can cause a real patient safety issue in other clinical areas of the hospital. In addition, the pumps might not be cleaned as properly as they should (Tucker, 2009).

Silos occur in a multitude of ways. Much like the Everybody, Somebody, Anybody, and Nobody story, silos can lead to ineffective communication when a workaround is put in place. A nurse or other healthcare worker might innocently create a workaround to accomplish their day's assigned work. This type of behavior makes it incredibly difficult to track workarounds that have been instituted, and they may inadvertently cause violations in standards of practice.

For instance, if nurses do not communicate with designated quality personnel, associated organizational metrics or quality indicators may never be achieved. Nurses in the acute care environment must be cognizant of compensable quality scoring. Each of the steps in the process of care makes a difference. If there is improper, inaccurate, or missing documentation of the established quality indicators, inappropriate information may be publicly reported. Erroneous information may also have a negative impact on financial reimbursement and public perception. This means money that is paid to hospitals through value-based purchasing plans might be less than expected, and the organization's reputation might negatively suffer in public reporting systems. System, people, and process communication are all vital to prevent silos from unintentionally damaging organizations. Today, informational knowledge is power, and communication is the way to unleash it.

## PRACTICE PEARLS

- Get to know the members of other departments and form key relationships.
- Stay current with evidence-based practices affecting nursing and the healthcare environment.
- Consider becoming an expert in a chosen nursing or other healthcare specialty.
- Ask for help from others when you need it.
- Always understand the *what* and *why* of your work.
- Keep leaders informed of what you need in order to accomplish your work.

## DISCIPLINARY SILOS

Silos in patient care areas can exist when nurses perform certain functions and tasks, nursing assistants perform other specific tasks, and other clinical disciplines perform only the tasks appropriate for their specialty. This personal or professional task-oriented mindset can cause disjointed patient care. Although limits relative to each care provider's scope of practice may affect who is capable or allowed to perform specific tasks related to care provision, siloed work without communication is of no benefit to the team or the patient.

Disciplinary silos can cause confusion or a lack of clarity, sending a distinct message to the patient and family. The message might be misinterpreted as non-communicative specialists only speak with each other through written word (in the medical record). This approach might unfortunately leave a patient or family member as the link to ensure each provider knows what the other provider is doing. A lack of communication and teamwork, either perceived or real, can cause a great deal of duplication (non-value-added work) and frustration for each individual involved. Patients tire quickly when repetitively answering the same questions for each discipline, and families lose trust when nursing information does not coincide with directives provided by the medical provider. In addition, patients and their family members often notice team conflict or a lack of common direction.

Nurses and other healthcare providers can burn out quickly when working in an environment that results from a lack of trust, no involvement in decision-making, and a lack of inclusion. Positive team behavior and optimal communication are necessary to create trust. Teams of care providers need trust to provide the best care. Teams that communicate effectively are also able to be proactive; thus, they handle issues before they arise and answer questions before they are asked. This can eliminate patient and family feelings of confusion.

Jennings (2008) identified that communication among nurses, both at the peer level and with leaders, decreases the amount of stress and burnout in nursing.

## PRACTICE PEARLS

- Communication is the most influential way to eliminate silos in healthcare.
- Be honest in all communication for effective collaboration.
- Speak positively to build successful relationships with others or "manage up" teammates.
- Be a good example—be the teammate you want your coworkers to be.
- Prepared caregivers can deliver care that appears seamless.
- Proactive teamwork creates excellence.

## ORGANIZATIONAL SILOS

Many of today's healthcare organizations have reorganized into larger systems due to the number of complex regulatory and accreditation changes in the healthcare environment, and some hospitals have actually closed. Of the 6,093 remaining hospitals in the US, 3,483 are organized in some type of system (American Hospital Association, 2022). Multi-hospital systems within a network have become much more common in recent years as organizations seek consolidation of services and aim to improve finances and avoid duplicative competition. Some of the affiliations are formal, while others are not. However, new challenges have surfaced between sites or within the same system, especially when caregivers do not manage patients the same way. Examples include variable documentation systems, not using common systems in a uniform way, not planning care based on the most recent evidence, and not defining standardized policies and procedures.

Nurses, as well as, other healthcare workers who work in system hospitals that do not work as effectively as they could or should can become frustrated with variances in procedures and practices that may not match the system policy to which they are held accountable. System policies typically represent the largest or most vocal hospital in the system, but often neglect to review the application of the policy to *each* hospital in the system. This specifically can negatively affect smaller organizations with fewer resources.

Litigation concerns and risk are often higher with such discrepancies because it appears a nurse simply did not follow policy. Although this may have been unintentional, it can create a great deal of stress for a nurse and their employer and can affect the nurse's future practice. Being involved in any type of legal situation is stressful and can cause a nurse to rethink their career choice. This may diminish a nurse's passion for the profession, resulting in tiring and fatigue for both themselves and their colleagues. If there is no intervention, the symptoms may progress. This kind of burnout is a result of system or process challenges that affect individual care providers and their ability to perform their jobs.

Risk and liability are shared among all care providers and the organizations in which they choose to practice. One landmark case from a Nashville, Tennessee hospital medical mistake had a surprising verdict in 2022, which sent shockwaves through the nursing profession. The former nurse was found criminally negligent for homicide and abuse of an impaired adult for giving the wrong medication in 2017 (Salovitz, 2022). Nurses now fear the threat of litigation for making a mistake. Most likely this will only escalate the known levels of stress already felt in a profession where "perfect practice" is next to impossible. It will also affect other caregiving providers and may discourage them from reporting errors, thus negatively affecting overall patient safety. You can read more about the story here: https://health.wusf.usf.edu/health-news-florida/2022-04-20/southwest-florida-nurses-react-to-guilty-verdict-in-tennessee-wrong-medication-death.

Healthcare organizations, as well as patients, experience silos in nearly every healthcare encounter. Many of the pay-for-performance initiatives and governmental payment structures have caused healthcare facilities to rethink how they provide care in an effort to achieve a higher percentage of reimbursement per patient. This system, while altruistic in theory to improve coordination and care, may have the opposite effect.

As value-based purchasing dictates program objectives and payments such as meaningful use and community assessments, organizations must become fluent in the new language. Most nurses and other healthcare providers do not have a common knowledge about these structures and how they might affect their employer's bottom line. Historically, nursing has not been held accountable for practice outcomes in a financially focused arena. While quality has always been important to both nurses and patients from an outcome perspective, it is even more so today. In addition, the government-sponsored programs also have the ability to levy financial penalties and taxes, which provide a new layer of heightened awareness and associated compliance. It may be time to consider building accountability for practice scorecards to inform personnel of their individual contribution to the unit's overall clinical quality performance.

If facilities do not comply with healthcare's rules and regulations as directed, they must develop plans of correction to achieve measurable metrics and do so within their budgetary constraints. The information also may become public. Regaining compliance is much more costly and difficult than complying with the outlined regulatory requirements and accreditation standards.

Although each of these functions alone can create positive outcomes for an organization and its patient population, they can also cause conflict. Nursing and healthcare is changing. What it takes to be a nurse or other clinical care provider today is quite different than in previous times. This rapid-fire change in practice(s) is particularly complicated by the five generations of people who now are expected to work together despite differing values, expectations of work, and more.

In addition, the care continuum for patients has been widened with a new focus on what happens outside of an acute episodic hospital admission. Organizations must develop systems to track efforts to prevent unplanned hospital readmissions to keep patients out of the hospital and thus, healthier. Hospitals have been forced to work closely with not only physicians and their clinics, but extended care facilities, skilled nursing facilities, rehabilitation facilities, and hospice organizations. Reimbursement may also be affected if some types of patients are readmitted with a similar or same diagnosis to an acute care facility within 30 days. Healthcare in general is drastically changing. This requires the removal of silos toward a new dawn of transparency. An opening is necessary in the historically built walls of communication in order to succeed in this different, fiercely competitive healthcare market.

## DEPARTMENTAL AND INTERLINKING SILOS

One example of how silos are interlinked and related to a clinical improvement project can be found in one hospital's efforts to decrease catheter-associated urinary tract infections.

***Case 1***

> A team of nurses began by breaking down each step in the process for urinary catheter insertion, maintenance, and removal. The nurses also searched for best practices and relevant evidence in the literature. Based on the variety of sources of information, they made a plan for improvement. To implement the newly defined standards, the nurses began performing a peer-review process to assess competency of insertion and audits for compliance of the new maintenance requirements. During the project's implementation process, the nurses realized that nursing students rotating through their organizational departments were being taught to insert urinary catheters in a way that differed from what the hospital had deemed to be best practice. This variation did not meet the new competency requirement. Because the school was associated with the hospital, there was an easy avenue with which to address the variation in practice. Had it not been addressed; the variation could have caused a great deal of stress and frustration to both practicing and newly hired nurses as they took the time to isolate the cause of the variation.

Schools of nursing are another example of an interlinking silo that can produce conflict and variation in practice. Departments often have differing practices versus a single nursing standard. This is why it is important for clinical site instructors to know the current standards of nursing practice, as well as organizational and departmental policy for the facilities where their students are typically deployed.

## EXTERNAL INFORMATION SILOS

Silos of information exist in the electronic information world, as well as in the physical world. One example is in pharmacies across the country. Pharmacies have experienced significant challenges in identifying practitioner diversion, inappropriate use of controlled substances, and medication reconciliation. Concerned parties include distributors, the Drug Enforcement Administration, Automation of Reports and Consolidated Orders System, as well as individual and corporately organized pharmacies.

Historically, each pharmacy and medical provider has been a silo. Typically, there was little communication and a lack of tracking information (Traynor, 2012). It was possible for medical providers to write prescriptions for the same patient, who might use several different pharmacies. There was no overlap or methodology to track duplication and drug usage or misuse.

Until the US government began seeking the assessment of criminal activity relative to narcotic abuse, pharmacies had no reason to follow the throughput of medications or track the process for distribution. This enabled those seeking to abuse the system, such as drug abusers and drug dealers, to devise intricate schemes to profit from the loopholes. Eliminating the silos of communication in the pharmacy arena has significantly reduced the downstream problems of abuse often seen in emergency departments and provider offices.

Now, patients who choose to abuse any part of the healthcare system are more easily identifiable. This has been a long-standing frustration for practicing medical providers and nurses. This type of encounter with patients significantly contributes to negative thinking and nursing burnout. The mental health system and the amount of drug abuse in the United States is a complex social and health problem. Read more about the US statistics related to drug abuse here: https://drugabusestatistics.org.

Healthcare system abuse by patients who take no responsibility for their own health causes nurses and other clinicians to feel stressed. Healthcare providers want to help others; however, it is difficult to provide interventions for health improvement or illness management for this type of patient. The frustration can be exhausting. It is a challenge for nurses and other clinicians to feel any sense of accomplishment with care provided to this patient population.

The Maslach Burnout Inventory (MBI) is a tool that has been used in healthcare to measure burnout in nurses. The elements identified as important and contributory to the symptoms of burnout are emotional exhaustion, depersonalization, and decreased personal accomplishment (Statistics Solutions, 2015; Vahey et al., 2004). Information about the MBI instrument can be found at https://prezi.com/bn2vlq3fjzj8/maslach-burnout-inventory-3rd-edition.

### PRACTICE PEARLS

- Seek satisfying work.
- Excellent communication keeps patients and caregivers safe.
- Do your part to eliminate silos.
- Learn both how the business of healthcare affects your practice and your how practice affects the business of healthcare.

## HUMAN FACTORS AND DESIGN THINKING IN HEALTHCARE

Healthcare delivery has become increasingly complex. Healthcare professionals frequently use tools, processes, and systems that *have not* been designed to facilitate efficient human performance—which in turn can lead to costly and preventable patient safety errors, decreased effectiveness, and a loss of patient-centered care (ECRI, 2022).

Human factors and design thinking in healthcare lends a scientific approach to better understand patient safety for more predictable and reliable outcomes. This approach leverages an understanding of how human performance and behavior may impact clinical outcomes. System performance is often based upon human actions and limitations. Using a human factors approach, healthcare could redesign systems, identify key processes at risk for failure, and potentially prevent patient safety–related medical errors, thus improving overall quality.

The Institute of Design at Stanford uses this model for a design thinking process (Stanford University Institute of Design, 2012):

1. Empathize: To gain an understanding by observing, engaging, watching, and listening to why the customer (a patient) does things.
2. Define: What is the problem to be solved?
3. Ideate: Collaborate to discover untapped areas for exploration to develop innovative solutions.
4. Prototype: Decompose the larger problem into testable chunks.
5. Test: Use the prototype to learn about the customer's (patient's) experience in the new design.

You can also read about the Mayo Clinic's Center for Innovation incubator for improvement in a case study here: https://www.cio.com/article/240945/design-thinking-for-healthcare.html.

IDEO is a leading global design innovation agency founded by David Kelley aiming to transform business with human-centered design. Human-centered design methodologies focus on the following principles:

1. Things exist for people to use.
2. Company culture impacts innovation.

Design thinking in healthcare centers on putting patients first. By putting user needs first, human factors can guide design. The design is then tested via three simple but specific questions:

1. What do we want?
2. Can we do it?
3. Can we afford it?

You can read more about IDEO's work in healthcare here: https://page.ideo.com/health and here: https://www.ideo.com/journal/can-digital-therapeutics-revolutionize-medicine. You can also read about how IDEO views the importance of workplace culture here: https://www.ideo.com/blog/why-workplace-culture-matters-and-how-to-build-a-good-one.

This is an example of an outside influence with creative and innovative thinking that has the potential to transform healthcare. Designing customer-focused environments, smooth healthcare encounters, and high-performing organizations are needed more than ever as the demand for services increases and the world changes with augmented technology. And, if those of us inside healthcare don't drive the necessary change, someone else will.

## CONFLICT: SURVIVAL OF THE FITTEST

Task lists for healthcare providers are getting longer. The amount of work to be done can easily cause providers to feel overwhelmed. Solo thinking, such as a "survival of the fittest" mentality, drives people to behave in a competitive manner rather than working as a team. This type of thinking and isolationist approach to practice creates a spirit of "dog eat dog"—also known as nurses eating their young (Cole & Cole, 2005, p. 43). Cole and Cole (2005) reported that training related to teamwork does little to no good when the organization's culture is not supportive. Cultures that support behaving in a positive manner embrace effective communication and transparency. Frequently, this journey begins with dynamic leadership at the helm in the organization and spreads, one caregiver at a time.

*Unintentional* silos of information have become the norm in healthcare. Systems are not interfaced, software changes, data is not presented in a useful way to be used as information, specialty providers have difficulty communicating with referring providers, and so on. When conflict exists in the workplace, often those involved are looking for someone to blame versus providing an effective solution to the problem. This knee-jerk reaction to hoard information gives power to the party who has it and diminishes the effectiveness of those who do not have access. It is not terribly uncommon to hear a nurse say, "He should do his own work," or, "If she were here, she would know the patient went to radiology," or, "That is not my patient."

Clinicians and units that do not work well together put patients at risk. An unhealthy environment of care leaves nurses feeling alone, angry, frustrated, and ultimately unsatisfied with their work, the environment, and the leadership. This can compromise both the patient's experience and the care provided. As frustrating and stress-invoking as inter- and intra-departmental conflict can be, conflict can have an even larger facility impact related to regulatory compliance.

***Case 2***

One hospital example includes a well-meaning quality/survey readiness nurse who forwarded all types of survey-related information on to the leadership. She neglected to filter the information nor provide any explanation of applicability for their assigned areas of responsibility. Although her efforts to keep the leaders informed (to ultimately achieve a successful survey result) were not malicious, she inadvertently angered many of the departmental leaders. The leaders had one expectation of an interpretation of the regulations and the quality nurse had another of providing the information, with an assumption that no translation was needed. The leaders felt they

> did not have time to sort through the mass of forwarded email or to read all of the information. In addition, the survey-readiness nurse was frustrated because the leaders never responded to her messages, and she felt they were ignoring her attempts to provide them the information they needed to be successful. In this case, conflict was caused by differing expectations, where communication was not clear and feedback was not offered in a proactive manner.

This example raises a number of questions: Was the quality nurse a fit for the position? Were her job expectations clear? Was she provided the appropriate training? Did she receive performance feedback on a regular basis? Unfortunately, this story ends in a negative outcome for the nurse because no one ever approached her about her style of communication. She merely lost her position in quality as a survey coordinator and was given an alternate assignment. What kind of precedent did this set? Unfortunately, it caused a higher level of mistrust and inter-facility conflict. The employees viewed the leadership as unable to fix a simple problem with communication when she was reassigned.

Stress, fatigue, and burnout can be created by silos, the work environment, organizational culture, suboptimal work processes, and position fit. Symptoms of dissatisfaction are evident with nurses who move from position to position. They are usually searching for something. Could the cycle be broken if instead they received honest performance feedback? Could the situation be improved by good leadership? Never in history was this more evident than during and post the COVID-19 pandemic. Nurses and other care providers left their positions in record numbers; totals not seen since 2000 (Hut, 2021). Some left for similar jobs in a different locale, some for a conflict in values, some for more compensation, some for other industries, and some just plain left the profession altogether. If many of the issues raised in this publication had been previously addressed with the first edition (in 2016 and beyond), would the outcome have been different?

A multitude of nurses and other healthcare workers stay in organizations that function as "secret societies" because they believe they can make a difference, are loyal employees, and believe the organization needs them. These organizations are fortunate, because nurses are the backbone of healthcare and are an invaluable resource to effective organizational performance. Decreasing stress, fatigue, and the potential for burnout in the work environment would inevitably decrease risk for a host of negative outcomes for all involved personnel.

## COMPETITION FOR LIMITED RESOURCES

Budgetary constraints in healthcare organizations result in limited resources. Every healthcare organization across the care continuum is attempting to work with fewer available resources. Capital expenditures have been difficult to secure, and the bottom line is that this affects infrastructure. Where organizations most often tend to fail is in an honest assessment of the departmental needs throughout the organization. The competition for resources is fierce and the money generally goes to new products, services, and buildings versus items in the infrastructure to provide daily patient care. Often the most vocal, or even the most revenue-generating, departments are the ones selected to receive the majority of capital budget items.

Not having the appropriate equipment or supplies for nurses to carry out their duties can be maddening. Precious time is often wasted looking for necessary items to complete care delivery. Because many items can be purchased at a discount in bulk, it makes sense to stock inventory at an organizational versus departmental level. Frontline healthcare providers have a responsibility to participate in designing effective systems for placement and replacement of capital and disposable items. Standardization of equipment and supply is not just good business, but facilitates movement of nursing staff among and between units. Standardization improves patient safety and care delivery. Nurses and other caregivers should be familiar with equipment and the environment, and should have the necessary inventory of supplies and tools to safely perform their jobs. Organizations should have a streamlined and efficient process for care providers to communicate needs for equipment, supply, medication, technology, etc. to care for the patients they serve.

**PRACTICE PEARL**

Tools + Talent = Success

## PERSONNEL SHORTAGES

With ever-increasing challenges for healthcare entities to perform, staffing often becomes a target. Labor is the costliest expense in nearly all organizations. Since the COVID-19 pandemic began, it has only escalated. Hut (2021) described how clinical labor costs have risen 8% per patient day since 2019. In addition, one particularly "vexing" aspect is that they are now paying more for less staff with costs per adjusted patient day 20.4% higher when compared to 2019. Overtime pay, contract workers to cover vacant positions, and creative incentives are challenging even the best-managed facilities.

In recent decades, securing the correct type of staff by skill and experience has become more challenging. This challenge was raised both in shortage and intensity during the COVID-19 pandemic. In addition, staffing ratios between nurses and patients have changed. Commonly, more assigned patients and less nursing staff has been the result. Some states have even legislated ratios or mandated staffing committees with smaller numbers of patients per nurse. Sadly, the ratio limits have not produced the clinical care outcomes predicted. And it is well understood that a diversified skill mix of varying care providers provide better and more timely care to satisfied patients. The good news is that when labor expectations are made clear, whether with ratios, committees, or joint leadership, the goals or targets to predict financial outcomes are understood by all.

The upshots of personnel shortages are concerns about recruitment and retention, patient safety, and sicker hospitalized patients requiring more skilled and qualified clinical staff. Projections for future demand of healthcare and the mismatch of projected clinically trained resources is daunting. Additionally, nursing leaders have expressed concern about nurses' training and bedside nurses being too task-focused, with little ability for critical thinking. Although this may be true, the preface for this concerning change in nursing performance is most likely due to the ever-increasing task list. Nurses have to give medications, educate patients about them, and follow up on their effectiveness. Nurses perform daily patient hygiene, ambulation, bathroom assistance, assessments, and provide physician support. Nurses often find themselves merely surviving the day instead of thriving in their role as nurse and lead communicator in the patient-healing process.

It is doubtful anything substantive will be done in the near future about the variability in nurse staffing and ratios. The supply is not expected to be able to meet the demand in health services for some time. In addition, Hut (2021) cited the Association of American Medical Colleges, which estimated a shortage of 37,800 to 124,000 medical physicians; the *American Journal of Medical Quality* estimated the nursing shortage at 510,000 *pre-pandemic;* and Mercer projected a shortage of support staff by 3.2 million for lower wage healthcare occupations by 2026.

Cost is only one driving factor; therefore, nurses and other healthcare providers must learn how to utilize the available resources to provide the best care. In studies conducted in nearly 125 Veterans Affairs (VA) facilities, the dual benefit of efficiency and teamwork for healthcare disciplines led to greater patient satisfaction (Meterko et al., 2004). Culture clearly affects outcomes. In a separate Taiwanese study by Chang et al. (2009), a similar result was found. If a healthcare organization can create a culture of teamwork, it is likely to have higher levels of job and customer satisfaction. Patients expect to be cared for by a team of attentive people working together to ensure healing and a return to previous health status.

Emerging roles in nursing, such as nursing informaticists, have become popular across the country. As organizations move to an electronic health or medical record, integrated records of various types of encounters are improving communication for providers and patients. Nurses have always held a vital role in communication. They are often the coordinators of care who facilitate communication between the various disciplines. This is necessary to achieve highly reliable and safe care for the best patient outcomes. Effective communication decreases stress for both patients and providers. While the electronic medical or health record is not designed to replace communication between healthcare providers, it is a key indicator of the kind of communication existing in an organization (Herman, 2014).

## THE PRESSURE TO PERFORM

The Affordable Care Act of 2010 has driven much of the recent change in the healthcare landscape. In 2014, the *Journal of Healthcare Management* published a study in which frontline staff were surveyed about why change in their organization was unsuccessful. The most common failure was poor implementation planning. Two other significant findings, in the top reasons for project failure, were ineffective communication (top-down) and little-to-no teamwork (Longnecker et al., 2014).

Communication and teamwork have continually surfaced as key elements to organizational success. Is it really this simple? Could all silos be eliminated? One of the leadership lessons in the *Journal of Healthcare Management* article (Longnecker et al., 2014) conveyed that leaders must lead by example. When organizations segment disciplines within the leadership structure, care processes become fragmented. It is more difficult for frontline staff to connect all the dots in the care continuum. It is challenging to understand each care provider's role and subsequent limitations. Nurses must learn how best to integrate ancillary peers into the cycle of work. Thus, the design of the organizational structure is crucial to eliminate silos and facilitate communication.

Cassady's lecture in 2013 described how teamwork, as a core element, is essential to the provision of better healthcare. Cassady (2013) also recommended teamwork be infused in each discipline's educational development to benefit communication. Cassady cited Patrick Lencioni's groundbreaking work showcased in the book *The Five Dysfunctions of a Team.* A summary and visual model of Lencioni's work is displayed in Figure 6.2.

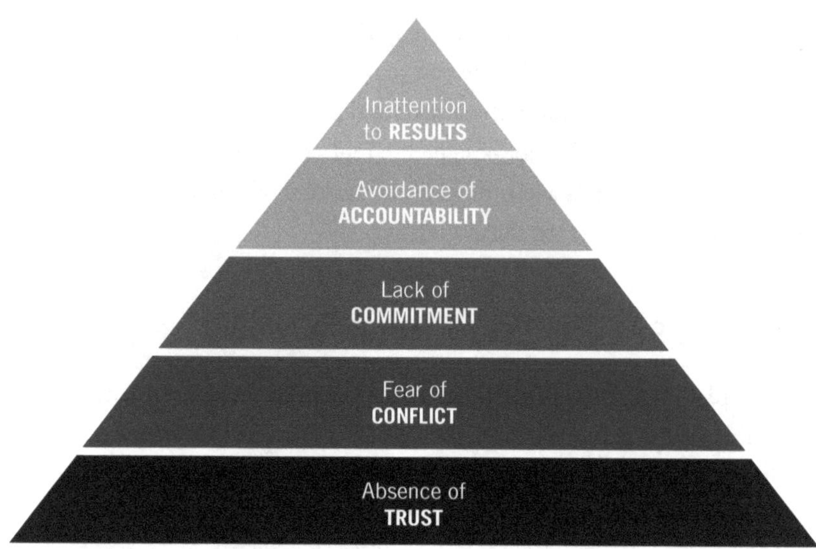


**FIGURE 6.2** The five dysfunctions of a team.

*Copyright © Patrick Lencioni, 2002. Used with permission.*

Creative organizations have been able to take teamwork beyond theory. Application is evident in organizational process, policy, and procedure, as in the following case study.

***Case 3***

> Baptist Health in Arkansas designed a care model using every distinct discipline in the healthcare organization. The model was designed to screen every incoming patient for necessary consults, regardless of discipline, based on patient needs. An example of a non-clinical discipline in the model included information technology personnel, who were instrumental in assisting clinicians with the practicalities of documentation in the electronic health record. This unique team approach led to higher levels of trust among the disciplines. The model also allowed the admitting nurse to design and appropriate specific care teams based on individual and unique patient needs.

As the disciplines worked to refine the model, communication improved, duplication decreased, and teamwork was enhanced. The team also learned that when frontline disciplines are included in the process, they have a better understanding of objectives and learn the organization's methods to reach its goals. Buy-in was better obtained for organizational resource alignment. Strong healthcare systems communicate clearly and share results openly (Cassady, 2013).

## PRACTICE PEARLS

- Buy-in is obtained though clear communication.
- When nurses and other healthcare providers are included in decision-making, they commit wholeheartedly to the outcome.
- Nurses who participate in shared governance lead others.
- Be a valuable participant in problem solving.

---

"Inter-professional collaborative practice happens when multiple health workers from different professional backgrounds work together with patients, families, caregivers, and communities to deliver the highest quality of care" (Gittell et al., 2013, p. 210). Any time organizations build collaborative team care models or practice patient-centered care, they are engaging in interprofessional collaborative practice. The researchers further defined relational coordination as a mutually reinforcing process of communicating and relating for the purpose of task integration. The call for organizations to implode and rebuild organizational design, structure, and functions in new cross-functional, team-focused work environments is now—because it is needed more than ever.

Consideration should be given to rebuilding every department and every process, from hiring to the management of conflict resolution. Concepts such as shared governance, interdisciplinary care models, and town hall meetings are great methods of sharing information for improved communication.

Shared governance is a model of professional practice founded on partnership among leaders and staff. Shared governance promotes collaborative efforts that lead to shared decisions, responsibility, accountability, quality, and safety (Porter-O'Grady, 1991). The promotion of shared governance includes interdisciplinary care models—inclusive versus exclusive groups of varied care providers.

Town hall meetings are an incredibly effective way to get in front of your team and ensure they are heard. The concept of town hall meetings is most likely taken from the political arena. A variety of formal organizations—such as unions, campaigns, and groups like the National Nursing Action Coalition—use town hall meetings. Town hall meetings provide clear direction about the objective of the group, session, or meeting and allow opportunity for statements and questions from those present. One strategy when a healthcare organization has a big announcement and wants to ensure the employees understand it is holding a series of town hall meetings to offer information, hear concerns, and most importantly ensure everyone understands the objective and is focused and committed to working toward the same goal.

In addition, the new age of technologic communication methodology should be leveraged to provide up-to-date communication briefs organization-wide. Twitter's initial word limitation was frowned upon by those who felt they had "more" to say, but as the world adjusted to this concise form of communication, it proved effective and successful. Despite initial pushback by many regarding the brief nature of online forms of communication today most people prefer their sought-after information in soundbites as opposed to long meetings. Organizations now have the ability to brief their entire organization quickly and easily (if they choose to) with similar communication methods using personal cellphones via privacy-compliant individual texts, automated systems using text messages and more (i.e., using the hashtag format #openthelines #informtheteam).

# CONCLUSION

We can no longer operate "business as usual" in the healthcare systems of today that have evolved over time. They are just too stressful—for patients and care providers. Healthcare must undergo radical change encompassing the patient experience and innovative strategies to provide better access and care. Nurses, as central communication conduits, must be willing to lead the charge by recognizing the value in becoming an active participant of the team and using their collective voice to drive needed changes in care delivery models and practice.

Healthcare entities must become the kind of organizations that breed healthy work cultures by breaking apart silos, encouraging free-flowing communication, and providing safe care with highly reliable outcomes. Thus, a decrease in stress and fatigue in healthcare work environments should result. The potential for the internal strain of silos to cause burnout for nurses and others who choose a career in healthcare should be banished for a better future. The next chapter investigates how the healthcare culture can exacerbate stress and burnout.

# REFERENCES


American Hospital Association. (2022). *Fast facts on U.S. hospitals, 2022.* https://www.aha.org/statistics/fast-facts-us-hospitals

Cassady, S. (2013). The Linda Crane lecture from silos to bridges: Preparing effective teams for a better delivery system. *Cardiopulmonary Physical Therapy Journal, 24*(2), 5–11.

Chang, W. Y., Ma, J. C., Chiu, H. T., Lin, K. C., & Lee, P. H. (2009). Job satisfaction and perceptions of quality of patient care, collaboration, and teamwork in acute care hospitals. *Journal of Advanced Nursing, 65*(9), 1946–1955. https://doi.org/10.1111/j.1365-2648.2009.05085.x

Cole, L., & Cole, M. (2005). The teamwork values statement. In Cole & Cole (Eds.), *People smart leaders* (p. 43). Oakhill Press.

ECRI. (2022, Spring). *Using human factors engineering & design thinking to improve clinical operations.* https://www.ecri.org/events/understanding-human-factors-design-thinking-clinical-operations

Felgoise, S. H., Branch, J., Poole, A., Levy, L., & Becker, M. (2019, September 1). Interprofessional education: Collaboration and learning in action. *Journal of the American Osteopathic Association 119*(9), 612–619. https://doi.org/10.7556/jaoa.2019.109

Gittell, J. H., Godfrey, M., & Thistlethwaite, J. (2013). Interprofessional collaborative practice and relational coordination: Improving healthcare through relationships. *Journal of Interprofessional Care, 27*(3) 210–213. https://doi.org/10.3109/13561820.2012.730564

Herman, B. (2014). Nurses take bigger role in health IT. *Modern Healthcare, 44*(45), 32–36.

Hut, N. (2021, November 30). *The COVID-19-induced surge in healthcare labor costs is testing hospitals and health systems.* Healthcare Financial Management Association. https://www.hfma.org/topics/hfm/2021/december/soaring-labor-costs-stemming-from-covid-19-test-hospitals-and-he.html

Jennings, B. (2008). Work stress and burnout among nurses: Role of the work environment and working conditions. In R. G. Hughes (Ed.), *Patient safety and quality: An evidence-based handbook for nurses* (Chapter 26, pp. 4–22). Agency for Healthcare Research and Quality.

Lencioni, P. (2002). *The five dysfunctions of a team: A leadership fable.* Jossey-Bass.

Longnecker, C. O., Longnecker, P. D., & Gering, J. T. (2014). Why hospital improvement efforts fail: A view from the front line. *Journal of Healthcare Management, 59*(2), 148–157.

Mayo, A. T., & Wooley, A. (2016, September). Teamwork in healthcare: Maximizing collective intelligence via inclusive collaboration and open communication. *AMA Journal of Ethics.* https://journalofethics.ama-assn.org/article/teamwork-health-care-maximizing-collective-intelligence-inclusive-collaboration-and-open/2016-09

Merriam-Webster. (2015). Silo. In *Merriam-Webster.com dictionary.* http://www.merriam-webster.com/dictionary/silo

Meterko, M., Mohr, D. C., & Young, G. J. (2004). Teamwork culture and patient satisfaction in hospitals. *Official Journal of the Medical Care Section, 42*(5), 492–498. https://doi.org/10.1097/01.mlr.0000124389.58422.b2

Porter-O'Grady, T. (1991). Shared governance for nursing: Part 1: Creating the new organization. *Journal of Association of PeriOperative Registered Nurses, 53*(2), 464–466. https://doi.org/10.1016/s0001-2092(07)69934-7

Salovitz, S. (2022, April 20). *Southwest Florida nurses react to guilty verdict in Tennessee wrong-medication death.* WGCU. https://health.wusf.usf.edu/health-news-florida/2022-04-20/southwest-florida-nurses-react-to-guilty-verdict-in-tennessee-wrong-medication-death

Stanford University Institute of Design. (2012). *A design thinking process.* https://web.stanford.edu/class/me113/d_thinking.html

Statistics Solutions. (2015). *Maslach Burnout Inventory (MBI).* http://www.statisticssolutions.com/maslach-burnout-inventory-mbi/

Traynor, K. (2012). Data silos impede progress against prescription drug abuse. *American Journal of Health-System Pharmacy, 69*(8), 628–632. https://doi.org/10.1093/ajhp/69.8.628

Tucker, A. L. (2009, August 1). *Workarounds and resiliency on the front lines of health care.* PSNet. https://psnet.ahrq.gov/perspective/workarounds-and-resiliency-front-lines-health-care

Tuckman, B. W. & Jensen, M.A. (1965). Developmental sequence in small groups. *Psychological Bulletin, 63*(6), 384–399. https://doi.org/10.1037/h0022100

Tuckman, B. W., & Jensen, M. A. (1977). Stages in small-group development revisited. *Group and Organisation Studies, 2*(4), 419–427. https://doi.org/10.1177/105960117700200404

Upwork. (2021, April 28). *The 5 stages of team development (including examples).* Upwork Global Inc. https://www.upwork.com/resources/stages-of-team-development

Vahey, D., Aiken, L., Sloane, D., Clarke, S. and Vargas, D. (2004). Nurse burnout and patient satisfaction. *Medical Care, 42*, II57-II66.

# 7

# THE SOCIAL MILIEU (CULTURE)

## OBJECTIVES

- Understand the importance of culture.
- Build a positive work environment.
- Understand the value of relationships in getting your job done.
- Explore how being engaged affects your satisfaction at work.
- Consider how nurses can lead the charge in creating patient-centered care models.

As healthcare professionals, we dream of finding the perfect job where we can care for the patients that give us the most professional satisfaction. If you are a person who loves a critical challenge and an adrenaline rush, you may want to work in an emergency department or a critical care unit. If you like having the ability to make long-term connections with patients, you may choose home care, a dialysis unit, or long-term care. One of the best reasons to choose healthcare, and nursing in particular, is the diversity in the profession and the multiple and varied opportunities for employment. Aside from the reasons you might have chosen healthcare, one factor that may significantly influence an employee's feelings about a particular work assignment is the work environment.

## THE IMPORTANCE OF A POSITIVE WORK ENVIRONMENT

The work environment has a major impact on an employee's job satisfaction. *Work environment* involves everything that is a part of the employee's work, such as their relationships with coworkers and department leaders, the organizational culture, and access to professional development activities. Taking into account commuting time, hours at work, and the time we spend thinking and worrying about our jobs, we spend more waking hours at work than we do at home or in life's other activities. The power of a positive work environment cannot be underestimated. The impact it can have on how people think about work and their resulting happiness with work is immense. The opposite, a negative work environment, has the potential to increase stress and cause burnout.

In 2001, the American Association of Critical-Care Nurses (AACN) was one of the first professional nursing organizations to make a commitment to actively promote the development of *healthy work environment standards.* The decision to develop these standards sprang from the organization's dedication to optimal patient care and the desire to promote an environment that supports excellence in nursing practice for acute and critical care nurses (AACN, 2005). Read about the association's most up-to-date work here: https://www.aacn.org/nursing-excellence/healthy-work-environments.

The AACN standards for establishing and sustaining healthy work environments include the following categories (AACN, 2015). Information has been added below each category that can be shared by all providers of healthcare.

**Skilled communication.** Nurses must be as proficient in communication skills as they are in clinical skills, including:

1. Being honest and transparent.
2. Avoiding gossip.
3. Using a mnemonic such as Situation-Background-Assessment-Recommendation (SBAR) when discussing a clinical situation. More information about SBAR can be found here, from the Institute for Healthcare Improvement: https://www.ihi.org/resources/Pages/Tools/sbartoolkit.aspx
4. Supporting new nurses and other healthcare providers by modeling good communication skills to help them successfully transition to the practice environment.

**True collaboration.** Nurses must be relentless in pursuing and fostering true collaboration:

1. Focus on developing teamwork with colleagues.
2. Utilize clear communication with peers and providers for patient safety.
3. Partner with patients to engage them in their current and future care plans.

**Effective decision-making.** Nurses and other healthcare providers must be valued and committed partners in making policy, directing and evaluating clinical care, and leading organizational operations:

1. Get involved in unit operations (unit councils), service lines, and collaborative improvement efforts with other disciplines.
2. When a practice issue is identified, research best practices and make reasonable evidence-based recommendations for change.

**Appropriate staffing.** Staffing must ensure an effective match between patient needs and nurse competencies:

1. Support staffing by acuity or complexity of patient care needs.
2. Work together (as a team) to support patient-care requirements during times of staff shortages.
3. Develop contingency plans for when demand for patient care exceeds the available resources.
4. Be creative in designing care delivery models within scopes of practice and regulatory standards.

**Meaningful recognition.** Nurses must be recognized and must recognize others for the value each brings to the work of the organization:

1. Recognize fellow nurses and other care providers who do a good job.
2. Distinguish other team members (who are not nurses) but support great patient care, including non-clinicians.
3. Engage all team members from the bedside to the boardroom in creating innovative and relevant reward and recognition systems to appeal to the varied generations in the workforce.

**Authentic leadership.** Nurse leaders must fully embrace the imperative of a healthy work environment, authentically live it, and engage others in its achievement:

1. Be a role model. Leaders must demonstrate transformational leadership skills to achieve the best results.
2. Help others take action by offering the ability to influence decisions about departmental or organizational processes.
3. Look for signs of increased stress levels and use available organizational and professional resources to mitigate them.

While this document is focused on nursing alone, these concepts are applicable across the healthcare spectrum. Most departments are now using SBAR or a similar handoff process, employee recognition, rounding, and departmental councils. This work is valuable as well as meaningful. It has purpose and creates positive results, despite challenging circumstances. The intention and subsequent action must outweigh the daily challenges with operations.

## DEVELOPING A POSITIVE WORK ENVIRONMENT

A positive work environment can only develop with support from leadership and employees who work together. HR Exchange Network (2021) discussed how a leader can affect the culture and how the culture of an organization affects a new leader joining an organization. They concluded that the entire purpose of leadership is to create a culture.

That's an interesting thought: The entire purpose of leadership is to create a culture. But do most leaders really understand that? It can be incredibly difficult to move a culture as a leader. Often, complacency is the norm. Those who have been in the organization and have outlasted previous leaders may be subversive with efforts to make organizational change, especially with new leadership. It requires a team of people at the helm who all adopt the same vision and are able to move the organization forward. And the organization's people are inspired by the leadership's vision to get onboard.

Leaders can develop the structure and a strong base for a positive work environment. Successful organizations support the structure and actively work with leaders to improve it. The importance of each person's role in creating a positive and healthy work environment should not be underestimated. What is permitted gets promoted, and it's the leader's job to manage team member behavior to shape the culture. Sometimes it requires managing others up or out of the organization. Benefits of a healthy work culture are evident when the focus is on patient safety and reliability, excellent teamwork, and the delivery of quality care (think about the human factor).

How do employees and leaders work together to create a positive work environment? Is it possible to harness the positive energy from each person's perspective? The HR Exchange Network (2021) posited that companies should reflect the ethics of the leaders who run them.

Each person needs to exhibit the qualities described in Table 7.1 to create a positive and healthy work environment (Poh, 2018).

### **TABLE 7.1** FIVE CHARACTERISTICS OF A POSITIVE AND HEALTHY WORK ENVIRONMENT

| | |
|---|---|
| Communication | Open communication addresses the need to be heard, feel valued, and want to belong in an organization.<br>Understanding the organizational mission, philosophy, and values clarifies the purpose of work.<br>Good two-way communication encourages the sharing of ideas for improvement. |

| | |
|---|---|
| Work-Life Balance | Recognize the potential for imbalance between work and life's priorities.<br>Active management strategies will reduce stress, fatigue, and the potential for burnout, thus improving job-related satisfaction. |
| Professional Development | Nursing requires lifelong learning.<br>Strong professional development activities should be available, and nurses as well as other healthcare providers should take advantage of the opportunities.<br>Equal priority should be placed on enhancing clinical expertise and interpersonal skills. |
| Recognition | Recognize peers by saying "thank you."<br>Look for what is going right in the work environment and reinforce positive behavior. |
| Strong Team Spirit | Teamwork is critical in healthcare. Patients receive the best care when each team member brings a high level of expertise and performance.<br>Team challenges facilitate learning. Common goals bring those with different perspectives and styles together. |

Finding ways to blend these five important criteria can create a positive and healthy work environment. Nurses and other team members will enjoy coming to work. Teamwork will be evident. Organizations that support professional development foster and encourage the growth of professionalism. Feelings of challenge, value, pride, professional competence, and confidence to solve complex problems will result. The most important improvements in the culture will be safe systems, a positive team, and good patient outcomes.

It's also important to note that in 2019, Picoult wrote an article for *Forbes* asking the question, "Are engaged employees a driver of success or a consequence of it?" His research led him to a study from Gallup and the University of Iowa in 2010. The research project included over 2,000 business units across 10 different industries. The findings were surprising—happy and engaged employees are indeed a precursor to business success, not a byproduct of it (Picoult, 2019). Could it be that if more healthcare organizations focused their efforts on the people side of the business, the finances would fall into place?

## PRACTICE PEARLS

- Walk the talk. People observe others and choose how to behave based on what is acceptable in the culture.
- Rewards and recognition must be consistent with organizational values.
- Become passionate about your work. Enthusiasm is contagious. People like to be around positive people and a part of success.
- Get "networked" for the best information sharing in the organization. The more people you know, the easier it is to get things done.
- Communicate clearly and honestly. Be straightforward.
- Communicate in a timely manner. Day-old information is not the norm for today's news.
- Help your organization's leaders improve the culture of your workplace—everyone will benefit from the success.

---

# HUMAN CAPITAL AND THE VALUE OF RELATIONSHIPS

The greatest asset in any healthcare organization is the people. No technology can replace the human touch in nursing and healthcare. Who to hire is one of the most important choices a leader will make because it affects multiple aspects of any organization. Many organizational leaders say employees are their greatest assets, but their actions are inconsistent with their words. It is disingenuous to say this if too few resources are chronically allocated, there is a lack of professional development, staffing is always too lean, vacancy rates are always too high, and so on. Staff feel devalued.

Because nurses are the largest workforce in healthcare, they have an opportunity to mold the future. Nurses can help create work environments where all team members feel valued. Nurses can and should be considered frontline leaders. Nurses can be organizational ambassadors just as they are patient advocates. Exit interviews show that most people do not choose to leave an organization because of the executives. They choose to leave because of behavior of their peers, the work environment, or the relationship with their direct supervisor (or lack thereof). Nurses can make a difference by working with leaders to develop an environment where everyone feels valued and included.

One of the questions asked in almost every employee satisfaction or employee engagement survey is, "Do you have a best friend at work?" Most people wonder what that has to do with anything related to the work environment and don't believe it is important to have a best friend at work. However, it is important to be able to trust the people you work with. Trust facilitates the development of friendships. Friends are loyal, supportive, and can be counted on for help in times of need. To develop close friendships, you have to be willing to share some of the intimate details of your life in confidence. People are more likely to leave a job when they do not have positive and strong relationships with their coworkers or departmental leaders.

Xu and colleagues (2019) explained that a nurse's social capital in the workplace consists of a series of relationships made up of interactions between other healthcare professionals. Specific attributes influence interactions, their relational network, trust, shared understanding, reciprocity, and social cohesion. When these attributes are healthy, the healthy relational network supports a healthy environment. This is further strengthened by active listening, effective communication, active group participation, and the support of leadership.

Hospitals, like many other organizations, have formal and informal leaders who have the ability to influence social capital. The role of the informal leader can be pivotal. This person can help improve and sustain the morale of a unit by serving as an ambassador for nursing or another healthcare profession. They help others integrate and stay active as members of the unit's social cohesion. Informal and formal leaders can foster an environment where all members feel that they belong, are appreciated, their role makes a difference, and their voice is heard.

This role should not be overlooked but be leveraged. The ability of informal leaders to motivate, encourage, and promote positive relationships has a direct impact on others in the work area. The title of manager or director does not in itself make a leader. Informal leaders can be transformational. They lead with an understanding that most everyone comes to work to do a good job. They are quick to help when there is knowledge to be shared. They are active listeners for a frustrated peer. They do this often without formal education or training. The unofficial leader leverages human capital to create synergy.

## A COMMITMENT TO A DIVERSE HEALTHCARE WORKFORCE

> To build a future workforce that effectively provides the health and health care that society needs will require a substantial increase in the numbers, types, and distribution of the nursing workforce, as well as an education system that better prepares nurses for practicing in community-based settings with diverse populations that face a variety of lived experiences. (Wakefield et al., 2021)

This call to action comes directly from *The Future of Nursing, 2020–2030* report and is a continuation of the 2011 *The Future of Nursing: Leading Change, Advancing Health* report published by the Institute of Medicine, which called for more racial, ethnic, and gender diversity among nurses in order to improve quality of care and reduce health disparities. Many ethnic groups are still underrepresented in nursing and other healthcare disciplines.

We know the benefit of having a more diverse workforce to match the wider population is important. Matching provider-patient ethnicity has been shown to speed the connection for gaining trust and activation needed for the patient to take ownership in their care and well-being. Secondly, there are untapped talent pools of potential healthcare providers who need to know that they are wanted, needed, and can be successful in fulfilling nursing or healthcare careers.

Like so many other endeavors, this requires industry to partner with academia. We need innovative thinkers who can tackle the problem in ways not seen before in times past. Recruitment and exposure to the benefits of a career in healthcare must begin in early life by reaching school-age children. Current healthcare providers from underrepresented groups can have a visible and valuable role in recruitment by community outreach.

Academic and community partners can assist the healthcare industry pipeline by providing and encouraging underrepresented students to take advantage of support programs to reinforce learning the basics of math, science, communication, and other relevant topics necessary for a career in healthcare. The same recruitment applies for healthcare teaching staff—recruit more underrepresented faculty.

Enhancing the diversity of the healthcare academic and professional workforce will take time. No strategy will be a quick fix. Shortages of healthcare personnel have persisted for decades for a variety of reasons: other career options in more lucrative industries, shift work, expensive academic preparation, economic turmoil, etc. As the demographics of the healthcare workforce begin to more closely match the population, there will be additional opportunities to eliminate overall health disparities.

## SHARP HEALTHCARE

In healthcare, there are some great examples of companies doing the right things. For example, Sharp HealthCare, based in San Diego, California, clearly values their human capital. Their healthcare system includes four acute care hospitals, three specialty hospitals, a number of medical groups, and their own health plan (Sharp, n.d.). This includes over 19,000 employees and 2,700 affiliated physicians. The organization made a decision in 2001 to dedicate their organization to transforming the healthcare experience, and this work continues today. Understanding the value of human capital, they started this movement with their employees.

The overall vision at Sharp was to "become the best place for employees to work, the best place for physicians to practice medicine, the best place for patients to receive care, and ultimately the best healthcare system in the universe." (Sharp, n.d.)

The model developed by Sharp HealthCare has three core components (Adamson, 2009, p. 22):

- Experience and performance improvement designed to actively engage team members, at all levels, in creating positive change related to the workplace experience and the customer experience.
- Accountability systems and structures ensuring alignment of goals across the organization.
- Learning and development that launched The Sharp University, a corporate university designed to provide education and development for leaders, team members, and affiliated physicians.

The results at Sharp HealthCare, secondary to their focus on employees, have demonstrated the value of employee engagement. Since the transformation began, the results have been astounding. One of the most important lessons to be learned from this example of transformation is that the more employees are engaged in their work, the more positive improvement is enjoyed. Sharp has engaged their workforce to reduce employee turnover, achieve higher patient and employee satisfaction, garner annual improvement in quality metrics, and improve market share and net revenue for the organization (Adamson & Rhodes, 2009).

In 2007, Sharp HealthCare received the Malcolm Baldrige National Quality Award for organizational excellence (Adamson, 2009). It is one of the most prestigious awards an organization can receive. The Malcolm Baldrige criteria provides a prized framework for measuring performance and planning in an uncertain environment. The structure is perfect for the healthcare environment, where there is controlled chaos and an uncertain environment.

In addition, each of the Sharp acute care hospitals have received the prestigious Magnet® designation (some more than once). The American Nurses Credentialing Center awards hospitals for excellence in nursing practices and quality care. You can read more about Magnet designation here: https://www.nursingworld.org/organizational-programs/magnet.

The Baldrige criteria can help any healthcare organization achieve and sustain the highest national levels of patient safety and loyalty; health outcomes in the areas of acute myocardial infarction, heart failure, pneumonia, and other conditions; physician and staff satisfaction or engagement, with a focus on registered nurses; revenue and market share; and community service (National Institute of Standards and Technology, 2010).

Today, Sharp's mission continues to focus on improving the health of everyone they serve. Read more about "The Sharp Experience" here: https://www.sharp.com/about/sharp-experience.

As this example illustrates, having a happy and engaged workforce has a positive impact on productivity and morale, reduces employee stress, and improves employee retention. So, what can you do to become an engaged employee who finds happiness and joy in your work? The decision to find happiness and joy rests with each individual.

## FINDING HAPPINESS AT WORK

Optimistic, hopeful, and happy staff members can convey those attributes to patients and other staff through developed relationships in the workplace. Work environments where patients and coworkers are cranky, pessimistic, and depressed do exist. The impact of attitude and effort always comes back to you. Are you not drawn to people who laugh, have hope, and care about others? Are you not happier when around patients who are involved in their own recovery, who exhibit hope and optimism, and who make you laugh? This is most likely the most valuable lesson in relationships, and it begins with you. You attract happy and positive people by how you exhibit the same behaviors and traits.

Dr. Martin Seligman is recognized as the father of the theory of positive psychology. Seligman spent the majority of his career studying depression and learned helplessness. However, after a number of years in practice, he changed his focus and his own thinking. In 2000, he began writing a book about happiness titled *Authentic Happiness* (2002). In his theory of authentic happiness, he included three elements: positive emotion, engagement, and meaning.

After development of the original authentic happiness theory, he received input from his students and fellow psychologists over the next 10 years. Seligman then expanded the theory and changed it to the well-being theory. The new theory added two elements to the previous three elements for a new total of five critical elements thought to achieve happiness and the ability to truly flourish in life. The revised theory of well-being includes these areas of measurement, which he terms "PERMA" (Seligman, 2011):

- Positive emotion (which includes happiness and life satisfaction)
- Engagement
- Relationships
- Meaning and purpose
- Accomplishment

The goal of positive psychology (in authentic happiness) is to increase the amount of happiness in your own life and in the world. The well-being theory posits a slightly different goal of expanding or increasing the amount of flourishing in your life and in the world (Seligman, 2011). Flourishing speaks to the quality of your life and the impact you have over your individual circumstances. Read more about Seligman's work with PERMA and well-being here: https://ppc.sas.upenn.edu/.

*Morale* is simply the collective happiness of the workforce. The workforce is comprised of individuals who can each decide to have a positive or negative effect on the whole. The success of any office, department, or service provider depends on the individual investment of people in how they think, how they act, and what they do. There is no success unless people make it happen.

It is often easier to think negatively and want to blame others for the current circumstances. However, much of the difficulty in life is a result of the atmosphere and who is in it. What is most difficult is realizing that you have the power to change your thinking and subsequent actions. The secret to happiness, success, satisfaction, and fulfillment is not doing what you like but liking what you do. This includes liking the surroundings, the people, and the work.

Being happy all the time is an unrealistic expectation. Happiness comes with learning the skills of living in the present, valuing each moment, and making the best of each situation. Certain experiences, job tasks, and people might make it easier to be happy. However, they do not have the power to influence your ability to be happy or unhappy.

## ENGAGEMENT FOR SATISFACTION (PERSONAL AND CUSTOMER)

Employees want to feel valued at work. In a global study by Insight Training Solutions (2022), 79% of people left their job due to a lack of feeling appreciated. Employee satisfaction plays a big part in the perception of patients and their satisfaction. Patients are beginning to look at data related to hospital or physician performance prior to selecting providers. When looking at the bottom line, organizations can see an increase in their profit margin when their employees are satisfied with their positions and organizations.

Healthcare industries frequently utilize customer service and quality improvement programs in an attempt to increase customer satisfaction and quality scores. While these programs are grounded in positive concepts, the culture of an organization has a tremendous impact on the staff and consequently on the patient. If you do not alter a negative culture, no program will make the desired improvements in patient satisfaction or quality. Since 2000, the Gallup organization has been tracking employee engagement. The year 2014 marked the lowest employee engagement reading (in the first edition of this book). Gallup noted that the number of workers who were actively engaged in their job was less than one-third, at 31.5% (Adkins, 2015). Over 50% of employees were not engaged; they appeared to have no passion for their work and were "just putting in time." The remaining 18% of employees were thought to be actively disengaged. Unfortunately, the disengaged group of employees usually demonstrated their unhappiness in an active fashion to other employees and undermined the work of the engaged employees.

Since the COVID-19 pandemic began, by 2021, only 21% of employees were engaged, with 19% actively disengaged (Gallup, 2021). Gallup has been using their proprietary Q12 survey to measure employee engagement for decades.

Read more about the consequences of employee engagement across the globe here: https://www.gallup.com/394373/indicator-employee-engagement.aspx.

The value of an engaged workforce has been shown to directly affect the success of an organization. Employee engagement can be a strategic advantage with lower costs, better productivity, and more. The competence and skills of engaged employees is reflected in enthusiasm, motivation, and loyalty to an organization. It has a major impact on the overall culture of the organization and the level of customer service provided by the organization. Teamwork, organizational support, living the stated mission and vision, and adherence to standards are critical to productivity, innovation, and the ability to create an exceptional patient experience.

One of the most well-known and earliest adopters of using an engaged workforce to drive organizational improvement and showing the difference it can make was Quint Studer at Baptist Health Care in Pensacola, Florida. The impact to customer satisfaction was amazing; the hospital virtually went from the bottom to the top. Studer developed his method, formed his own company, and has since helped hundreds of hospitals implement evidence-based leadership systems. These leadership systems have helped organizations attain and sustain outstanding results in improved organizational performance and patient-care outcomes. In 2010, the Studer Group won the Malcolm Baldrige National Quality Award, and they have coached 10 of the 18 Malcolm Baldrige Award recipients in healthcare. In 2015, the Studer Group was acquired by Huron Consulting Group.

The global COVID-19 pandemic created a rapidly chaotic environment that greatly affected the social milieu. Healthcare providers from all disciplines had to determine quickly how to serve a specialized patient population who had to be segregated from their "routine" patient population. The segregation provided both patient and worker safety. The addition of layers of personal protective equipment complicated caregiving and exponentially increased cost.

Some caregivers succumbed to the virus, which created additional shortages of personnel—either temporary or permanent. The emotional toll the global COVID-19 pandemic took on caregivers was unimaginable. Many caregivers even crossed specialties to assist other caregivers without reservation.

All healthcare providers "leaned in" to the legislative conversations about vaccines and prevention from both the government and public health. However, the politization of the conversation lead to much mistrust in the public. Many weren't sure who or what to believe.

Still today, in 2023, we see mutual support among healthcare disciplines on the front lines, and we have drastically raised the bar on awareness of the emotional toils of providing healthcare. This crisis provided an opportunity to show our true collaborative nature in healthcare. It could be compared to the cultural learnings of patriotism and faith after the 9/11 tragedies in 2001. It has forced each of us to examine what is really important to us, what pulls us through difficult times, and what brings contentment and joy in our work. Mutual respect, collaboration, and teamwork are the social milieu of healthcare. We must begin to figure out how to build on our learnings of the past few years and then maintain it.

## PRACTICE PEARLS

Determining whether you are an engaged and happy employee requires self-reflection about your state of being. Here are a few important questions to ask yourself:

- What things do I do at work that might be perceived as negative?
- What physical or verbal attitudes might be perceived as negative?
- What puts me in a bad mood at work? How do I contribute?
- What puts me in a good mood at work? How do I contribute?
- Do I make a difference at work, and is that difference positive or negative?
- Employee satisfaction can directly impact customer satisfaction.
- Recognize that when healthcare providers are saving lives in extreme circumstances by optimally working together, we achieve the best patient outcomes.

---

Awareness and self-reflection are the first steps toward making change. Improvement and a path of self-discovery can be rewarding. Making a conscious decision to influence your own happiness and joy in your work can yield other collateral benefits. It may include improved relationships both at and outside of work, a sense of calm, and feelings of less stress.

Taking responsibility for negative feelings about work and changing your thinking or reaction to the negativity can provide relief from stress and fatigue and can lessen the potential to reach burnout. How a person perceives a given situation is a predictor of subsequent action, not necessarily an appropriate assessment of the situation itself. We must be careful of others' ability to influence our behavior through their negativity.

It is well-known that customers who are satisfied will be passive but loyal advocates. Dissatisfied customers are known to be active complainants who will share their customer experiences with many others. Estimates of how many people become unaware of negative perceptions or experiences are growing with access to social media and other online platforms to post their experiences on Yelp, Google, and others.

The importance of customer satisfaction has always been important to hospital and healthcare providers. This is a people business. An unsatisfied customer can have a negative impact on reputation and is more likely to consider legal recourse. The importance of scoring well has escalated for hospitals on the Hospital Consumer Assessment of Healthcare Providers and Systems (HCAHPS). The survey has received increased emphasis since the establishment of the Patient Protection and Affordable Care Act of 2010 (more commonly known as Obamacare).

The "pay for performance" payment scheme that resulted from this law reduced the Medicare diagnosis-related group payments for all hospitals (Medicare.gov, n.d.). Savings are redistributed at a later date according to individual hospital performance. The public can now search for quality data and hospital performance via the Hospital Compare website at https://www.medicare.gov/care-compare/?providerType=Hospital.

The first publicly reported surveys for rating inpatient care began in 2008 (Centers for Medicare & Medicaid Services [CMS], 2021). The purpose of the survey is to produce standardized information about patients' perspectives of care that allows objective and meaningful comparisons of hospitals on topics that are important to consumers (CMS, 2021). The HCAHPS survey today is composed of 29 items, and 19 items encompass critical aspects of the hospital experience (such as communication with nurses, communication with doctors, responsiveness of hospital staff, communication about medicines, discharge information, care transition, cleanliness of the hospital environment, quietness of the hospital environment, overall rating of hospital, and recommendation of the hospital).

In the beginning, 70% of the Total Performance Score (TPS) was determined by Clinical Process of Care outcomes, and 30% was from Patient Experience of Care scoring. By 2015, the TPS was comprised of the Clinical Process of Care domain score (weighted as 20% of the TPS), the Patient Experience of Care domain score (weighted as 30%), the Outcome domain score (30%), and the Efficiency domain score (20%). Although measurement has shifted into other areas such as readmissions, patient experience still accounts for a large percentage of the possible negative or positive financial impact (CMS, n.d.).

In looking at the issue of pay for performance, labor costs have continued to escalate in healthcare. In part, this is directly related to shortages of key personnel. Fierce recruitment strategies with sign-on bonuses and increased pay rates both for permanent and temporary staff have only exacerbated overall healthcare costs. Unfortunately, when nurses and other care providers do not feel valued, they will seek an employer that offers more. This may be a sign-on bonus with another permanent employer or work with a temporary or travel agency where one can expect a higher rate of pay. Seasoned employees in an organization are frequently asked to orient new employees or temporary staff and/or take on more responsibility, frequently without compensation. The additional responsibility comes with additional stress, which can also lead to burnout.

In addition, today's inflation is pushing healthcare employees to organizations and temporary agencies that can provide higher wages. If work is challenging wherever you go, why not go where the money is the greatest? Organizations really need to be attentive to engagement now more than ever for both recruitment and retention. They need to focus resources to keep long-term loyal employees with unique organizational knowledge and ensure their culture is too good to leave.

## THE PLANETREE MODEL FOR PATIENT CENTERED CARE

Those who work in hospitals know they must be responsible to take care of sick or vulnerable patients. The need to improve patient experience scores can be so frustrating. Organizational strategies are frequently viewed as superficial and don't yield improved results. Healthcare providers are challenged with a number of systems beyond their direct control, which may present obstacles in providing care. Examples include cumbersome discharge processes, late provider rounding, physicians not communicating with patients and families, as well as complex family issues. Improving patient experience scores is a complex task that requires all members of the team to be on the same page (so to speak). It can be very complicated in the inpatient hospital setting. Movement toward a patient-centric model, which focuses on patient needs and includes all members of the healthcare team, is a good place to start.

The Planetree model for patient-centered care, created by patient Angelica Thieriot, was one of the first such patient-centric models created. Thieriot dreamed of what a hospital could be if a patient were treated like a whole person with their body, mind, and spirit being supported, and where the importance of caring, kindness, and respect were as important as technical skills (Frampton, 2009). The goal of the Planetree model was to change the hospital environment from a provider-centric one, which historically has been designed for the convenience of the practitioner, to an environment centered *around* the patient. It focused more on personalized care and promoted patient engagement in that care (Frampton, 2009).

> Today, Planetree, Inc. is a mission based not-for-profit organization that partners with healthcare organizations around the world and

> across the care continuum to transform how care is delivered: from the vision of one patient to a global reach extending over 6 continents and touching the lives of millions. Planetree is uniquely positioned to represent the patient voice and advance how professional caregivers engage with patients and families with over 40 years of experience. By applying the Language of Caring guided by a foundation of four principles, caregivers can improve the patient experience and create a culture of caring. (Planetree, 2022)

Thieriot described her original experience as follows:

- Sound medical care
- Institutional, impersonal, and alienating environment
- Bare white walls, excessive noise, nightly disturbances, and limited visitation
- Inadequate access to information related to her care and treatment

The first Planetree model unit opened in San Francisco on a 13-bed medical-surgical unit in 1985. Since then, the Planetree model members have continued to develop best practices to move organizations to a more patient-centered model of care. Planetree, in 2014, identified 10 components of today's contemporary model:

- Human interaction
- Family, friends, and social support
- Access to information
- Healing environments through architectural design
- Food and nutrition
- Arts and entertainment
- Spirituality

- Human touch
- Complementary therapies
- Healthy communities

You can learn more about the Planetree model at https://planetree.org/certification/about-planetree/

During the global COVID-19 pandemic, many of the human interaction and family support components of care were erased out of necessity and fear. Healthcare employees were resourceful and creative in finding ways to bring families together despite the virus that kept them apart utilizing the latest available technology. While this wasn't a suitable replacement for human contact, it was important for patients to be able to connect with their loved ones. At times, it was extremely hard on caregivers when family members were not allowed to be present. It shifted much of the "caring" responsibility to caregivers in addition to the bevy of crucial clinical tasks. And it took an immense emotional toll. The added stress was unbearable for some. It highlighted the extraordinary importance of the family unit as a significant part of the healthcare team for decision-making, planning, and execution of care.

## THE NURSE'S ROLE IN PATIENT-CENTERED CARE

What is the nurse's role in moving the hospital to a more patient- and family-centered care environment? How does nursing philosophy add to the caring environment? Faubion (n.d.) looked at nursing philosophy and identified four key components to help individual nurses identify their *personal* philosophy. The first component is that of *role* and how it applies to the responsibility of patient care and the profession. The second component is *knowledge*. Nurses are responsible for their practice and ongoing education to enable them to critically think through changes in patient condition and apply clinical judgment and reasoning. *Values* are the third component in nursing philosophy and may be personal and/or professional. Values have an impact on how nurses practice and acts concerning their responsibilities. *Process* is the final component and relates to knowledge. A nurse must be able to put all the pieces together to provide the best possible care for their patients, which in turn provides the best outcome.

The nurse is often the one professional who spends the most time with patients. They are truly patient advocates. They communicate, collaborate, and negotiate on behalf of patients. They help to translate concerns between multiple medical providers and patients. The nurse has an opportunity to provide care to the patient and family with compassion, the ability to focus on quality and patient safety during their interactions, and the ability to reduce patient anxiety about their care by providing education. Nurses can develop a trusting relationship with patients and family.

Patient experience is always going to be a high concern for nurses and other healthcare providers. The nurse will likely be the person to establish the strongest relationship with the patient and family. Many times, the nurse will mediate misunderstandings, apologize for the behavior or actions of others, and share the truth. Nurses need to take the lead in creating a healing environment. Healthcare leaders, other clinical providers of care, and healthcare organizations need to facilitate excellent patient experiences in a positive culture in all the areas of healthcare.

# CONCLUSION

The importance of culture with a positive and healthy work environment cannot be overstated in improving job satisfaction—it is critical for the retention of all healthcare workers both in organizations and in specific professions such as nursing. Engagement of all team members is crucial for organizational success. Every nurse, whether a staff nurse or a nurse leader, has the power to influence and impact the work environment in a positive or a negative way.

And each individual healthcare worker has the ability to choose their level of engagement in the work environment.

After reflecting on the power of a positive work environment and the benefits of working with an engaged workforce, think about how you can begin to make a difference. The concepts detailed in the children's book *Random Kindness and Senseless Acts of Beauty* (Herbert & Pavel, 2014) outline the idea that we are all *in the circle* together. Each person can become an agent of goodness and beauty if they so choose (Herbert & Pavel, 2014). The COVID-19 pandemic highlighted many of the existing weaknesses in the current healthcare system. And, the idea of us all "being in it together" was found to be true; we needed each other then and we need each other now.

Senseless acts of beauty could be viewed as those things that are above and beyond the normal work expectations. It is not necessarily about doing more work, but doing work well. It is about showing unexpected appreciation and compassion to others. This could be as simple as writing a sincere note of praise or thanks, bringing food to share with coworkers, putting a flower in someone's mailbox, or making a decision to sincerely compliment five people during the day. The ideas are endless. People look forward to committing to and receiving senseless acts of beauty, and that is something we could all use now after experiencing the last three years of turmoil.

## PRACTICE PEARL

Consider a senseless act of beauty campaign. It could lead to a new and improved culture and bring the "beauty" back to nursing and healthcare.

So, how might the work environment be changed? The more engaged an individual is in their environment, the more likely they will be able to influence and impact decisions. The best outcomes occur when collaborative multidisciplinary teams interact. No nurse or other team member works alone in healthcare. Collectively, nurses can have a very powerful voice, and they hold one of the most important healthcare team roles as a patient advocate. Healthcare workers must be engaged to think creatively to influence others by leading change in creating better patient-centered models of care for the future. The next chapter takes a look at the clout of allies and why relationship-building in healthcare is crucial.

## REFERENCES

Adamson, G. A. (2009). *The complete guide to transforming the patient experience.* HCPro.

Adamson, G., & Rhodes, S. (2009). *The complete guide to transforming the patient experience.* HCPro.

Adkins, A. (2015, January 28). *Majority of U.S. employees not engaged despite gains in 2014.* Gallup. http://www.gallup.com/poll/181289/majority-employees-not-engaged-despite-gains-2014.aspx

American Association of Colleges of Nursing. (2022). *Nursing fact sheet.* https://www.aacnnursing.org/News-Information/Fact-Sheets/Nursing-Fact-Sheet

American Association of Critical-Care Nurses. (2005). *AACN standards for establishing and sustaining a healthy work environment: A journey to excellence* [Executive summary]. https://www.aacn.org/~/media/aacn-website/nursing-excellence/healthy-work-environment/execsum.pdf?la=en

American Association of Critical-Care Nurses. (2015). *Healthy work environments.* http://www.aacn.org/wd/hwe/content/hwehome.pcms?menu=hwe

Centers for Medicare & Medicaid Services. (n.d.). *Hospital compare.* https://www.medicare.gov/hospitalcompare/search.html

Centers for Medicare & Medicaid Services. (2021, March). *CAHPS hospital survey, quality assurance guidelines.* https://www.cms.gov/files/document/hcahps-qag-v160.pdf

Faubion, D. (n.d.). *50 nursing philosophy examples + how to write your own.* https://www.nursingprocess.org/nursing-philosophy-examples.html

Frampton, S. (2009). Creating a patient-centered system. *American Journal of Nursing, 109*(3), 30–33. https://doi.org/10.1097/01.NAJ.0000346924.67498.ed

Gallup. (2021). *Employee engagement.* https://www.gallup.com/394373/indicator-employee-engagement.aspx

Herbert, A. A., & Pavel, M. P. (2014). *Random kindness and senseless acts of beauty.* New Village Press.

HR Exchange Network. (2021, February 1). *Ways leadership affects culture and culture affects leadership.* https://www.hrexchangenetwork.com/hr-talent-management/articles/ways-leadership-affects-culture-and-culture-affect

Insight Training Solutions. (2022). *The relationship between employee satisfaction and the patient experiences.* https://insighttrainingsolutions.io/relationship-between-employee-satisfaction-and-patient-experience/

Institute of Medicine. (2010). *The Future of nursing: Leading change, advancing health.* National Academies Press. https://www.ncbi.nlm.nih.gov/books/NBK209880/pdf/Bookshelf_NBK209880.pdf

McLaughlin, J. (n.d.). *What is organizational culture? Definition and characteristics.* http://study.com/academy/lesson/what-is-organizational-culture-definition-characteristics.html

Medicare.gov. (n.d.). *Linking quality to payment.* https://www.medicare.gov/HospitalCompare/linking-quality-to-payment.html?AspxAutoDetectCookieSupport=1

National Institute of Standards and Technology. (2010, March 25). *Baldrige performance excellence program.* http://www.nist.gov/baldrige/enter/health_care.cfm

Picoult, J. (2019, November 11). Are engaged employees a driver of business success or a consequence of it? *Forbes.* https://www.forbes.com/sites/jonpicoult/2019/11/11/are-engaged-employees-a-driver-of-business-success-or-a-consequence-of-it/?sh=51d5022c4ad7

Planetree.org. (2022). *About.* https://planetree.org/certification/about-planetree/

Poh, M. (2018). *5 characteristics of a positive work environment.* LinkedIn Pulse. https://www.linkedin.com/pulse/positive-work-environment-biswarup-ray/

Seligman, M. E. P. (2002). *Authentic happiness: Using the new positive psychology to realize your potential for lasting fulfillment.* Simon & Schuster.

Seligman, M. E. P. (2011). *Flourish: A visionary new understanding of happiness and well-being.* Free Press.

Sharp. (n.d.). *The Sharp experience.* http://www.sharp.com/choose-sharp/sharp-experience.cfm

Szyndlar, M. (2022, July 29). *Customer satisfaction: Why it's important in 2022.* Survicate Blog. https://survicate.com/customer-satisfaction/importance-customer-satisfaction/

Wakefield, M. K., Williams, D. R., Menestrel, S. L., & Flaubert, J. L. (2021). *The future of nursing 2020-2030: Charting a path to achieve health equity.* The National Academies Press.

Xu, J., Kunaviktikul, W., Akkadechanunt, T., Nantsupawat, A., & Stark, A. T. (2019, December 2). A contemporary understanding of nurses' workplace social capital: A response to the rapid changes in the nursing workforce. *Journal of Nursing Management, 28*(2), 247–258. https://doi.org/10.1111/jonm.12914

# 8

# THE CLOUT OF ALLIES

## OBJECTIVES

- Consider how to build alliances with coworkers and staff.
- Learn to promote teamwork across boundaries.
- Explore how to maximize resources through teamwork.
- Understand the factors that help and hinder positive change.
- Consider the best change process for your organization.

An *ally* is defined as "a person or organization who associates, connects, or unites for some common cause or purpose" (Dictionary.com, 2022). Healthcare professionals, and nurses in particular, have a number of opportunities to build allies and connect with others for a common purpose: delivering great patient care and excellent customer service. Alliances are the relationships built between those where there is mutual benefit for each.

Cultivating quality relationships takes time and skill. Providing care to patients is a "team sport," and no single provider can do it alone. Effective communication is a precursor to teamwork. Miscommunication, misunderstandings, or a lack of effective communication can all produce unintended interpersonal conflict, as well as compromise care. Conflict causes stress. In some cases, this can be avoided if the care providers attend to building solid relationships and establishing clear lines of communication.

Healthcare is inherently stressful. After all, we are taking responsibility for the lives of others as we assess, diagnose, write orders, implement orders, monitor, provide education and direction, and send people off to live their lives according to the recommendations we have made. What if something goes wrong? What if we made a mistake in the interpretation of lab values? What if there is more going on with this patient than we realized? Each of these questions are stressful to consider. The "clout of allies" expands each individual provider's reach. Instead of the glimpse in the clinic or the hospital room, a provider with an allegiance to a healthcare team will have input from each aspect of care, and together, that team will have a much clearer picture of the disease process or environmental complications that can cause a patient to succeed or fail in their treatment plan. Let's face it, this could be the difference between life and death.

## BUILDING ALLIANCES

Healthcare facilities across the nation have varying elements of team building or teamwork: negative, positive, and somewhere in between. Nurses have a great deal of influence, and they often do not give themselves the credit they deserve. As the most present members of the healthcare team, nurses play a leading role. Nurses intuitively facilitate teamwork between many care providers. And nurses are accustomed to taking an active role to lead teams of diverse individuals. However, nurses are not always on an even playing field, respected for their expertise, or allowed to fully participate as an equal partner in care delivery. Healthcare is a collaborative effort between clinical and non-clinical people. Inherently, caregivers want to work together with a shared objective(s) for treating the patient's condition. Nurses often have a dual role of being a member of the team and the "air traffic controller" to ensure the patient's care follows the plan. The nurse uses the art and science of nursing to provide, facilitate, and influence the patient's care with the patient, family, and other team members.

The following story offers an illustration.

## WHEN WEDGES BETWEEN EMPLOYEES ENCOURAGE MISCOMMUNICATION

Still relatively new, a nurse was reviewing electronic medical records (EMR) of patients who were admitted the previous evening for a newly deployed care model that included completing admissions with a multidisciplinary team. The nurse was assessing the records for completeness and accuracy, adding consults as needed, ensuring quality measures were implemented, communicating with the admitting nurse, and encouraging follow-through on any missing elements. The nurse noticed that one heart failure patient did not have an echocardiogram and was not on a beta blocker. She then placed a "sticky note" on the chart for the bedside nurse. The EMR system had one color of sticky notes for nurses and a different color for medical providers. Apparently within the next few hours, one of the care providers on the team (a pharmacist) obtained more information about the patient's status. He appropriately added medications to the list, which included a beta blocker noted in a previous visit. However, he did not remove the sticky note.

> The nurse caring for the patient received a phone call from the cardiologist, who proceeded to tell her that she was never to leave notes for any of his patients. He went on to say that he knows his quality measures, he is the best in meeting them, and he did not need any help from her. He also said he saw the note and thought the patient might have been re-hospitalized for not taking a beta blocker. Once he saw the medication list, even he was confused. He then proceeded to tell her she did not know about medications, and if she was too stupid to know them, she should not be commenting on the list.
>
> The nurse tried to explain the new care model and the purpose of the note. Dr. Cardiologist stated he was not interested in the nuances of the process change and cut off the nurse's sentences as she was speaking. He continued to condescendingly accuse her of not knowing the patient's medications. Finally, he got quiet and the nurse simply said, "I hear you." He was silent for only a moment, repeated it all again, and then hung up.
>
> The nurse cried because Dr. Cardiologist made her feel incompetent in her new role. She was also angry because he called her personal cellphone, and she knew that he could only get the number by asking someone in nursing for it. She felt betrayed by her colleagues and, in her mind, the nurses were all gathered around the nurses' station laughing at how Dr. Cardiologist had just chewed her out.
>
> Fortunately, the nurse felt better as time in the role passed. She later received a surprise phone call from the chief medical officer letting her know that Dr. Cardiologist had been to see him. She was instructed not to make him angry anymore—without even hearing her side of the story.

This story's ending is unfortunate, but it is not all that uncommon. Bad behavior among and between healthcare providers does exist and can cause a great deal of unnecessary stress in the environment. Being a nurse and taking care of sick patients is enough stress without layering on more from others' bad behavior. However, as nurses learn to avoid the pitfalls relative to ineffective communication or gaps in communication, healthy and positive alliances can be formed. It is wise to build strategic alliances with others before they are needed. Then, once "the going gets tough," nurses have those on the team they can rely on for assistance.

Some call building alliances at work "networking" or "creating good karma" (Schindler, 2014). Schindler advised that it is never a bad idea to create connections with people who you can help and who might be able to help you; the reasons are pragmatic besides just being a nice person. Nurses are usually nice people and generally easy to get along with. Repetition of good communication practices builds trust. People know what to expect from one another. Allies might even become friends. Figure 8.1 shows how trust is the foundation for building alliances.

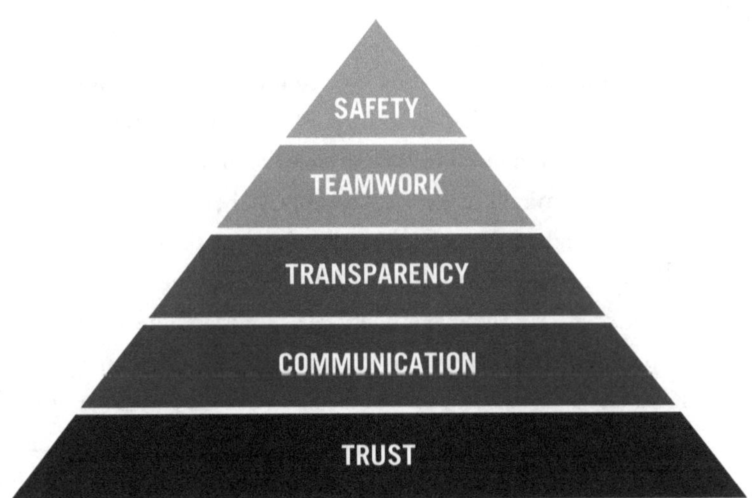


**FIGURE 8.1** Without trust as the bedrock, you cannot build alliances and reap all their benefits.

## PRACTICE PEARLS

- Consider doing something nice or helpful for someone else before you need something yourself.
- Share new information when you receive it.
- Work to improve the communication process with teammates.

---

## ELEMENTS OF TEAMWORK

Cole and Cole (2005, p. 43) cited the most important elements of teamwork in a four-legged table model—communication, cooperation, trust, and respect:

- **Communication:** A must-have when it comes to teamwork. Every team has a leader, whether formal or informal, and that leader must be a great communicator. The same is true in healthcare. Any leader unable to communicate clearly, appropriately, or confidently may remain a leader by position but will not retain the respect of a following. The Joint Commission (2022) has identified communication as one of its critical patient safety goals for years. The ability to get important information to the appropriate person in a timely manner has a direct impact on patient outcomes. Should a nurse or other healthcare professional need to contact a provider who has been disrespectful and condescending in the past, they may be hesitant to do so.
- **Cooperation:** Great communication plus cooperation yields teamwork. In healthcare, people rely on one another for their expertise. This ultimately benefits the patient. The national scope and standards of practice in nursing lists collaboration as a standard element of teamwork. It states:

  > The registered nurse collaborates with the healthcare consumer, family, and others in the conduct of nursing

practice...partners with others to effect change and produce positive outcomes through the sharing of knowledge of the healthcare consumer and/or situation. (O'Sullivan et al., 2010, p. 57)

- **Trust:** This is perhaps the most important part of the four-legged table. Trust is the main support or foundation. Without it the relationship, system, or project might tumble. Trust is the opposite of fear. There are not many people in this world who thrive on fear. What is often ignored in healthcare cultures are the silent acts of interaction (or a lack thereof) that break trust in workplace teammates. Elvis sang the song "Suspicious Minds," which said: "We can't go on together with suspicious minds, and we can't build our dreams on suspicious minds" (James, 1968). This philosophy also applies to healthcare because trust is vital to an organization's success; it is the foundation of teamwork. An excellent example of trust established between leaders and staff is found in a shared governance model. Shared governance creates a framework for a healthy work environment that allows nurses and other healthcare providers to embark on serious organization-wide procedural change and for all the right reasons. A shared governance organization encourages and supports evidence-based suggestions for improvement and supports change. Read more about Tim Porter O'Grady's shared governance model here: https://www.nursetogether.com/shared-governance-what-exactly-it.
- **Respect:** This is the final leg of the teamwork table. It does not have to be present for teamwork to exist, but it does have to be present for proactive teamwork to exist. Respect is a noun, which means it is a *thing.* It is a feeling or an emotion. Respect is how a person feels about others and how others feel about them. The actions a nurse takes on a daily basis can show respect. The responses a nurse exhibits can show respect. The support a nurse gives can show respect. Not showing respect is most often an act of omission, a passive-aggressive display of disapproval of another person's

> character, or is exhibited by what they do or do not value. Finally, respect is just common human decency. Respect is displaying proper manners, exuding kindness, and recognizing equality. Together, healthcare providers can build alliances among diverse groups of people who have the potential to achieve amazing things. Nursing is at the core of this positive progression.

In addition, collaboration is part of nurses' standard of professional practice and is synonymous for *cooperation*. Ideally, collaboration does not mean *not* standing up when necessary, compromising ethical standards, or skirting evidence-based practice. Cooperation is also not being a "yes-man" but rather asking the question "why."

## REMOVING BARRIERS TO IMPROVE TEAMWORK

As previously noted, the opposite of trust is fear, and teamwork is built on a foundation of trust. It is perfectly acceptable to view trust as an iterative process, waxing and waning at different times. Teammates need to know what to generally expect from each other; time in a specific environment and consistent experience with others contribute to the development of trust. Teamwork is built on trust, and trust is built on transparent communication. Inconsistency in performance creates distrust and the feeling of never knowing what to expect.

Healthcare leaders need to advocate and support healthy work environments that exude transparency, open communication, teamwork, and effective collaboration. Proactive planning in care design for optimal teamwork is critical to organizational success and patient safety. A culture of questioning should be the norm. Any time you face an uncertain situation or unfamiliar order or task, ask questions. An important role for caregivers is to advocate for a patient. Asking questions is core to patient advocacy. A safe environment embraces inquiry, active collaboration, and teamwork and facilitates learning. When a nurse or other healthcare provider does not ask necessary questions, it may be a symptom of a bigger organizational or cultural problem.

The culture of an organization is directed by the leadership, whether they intend to direct it or not (Martin, 2006). Cultural anomalies, challenges, and barriers are commonly found in most organizations. Barriers can be invisible to others and can be "covert," such as seat selection or preference in a meeting, what to do while a medical provider is making rounds, or where to sit at the nursing station. Cultural norms can be deeply embedded where everyone knows the unwritten rules (except if you are new to the team); some behaviors may be overt in exuding power and authority to undermine collaboration and teamwork. Behaviors opposed to building effective alliances or teamwork can also be found in organizations, such as bullying and lateral violence. Both silence individuals and groups; neither should be tolerated by leadership in nursing and healthcare. The culture should be transparent and solely patient-focused. Disruptive behavior has the ability to impact patient care by impacting optimal teamwork.

Why might you be afraid to ask a question? Rohde (2015, p. 3) supports problem-solving in high reliability organizations and spoke about the need to review organizational problems and sort the "what" of a problem from the "why" of a problem. Only when we understand "why" problems occur can we fix them. Otherwise, we cannot fix "what" might be the problem. Nurses and other healthcare team members must feel comfortable asking the right questions. One responsibility Nance (2008) noted of highly reliable organizations is that they create environments that are safe places to ask questions. Asking a question should never be an obstacle; it should be an expectation.

Healthcare needs to globally adopt a helping culture and exude a service orientation. Organizations that simply get by and practice mediocre service will be a thing of the past. Consumers of healthcare have become purchase-savvy. Technology has enabled patients to access information, engage with their providers, and make educated decisions about where they will receive the best care.

Good practices build trust and trustworthy organizations; just as organizations build trust, so must all healthcare providers. Nurses must commit to being consistent in delivering quality communications to provide valid, important information that allows other teammates to do their best work. Consistency with effective communication makes nurses trustworthy; trust builds teams and forges alliances.

## MAXIMIZING RESOURCES TO CREATE CHANGE

*"When change comes up against culture, culture always wins."*

–Author unknown

Culture change is hard work and requires a change in thinking. Organizations must start by assessing the possibilities and then drive change to maximize resources. One of the most commonly used change theories is Lewin's theory of change. It speaks of unfreezing, changing, and refreezing, and it can aptly be applied to most any situation.

Lewin's (1948) change strategies follow a three-step process that is familiar to most people. It has been popular since the late 1940s and early 1950s. The steps are as follows:

- **Unfreezing:** Lewin stated that for change to occur, the current equilibrium must change. Lewin calls this process *unfreezing.* It is a time for building trust and helping everyone recognize the need for change. Lewin refers to a need for thawing attitudes and using the thaw or unfreezing time to identify problems (the "whys"). Then, engaging in creative problem-solving comes easier to develop solutions or fixes for the problem.
- **Changing:** The second phase of Lewin's change theory is about *moving.* This is a simple yet clear directive. Moving tells the change agent exactly what to do. Move and make the change! This can mean

a multitude of different things to different people. As a nurse working to improve teamwork, it may mean move out of your comfort zone and open up your world to include the team around you. Start slowly by adding other nurses to your team and let teamwork develop around you to get through the day. Then, begin to engage other disciplines and build interdepartmental teamwork.

- **Refreezing:** The last phase of Lewin's change theory is the predictable yet surprising—*refreeze.* It is amazing to think that we might want to freeze anything in this world of fast-moving change. It seems that we might require a more "stay on your toes" final phase, knowing that change will most likely be required again. However, refreezing is a necessary step because it is the follow-through; it is required for the change to stick. Process changes frequently require policy changes and follow-up audits to evaluate the success of the change (Sullivan & Decker, 2001).

And don't we know it in healthcare! Think of the continuous stream of regulatory changes that must be accommodated in any healthcare organization. It's not a question of *if,* but *when.* The *why* is often determined by "outsiders" and imposed (e.g., changing quality metrics, pay for performance, patient satisfaction measures).

Leaders can use Lewin's theory to assist with organizational change, while nurses and other care providers use it to design and implement local change within the immediate work environment. Peer-led change (started by one brave person) can become a change largely recognized by and adapted in a unit, department, or beyond. When successful, it can be easily spread among peers or be replicated in other areas. Think of all of the workarounds staff develop to get things done. As long as they don't violate any standards of practice or general policy and are communicated at large—this can become a good thing. Staff need to be allowed to innovate and make decisions at the point of care for the right reasons. This type of communication and change has the potential to go viral in an organization, especially when it is led by the people, for the people. Leadership's role is to foster and support innovation, which can lead to improved patient care, improved efficiency, and cost savings.

## DRIVING VERSUS RESTRAINING FORCES

Lewin is known for a "change concept," which he calls a *driving force.* Driving forces are those that push us in a direction that encourages or facilitates change. A nurse or other healthcare provider seeking to make improvements in their practice strives to achieve change, and this can be viewed as a driving force. Outcomes-focused payment reform is a driving force. When organizations and providers no longer receive financial reimbursement because patient outcomes are not reaching the acceptable quality thresholds, a driving force exists.

Money is often the most stimulating driving force individuals or an organization can use to push change forward. This strategy works particularly well when engaging an organization's leadership and medical providers for behavioral change. When trying to instill change among peers, a driving force can be the biggest complaint existing in real time in a unit. This could be something as broad as "we never have enough staff" or "we don't have the correct supply." Change management is a shared responsibility between all members of the team. Informal leaders can influence change both with their peers and others to positively impact change. Nursing and healthcare are dynamic professions that require ongoing evaluation of clinical practice and support from systems and structures.

Nurses can be a driving force by thinking back to the engrained nursing process and asking the right questions about "why." Answering questions about "why" and "what are the causative factors" will provide evidence to drive conclusions. The answers to these questions provide clarity about processes that might need focused attention. Identifying a work process or project that requires change is an excellent opportunity for a team to begin to relate to each other as they work through the issue. Identifying potential solutions, performing controlled experiments, and navigating the change process together builds goodwill among team members. Learn more about using "The 5 Whys" for problem-solving, root cause analysis, and developing countermeasures for problems here: https://www.mindtools.com/pages/article/newTMC_5W.htm.

*Restraining forces* are those that counter the driving forces (Kritsonis, 2018). Dr. Cardiologist and his reluctance to allow nursing involvement in the quality monitoring process would be a restraining force. Anytime there is barrier to the progress of change, there is a restraining force. Leadership can indirectly promote restraining forces rather than driving forces when they utilize authoritarian or autocratic leadership styles. These styles of leadership are often intended to be very positive as the leaders work toward providing clear directives and ensuring everyone understands the objectives.

Unfortunately, when the style of leadership is not adjusted (situational leadership) based on group feedback, autocratic or authoritarian styles can be viewed as negative. Creativity, group dynamics, and group influence are often rejected, and employees begin to feel that their input or opinions are without worth. Thus, employees quickly stop driving forward and begin to revert to the status quo. This reversion to reflect and "complete the task list, clock out as soon as possible" attitude of work ethic is detrimental to organizational culture.

Visionary, coaching, and transformational leadership styles tend to encourage nurses and other care providers to rise to a high-level practice for participation in process change and improvement. Participatory and inspirational leadership is necessary for true, impactful change; it is the essence of teamwork. There is no substitute for the power of one—change can start anywhere, and all healthcare providers need to think of themselves as a leader. It is important for nursing and all healthcare professions to embrace change and embark on a journey of excellence because healthcare is rapidly changing.

*Equilibrium* exists when driving forces become equal with restraining forces and no change occurs (Kritsonis, 2018). Dr. Cardiologist stopping the nurse in her tracks and deterring her continued monitoring of records for potential errors had the potential to create equilibrium, with no change at all. Many nurses complain about always having to start something new at work. Often, they start something new, and within a few weeks or months revert back to the old way of doing things without ever having achieved what the change was intended to achieve. Sustainability for change is always difficult, takes focus and hard work, and needs constant review and monitoring. It is nearly always worth the effort.

## PRACTICE PEARLS

- Learn to use the concepts of change to facilitate positive cultural change: driving forces, restraining forces, and equilibrium.
- Become a disruptor to the status quo!
- Help others and begin to seek their support in return.
- Be grateful.
- Be participatory.

## THE CHANGE PROCESS

It is not unheard of to strongly believe in something and have complete buy-in of the need for change but not be able to achieve the change. Weight loss is a perfect example. Many attempt it, but it is difficult to sustain behavior, assess accurate metabolism, and make major lifestyle changes. Most everyone understands the basic concepts of how to lose weight, but they cannot lose the weight or keep it off. Weight loss is complicated. It requires a great deal of focus, experimentation, measurement, and constant work to just keep at it. It also requires preparation and planning, some analysis, and dedication to making the necessary changes. It usually is a much longer versus a shorter process. Similarly, sometimes change does not succeed because the circumstances necessary to achieve the desired change are simply not present.

Organizational change can be the same way. A healthcare entity can have the best participative leadership, best-paying patients, kind providers, easiest electronic medical record system, and a great spirit of teamwork. However, if all the nurses or other healthcare providers were educated at the same school and they have not been taught proper practice, clinical outcomes might suffer. Although this is an extreme example, which would most likely never occur, it does make the point. Nurses and other clinicians can sometimes be their own worst enemies. It takes great leadership to create a culture of open and honest transparency, encouraging participation in problem identification and resolution to promote positive change.

Generally, nurses and other healthcare providers are smart people, and once they understand the need for change, they almost always are willing to participate in the change. An organization's culture defines its *true* relationship with those who choose to work there, especially during the change process. Culture includes behavior on display from stated guidelines and employee engagement. The results of any change process can be influenced by engagement. Leadership support is needed for employees to believe there is an open and honest environment to bring innovative ideas for improving systems that can lead to better patient care.

## MOVING BEYOND JUST GOOD

In the bestselling book *Good to Great* (2001), Jim Collins explained why good is the enemy of great. Organizations that are built for excellence typically achieve it. Organizations that are good, even really good, at what they do can rarely reach greatness. Greatness requires a conscious decision by brave leaders to move forward, where merely good organizations are satisfied with the current status. Often, greatness comes from the work of just a few. While it may be amazing to work for a great organization, nurses have the power to influence the ability to become a great unit inside of a good organization.

Good teamwork can decrease communication frustration and enhance the patient-care experience for everyone while increasing the efficiency and efficacy of provided care. Finally, be sure to include the patient in decision-making. As with any major objective, improving patient outcomes requires buy-in from the person whose outcome is being measured. In this case, it happens to be the patient.

## ENSURING A CULTURE OF SAFETY

When times get tough, healthcare leaders and the entire team need to be able to openly discuss mistakes. Not to do so is often the first seed that might erode a positive team or culture. Holding in or onto feelings of resentment or enmity might stew (on any side of conflict), is unhealthy, and unfair when attempting to provide a culture of excellence. In the event you find yourself in such a circumstance, use your available resources: your immediate supervisor or another leader, an organizational development ally, human resources personnel, or another trusted liaison to help mediate conflict and find resolution.

Leaders can help with this by assessing team dynamics: How well do the shifts communicate with each other? Is there a particular provider everyone wants to avoid? Do staff desire to work one weekend over another related to their peers scheduled on that weekend? Are there team members who are isolated by others during a shift?

As we've stated earlier, the nursing profession and providing healthcare is a team sport. Paying attention to the dynamics, getting ahead of problems before they amplify, and managing conflict as soon as possible can all prevent errors and unfavorable patient outcomes.

### PRACTICE PEARLS

- Never withhold information.
- Always give accurate information.

- Admit mistakes and apologize.
- Be open to feedback.
- Make decisions based on what is best for the greater good.
- Do what you say and say what you will do.
- Be honest and listen attentively.
- Pay attention to the work environment to identify and manage conflict as soon as possible. (Don't be afraid to ask for help, if needed; we're all in this together.)

---

## DISRUPTIVE INNOVATION IN HEALTHCARE

American Family Care Centers (2022) has provided primary, urgent, and occupational care for the last 40 years in a variety of locations. They noted five trends in disruptive healthcare innovation to watch:

### 1. DIRECT PRIMARY CARE

Rather than the traditional fee-for-service model based on medical insurance, consumers are choosing to be part of a practice for a monthly fee that offers 24/7 availability with a care provider. These providers have leveraged technology using patient portals for electronic health records and may use texting or electronic messaging systems for expert medical consultative access and communication with their members (patients). This model allows consumers without emergent medical conditions to bypass the usual routes for care such as urgent care centers at a much lower cost. Many of the services provided are included in the monthly membership fee.

## 2. TELECARE AND TELEHEALTH TECHNOLOGY

The COVID-19 pandemic expedited care providers shifting to other means (besides in-person appointments) to be able to communicate and care for their panel of patients. This methodology has been utilized for years in rural areas for expert consultation in larger geographic settings when specialty medical consultation was needed. It is expected that newly introduced medical devices will allow patients to monitor themselves and connect via technology with their care providers. One example is Kardiamobile (https://www.kardia.com/kardiamobile), which people can use for their own clinically validated, personal EKG monitoring. Before the pandemic, only 43% of healthcare providers used telehealth options. Since the pandemic began, adoption has shot up to 95%.

## 3. ELECTRONIC HEALTH RECORDS

Electronic health records have been an expanding part of patient care over the last couple of decades. This new data mine will be useful for leveraging research, using artificial intelligence, and facilitating new product development in the future.

## 4. ARTIFICIAL INTELLIGENCE AND MACHINE LEARNING

Artificial intelligence and machine learning are growing in healthcare with the use of predictive analytics and patient services. Using this technology for patient intake, scheduling, billing, and chatbots to answer basic questions is becoming commonplace.

## 5. TRUE PATIENT-CENTERED CARE IS THE FUTURE OF HEALTHCARE

Empowering people to take charge of their health versus being a passive recipient of healthcare is the wave of the future. Care providers are not with patients 24/7. They can make recommendations for improved health based on their expertise, but it is up to the patient to execute and monitor the plan for improved health outcomes. This includes the use of digital therapeutics, a fast-growing new electronic health specialty, where technological devices are used by consumers (patients) via evidence-based software solutions. This allows people to become actively engaged in monitoring and managing their health (think chronic conditions such as diabetes, mental health, heart disease, and more) by making changes to their current behavior and lifestyle practices.

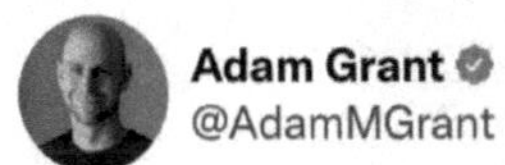


Toxic cultures define success as winning a cutthroat competition. They reward people for stabbing others in the back.

Healthy cultures define success as making a contribution. They reward people for having others' backs.

Good organizations elevate those who elevate others.

You can learn more about digital therapeutics here: https://www.mckinsey.com/industries/life-sciences/our-insights/digital-therapeutics-preparing-for-takeoff.

These are only a few examples of what the future in healthcare will bring. They are many innovations underway in professional medical devices; therapeutics; pharmaceuticals; personal health monitoring; health, wellness, and well-being initiatives; and more. The future holds exciting promise for changing the face of the current healthcare system from a "sickcare" system to one embracing health and wellness.

# CONCLUSION

Healthcare organizations of the future need to change the accepted norms in social or workplace culture. Innovation with operations will be crucial as consumer preferences change. Digital engagement is a must.

Any gathering of employees—including daily huddles, break room gatherings, social gatherings such as hospital picnics or tailgate parties, staff meetings, and leadership updates—is an important venue to communicate a new message of radical culture change. We will also have to use our creativity to engage others when in-person meetings are not feasible (as during COVID-19). As much as people loathe electronic means for meetings, they were effective. Secure texting, portals, electronic mail, and more will become commonplace to access information and to communicate.

You should grasp every opportunity to reinforce the expected behaviors (e.g., open and honest communication, respect, transparency) that promote healthy alliances, teamwork, and ultimately good care and patient safety. It has been said (although no one really knows by whom) that a person must hear something seven times to remember it. People bathed in a message of positive culture will eventually get "clean." The next chapter explores quality and safety in relation to stress, fatigue, and burnout.

# REFERENCES

American Family Care Centers. (2022). *Disruptive innovation in healthcare—5 trends to watch.* https://afcfranchising.com/blog/disruptive-innovation-in-healthcare-5-trends-to-watch/

Cole, L., & Cole, M. (2005). *People smart leaders.* Oakhill Press.

Collins, J. (2001). *Good to great.* HarperBusiness.

Dictionary.com. (2022). *Ally.* http://dictionary.reference.com/browse/ally

James, M. (1968). *Suspicious minds* [Single]. Scepter Records.

The Joint Commission. (2022). *Hospital National Patient Safety Goals.* https://www.jointcommission.org/-/media/tjc/documents/standards/national-patient-safety-goals/2022/simple_2022-hap-npsg-goals-101921.pdf

Kritsonis, A. (2018). Comparison of change theories. *International Journal of Scholarly Academic Intellectual Diversity, 8*(1) 1–7. https://globalioc.com/wp-content/uploads/2018/09/Kritsonis-Alicia-Comparison-of-Change-Theories.pdf

Lewin, K. (1948). *Resolving social conflicts: Selected papers on group dynamics.* Gertrude W. Lewis (Ed.). Harper & Row.

Martin, M. J. (2006, Spring). "That's the way we do things around here": An overview of organizational culture. *Electronic Journal of Academic and Special Librarianship,* 7(1). https://southernlibrarianship.icaap.org/content/v07n01/martin_m01.htm

Nance, J. (2008). *Why hospitals should fly: The ultimate flight plan to patient safety and quality care.* Second River Healthcare Press.

O'Sullivan, A., Barcott, J., Bonalumi, N., Collins, S., Darling, L., Davis, G., & Diamond Zolnierek, C. (2010). Standards of professional performance. *Scope and standards of practice: Nursing* (2nd ed., p. 57). Nursesbooks.org.

Rohde, K. (2015, April 10). *Occurrence reporting: Building a robust problem identification and resolution process.* Arkansas Patient Safety Conference. Lecture conducted at the Arkansas Organization of Nurse Executives (AONE) and Arkansas Association for Healthcare Quality (AAHQ), Little Rock, Arkansas.

Schindler, E. (2014, May 23). *Building alliances at work—Getting help before you need it.* https://schindler301.rssing.com/chan-25199534/article11.html

Sullivan, E. J., & Decker, P. J. (2001). *Initiating and managing change.* In E. J. Sullivan, P. J. Decker, & Jamerson (Eds.), *Effective leadership and management in nursing* (p. 250). Prentice Hall.

# 9

# PLANNING INTENTIONAL QUALITY AND SAFETY

## OBJECTIVES

- Consider how intentionality affects workplace decisions and stress.
- Consider how to manage patient risk.
- Explore reliability science.
- Understand the role of nurses and other healthcare providers in intentional quality and safety.
- Explore how to influence state and national policy.

# WHAT IS INTENTIONALITY?

Our first experiences with intentionality are typically in school. Although our parents intentionally feed us, care for us, and play with us for bonding purposes, there is very little agenda-driven interaction to guide the encounters. When we get to school, things are different. Most likely, this is one of the first places we learn about the consequences of feeling stress.

There might be a test to pass at the end of the week, and we have to learn primary colors, count to 10, and be completely bathroom-independent in order to advance from preschool to kindergarten. Epstein (2007) speaks about the importance of intentional teaching, which does not happen by chance. It is *planful* (full of plans), thoughtful, and purposeful. Intentional teachers use their knowledge, judgment, and expertise to organize learning experiences for children. When an unexpected situation arises (as it always does), these teachers can recognize a teaching opportunity and are able to take advantage of it.

Being an intentional teacher requires a wide range of knowledge and a recognition that learning occurs sometimes from adult-guided experiences and other times from child-guided experiences (Epstein, 2007). Epstein (2007) lists the characteristics of an intentional teacher: having high expectations, planning and managing, valuing a learning-oriented classroom, offering engaging activities, posing thoughtful questions, and providing feedback. Choosing a career in nursing and the healthcare industry allows practitioners to experience each of these characteristics as learners in the field and then subsequently as care providers and teachers.

As adults, most of our learning comes from life experiences. Any formal education we receive is often hand-selected to meet the intentional career or vocational plan we have for our lives. The word *intentional* is much like the word *purposeful*. In the best-selling book *The Purpose Driven Life*, Rick Warren notes that what we pay attention to in our lives flourishes. If we nurture sadness by refusing to leave the house or rejoin society after the death of a spouse, we might spiral into a deep depression. If, on the other hand, we nurture friendships that offer support after the death of a spouse, we build stronger relationships and process grief more effectively (Warren, 2002).

Lifelong and intentional learning are key to a healthcare professional's practice. Dr. Carol Dweck (2016) describes two mindsets: a growth mindset and a fixed mindset. A person with a growth mindset knows they can change over time using introspection to learn from life experience and challenges. Taking calculated risks and failure is less threatening with this mindset. The person with a growth mindset accepts and uses experiences and life challenges as learning opportunities. A person with a fixed mindset has difficulty working through their life experiences or challenges because they perceive their ability to make changes as futile.

Success in life's various elements, whether career, family, faith, physical, or emotional health, is rarely incidental. Success most often comes from intentional planning and thoughtful attention to detail. Nurses, as well as other care providers, must have intentional focus when it comes to providing care for patients. Healthcare providers naturally and intentionally strive for high-quality and optimal safety to help patients achieve the best clinical outcomes. To be intentional is to be purposeful, focused, and determined. Healthcare providers who are unable to focus and prioritize will struggle with higher levels of stress throughout their careers. Healthcare is a fast-paced and changing industry. It often requires rapid-fire decision-making with limited information. Knowledge of a multitude of subjects—science, math, technology, medicine, and more—are necessary to prepare for the challenging work environments of today. A self-actualized provider continues to learn and grow as they progress in their career journey.

Much like learning an instrument, you must practice a little bit every day to retain enough information to be able to advance the selected skill (Warren, 2002). Nursing and healthcare are careers with many opportunities for practice, learning, and growth. You can change specialties, learn new skills, practice in a variety of work environments, and receive formal advanced education. Being bored or unchallenged is certainly not an excuse for burnout in nursing or healthcare; opportunity to advance in the healthcare professions is abundant for those who are willing to stretch themselves.

Hospitals and healthcare organizations that achieve national renown for stellar outcomes in quality and safety are organizations that place intentional focus on those elements, as evidenced by their efficient systems and organizational design:

> In an interview with the chief nursing officer of Saint Joseph Hospital West in Lake Saint Louis, Missouri, she was asked, "How does your organization achieve a 'Truven Top 100 Hospital' ranking so consistently?"
>
> She simply replied, "We did not even know we were on the radar for recognition. We simply work to ensure quality and safety are the best that they can possibly be." (J. Pestle, personal communication, January 1, 2014)

This is an excellent example of intentional focus for the right reason. St. Joseph Hospital West was not only successful in meeting the objective they set out to achieve (excellent quality and safety), but it earned the hospital national recognition. Intentionality can be powerful.

## PRACTICE PEARLS

- Be intentional about learning new knowledge and skills.
- Learn to realistically prioritize short-term work to be done each day and longer-term career goals.
- Focus.

# PATIENT SAFETY, TRANSPARENCY, AND MANAGING PRACTICE RISK

Many organizations strive to attain a culture of safety. The World Health Organization (WHO, 2022) provides patient safety organization (PSO) campaign resources such as safe surgery, the safe childbirth checklist, clean your hands campaign, and so on. You can find the WHO's most recent publication about patient safety (from 2017) here: https://apps.who.int/iris/handle/10665/255507. The Joint Commission seeks to identify how safe an organization is by asking specifically what the facility does to promote patient safety. State hospital associations have devised patient safety organizational programs that are open to hospital participation. Nurses and other healthcare providers need to be aware of the variety of national and regional quality and safety programs. Healthcare organizations are expected to make the environment as safe as possible. This also includes those providing care. Because nurses are the vast majority of healthcare providers in most organizations, nurses must clearly understand and apply quality and safety concepts in their daily work. Applying this type of concept to our work environment is done through policy, standardized protocols, and efficient work processes; these create a structure to guide care to ensure reliability in patient outcomes.

The era of focus on safety in healthcare began in 1999 with the Institute of Medicine (IOM) report titled "To Err Is Human." Revealing details about operations and the business of healthcare not putting patient safety first or as a top priority were included. Per the 1999 report, medical errors caused between 44,000 to 98,000 deaths in hospitals each year. Deaths from medical errors are those defined as "could have been prevented" (Kohn et al., 2000, p. 1). With the national release of this information, healthcare providers have been vigilant to promote—with clear intention—the prevention of medical errors.

Rodziewicz et al. (2022) concluded that medical errors are a major cause of death and a serious public health concern. They believe part of the solution to reduce medical errors is to maintain a culture that works toward recognizing safety challenges and implementing viable solutions rather than harboring a culture of blame, shame, and punishment. A true culture of safety that focuses on system improvement is imperative for all types of healthcare organizations.

> Health care professionals experience profound psychological effects such as anger, guilt, inadequacy, depression, and suicide due to real or perceived errors. The threat of impending legal action may compound these feelings. This can also lead to a loss of clinical confidence. Clinicians equate errors with failure, with a breach of public trust, and with harming patients despite their mandate to 'first do no harm.' (Rodziewicz et al., 2022)

## INTENTIONAL PLANS AND CHECKLISTS

In an exposé comparing healthcare to aviation, John Nance (a former pilot and attorney) explained why hospitals should fly. The ultimate flight plan must include intentional systems designed to prevent error at all costs (Nance, 2008). A patient-safety orientation and quality care delivery program must have precise elements for safe practice. In aviation, Nance described how checklist protocols are applied to standard work processes. The same philosophy could be applied to the variation existing in current healthcare systems. Step-by-step processes or protocols decrease the need to memorize or recall every step of a process in an emergent situation. Having to remember a great deal of information at a moment's notice can in itself be very stressful, and checklists can relieve that stress.

A physician used the comparison of the idea of being "near perfect" in comparing those in healthcare to a professional baseball player. Baseball players with a batting average of .300 or higher are highly sought after. Batting average is determined by dividing *hits* by *at bats*, and Major League Baseball

(MLB) cites .250 as the average for all those playing in the league (MLB Advanced Media, 2022). Those who work in healthcare are expected to have a batting average of 1000, which means that they would always get a hit and never make an error. Is this realistic? We can use systems that assist us in being as "error-proof" as possible, but they must be designed this way. We also need to remember that we are not infallible as people and must learn to lean on reliable resources in care delivery.

Although PSOs are often organizations coveted by non PSO-hospitals across the nation, nurses in those facilities can identify with significant pressure for near-perfect performance. The implication that an organization has achieved a foolproof system (to prevent errors) can lead nurses to fear reporting errors that do occur. Fear of punishment or retribution makes all healthcare providers wary of reporting errors. However, nurses and other healthcare providers must remain vigilant because rarely is any process completely foolproof. The potential for human error cannot be completely eliminated. Being honest about error reporting helps prevent future errors.

## PRACTICE PEARLS

- Never rely on memory alone, and don't bother to memorize what you can look up.
- Use "tip sheets," pocket-size knowledge booklets, and checklists when possible.
- Patient safety is everyone's job: Be honest and transparent.
- Be intentional about the care you provide; it should be safe and of high quality.

---

These key strategies are basic to achieving a healthcare entity embedded with a culture of patient safety. "Back to basics" is a saying often used when something goes awry. To solve problems in healthcare, it is imperative to start with the beginning of a process and look at each step along the way for relevance and accuracy (root cause analysis). Historically, changes have been applied to current practices or processes without taking the time to break down what currently exists, what needs to change, and what is the best approach to achieving the desired result. The American Society for Quality (ASQ, 2022, para. 1) describes *root cause analysis* as:

> A factor that caused a nonconformance and should be permanently eliminated through process improvement. The root cause is the core issue—the highest-level cause—that sets in motion the entire cause-and-effect reaction that ultimately leads to the problem(s). Root cause analysis (RCA) is defined as a collective term that describes a wide range of approaches, tools, and techniques used to uncover causes of problems. Some RCA approaches are geared more toward identifying true root causes than others, some are more general problem-solving techniques, and others simply offer support for the core activity of root cause analysis.

Patient safety organizations frequently utilize the skills of consultants or employees trained in Six Sigma, Lean, or a combination of process-improvement strategies. Root cause analysis is one of these types of improvement methodologies. These specialized skills are an ideal match for organizations that want to improve their safety culture. Participation in process-improvement initiatives is a good way for nurses and others to learn additional problem-solving methodologies that can aptly be applied to a number of different kinds of problems.

These tools serve to help healthcare organizations to continuously improve on their core competency: to provide the safest, highest-quality patient care known at the time. This is likely the reason most of us went into the healing arts in the first place. Measurement of whether or not nurses, providers, and others are reaching the goals they set varies; more and more organizations are subscribing to one framework or another, to measure and in some cases be rewarded for improving or achieving benchmark performance. These results may be publicly available in your organization in a balanced scorecard or improvement dashboard format.

Some of the more common frameworks seen in the healthcare industry or to be seen in the near future include Magnet® designation, the Malcolm-Baldridge criteria, and the Shingo Model. Organizations use these methodologies to set priorities, as well as focus energy and resources to strengthen operations. They also ensure employees and other stakeholders are working toward common goals by establishing agreement around intended outcomes or results. This allows continual assessment and adjustment for the organization's overall direction in response to a changing environment.

## MAGNET

Magnet designation is the ultimate credential for high-quality nursing, and yet as of October 2022, only 9.86% of hospitals are designated as Magnet facilities, according to the American Nurses Association (ANA Enterprise, n.d.). Developed and administered by the American Nurses Credentialing Center (ANCC), Magnet is considered by many to be the leading identifier of successful nursing practices and strategies worldwide (ANCC, n.d.-a). Magnet hospitals report higher percentages of satisfied registered nurses (RNs), lower RN turnover and vacancy, improved clinical outcomes, and improved patient satisfaction (ANCC, n.d.-b).

Originally conceived in 1983, the framework consists of 14 forces of magnetism, more recently simplified into five model components (ANA, 2017):

I. Transformational Leadership

II. Structural Empowerment

III. Exemplary Professional Practice

IV. New Knowledge, Innovation, & Improvement

V. Empirical Quality Results

## MALCOLM BALDRIGE CRITERIA FOR PERFORMANCE EXCELLENCE

The Baldrige performance excellence criteria is a framework made up of seven categories (ASQ, 2022):

1. **Leadership:** How upper management leads the organization and how the organization leads within the community
2. **Strategy:** How the organization establishes and plans to implement strategic directions
3. **Customers:** How the organization builds and maintains strong, lasting relationships with customers
4. **Measurement, analysis, and knowledge management:** How the organization uses data to support key processes and manage performance
5. **Workforce:** How the organization empowers and involves its workforce
6. **Operations:** How the organization designs, manages, and improves key processes
7. **Results:** How the organization performs in terms of customer satisfaction, finances, human resources, supplier and partner performance, operations, governance and social responsibility, and comparison to its competitors

The intention behind the Baldrige framework is to provide a holistic assessment of an organization from goal setting to strategic plan development to performance tracking and improvement, and how an organization responds to both internal and external forces. Organizations are able to apply for the Baldrige Award and are judged by an independent board of examiners.

## SHINGO MODEL

A final framework that is gaining popularity in the healthcare sector, at least on the West Coast, is the Shingo model. Marketed as a new way of thinking, it endeavors to build a sustainable culture of organizational excellence through cohesive and aligned culture, principles, systems, and tools, all in the relentless pursuit of excellent performance. You can see the Shingo model here: https://shingo.org/shingo-model/.

Relatively few healthcare organizations have achieved a level of recognition from Shingo. However, with the focus on culture linked to the use of data and outcomes, it is likely we will see more organizations using this framework in the future. This may become especially important as more and more healthcare institutions are on the brink of financial disaster after the global COVID-19 pandemic.

## WHY ARE THESE IMPORTANT TO NURSING AND HEALTHCARE?

The answer is simply that *mood follows action*. While it's nearly impossible to control your thoughts and feelings, it is possible to control your behavior in response (Stulberg, 2017). Times of chaos, times of repetition, and times where we see opportunities for change are actually times for us to embrace our voice and participate in change efforts that we may find inconvenient, overwhelming, unnecessary, etc.

This lesson comes from a delightful short book, *Too Soon Old, Too Late Smart,* written by a retired psychiatrist. In it he writes,

> We are always talking about what we want, what we intend. These are dreams and wishes and are of little value in changing our mood. We are not what we think, or what we say, or how we feel. *We are what we do.* (Livingston, 2009, p. 7)

To listen to the negative voices around us and in the media facilitates hopelessness in times of despair. It can be magnetic and pull us further into being a victim of stress, fatigue, and burnout. We have the potential to become listless and depressed. We must challenge ourselves to find ways of reconnecting to passion and purpose for the professional care we provide, encompassing the outcomes our organizations strive to achieve and creating more honest platforms for difficult conversations. We must embrace the lessons learned from engagement with frontline providers.

## PRACTICE PEARLS

- Consider why you made a decision to enter healthcare or the healing arts field. Think about how your purpose drives practice and the intended outcomes.
- Are your passion, purpose, and outcomes aligned with the organization you serve?
- Compare your performance with others (benchmarking). This can be personal, professional, or organizational.
- Learn about the framework or tools your organization uses to measure and improve operational performance. Why are the chosen tools used?
- Find ways to get involved in practice and performance decisions. This can be with a small improvement initiative within your own unit/department/division or on a larger level (local, regional, state, or national).

- Being informed, engaged, and involved can help feed your *wellpower* by decreasing the feelings of despair that may come from messages we hear day-to-day.

---

# THE HEALTHCARE PROVIDER'S ROLE IN SAFER AND HIGHER-QUALITY SYSTEMS

How do nurses, other healthcare providers, and organizations ensure high-quality and safe patient care? Technology can be utilized for building safer systems. Most healthcare facilities now have an electronic health record (EHR). Checklists and standardized protocols can be embedded into the EHR for more consistent decision-making and to reduce practice variation. They also make the plethora of clinical data much easier to evaluate on a larger scale.

Before a procedure begins, a series of questions are discussed among the surgical team. The information is generally entered into the medical record, which only allows the user to proceed if all safety checks and balances have been completed. This standardization has prevented many medical errors, which include wrong-site surgeries, incorrect procedures or anesthesia, and incorrect patient-procedure matches. Following this type of checklist can be simple and it is important; following it step-by-step every time ensures a more predictable and safer outcome. Since implementation in the surgical arena, this methodology has also been adopted in other areas where invasive patient care procedures are conducted. The nurse's role to advocate for the patient is demonstrated in the time-out process.

Each person who is involved in the delivery of healthcare must understand their role in patient safety; no position should be exempt. Many organizations conduct daily safety meetings, either in person or via technology. This approach communicates the importance of patient safety and leader responsibility; it also ensures accountability as departments or disciplines are required to report their status. This also raises awareness for all departments of the challenges other areas experience and focuses the leadership on solutions for existing problems and prevention of potential problems. Because healthcare organizations are not silos, each department/discipline influences the functions of others. Examples include patients waiting in the emergency department for placement on an inpatient unit; surgical procedures that may be delayed due to a lack of operating room equipment or supply; patients awaiting discharge but needing a ride; the number of indwelling catheters, surgical site infections, patients in restraints, or patients who fell in the last 24 hours. This pertinent clinical or operational information can all help the organization and its leaders predict and plan the day.

Safety is everyone's job. If we notice breaks in protocol, such as a lack of handwashing, not labeling specimens in the presence of a patient, or an incomplete timeout, healthcare providers need to be able to speak up. If protocol is not followed in the cleaning of a room, it may impact the patient outcome. Each person needs to understand the importance of and their responsibility for patient safety and needs to feel empowered to speak up. For example, a surgeon seen wearing a surgical gown in the hallway outside of the surgery department should be reminded to remove the gown. If a coworker does not wash their hands per protocol, it should be brought to their attention. Cultures that support safety also support civility where all staff are seen as *equal* team members regardless of rank, position, or tenure.

## SYSTEMS THEORY IN HEALTHCARE PREDICTABILITY

When we hear about a patient safety event, the first thought for some people is, "What happened?" or "What did the provider do wrong?" rather than, "What steps in the system or process failed?" Today, fortunately more healthcare entities are moving away from immediately blaming the last person who cared for the patient to an approach that looks at the steps in a system that failed to protect the patient. The "To Err Is Human" publication called for healthcare to use a system engineering approach and principles to prevent and solve patient safety problems (Kohn et al., 2000).

Dr. James Reason's Swiss cheese model (Reason, 2000) is an excellent example of an approach that evaluates the steps in a complex system that have a likelihood of failing. Using Reason's Swiss cheese example, patient safety issues are prevented by placing barriers to block harm before it reaches the patient. Each slice of cheese represents a type of barrier such as policies and procedures, staff competency, equipment, safety culture, etc. When the holes in the Swiss cheese line up, the barrier to protect the patient can then go through the hole to reach the patient and cause harm. The systems approach to addressing patient safety events focuses on identifying "holes" where the barrier could or has failed and is a contributing factor to the event.

The Swiss cheese approach can be used to address an example safety event where staff did not hear the audible alarms that are intended to notify them of the patient's worsening heart rate and blood pressure. Following the safety event, the investigation identified that the hospital inpatient beds were full, so the patient was admitted and placed into a room used to perform dialysis. The room was built with the intention of the dialysis nurses always remaining in the room with the patient. Thus, the alarms for the monitoring equipment were never checked to determine if they could be heard in the hallway when the door was closed. In addition, the monitoring equipment alarms were never connected to the nurses' station to alert staff of low or high blood pressure or heart rate. The hole in the Swiss cheese related to technology lined up with the hole for policies that guide staff to where they can place patients for treatment when the regular patient rooms are full and the hole for the hospital to proactively determine that alarms can be heard when the door is closed, regardless of whether the room is used for dialysis.

Responsibility and accountability for safe care are fundamental for all healthcare providers. Each has a duty to proactively identify failures in the systems we use each day to treat patients. Nurses are often the first line of defending the patient from harm. By looking at the steps in the system that are weak or vulnerable, actions can be implemented to prevent safety events.

A culture of safety in healthcare is *still* evolving. Most institutions are experiencing significant change, especially since the untenable challenges of the global COVID-19 pandemic. The good news is, the forward progression for a culture of improved quality and higher system reliability has not been deterred. Transparency for doing the right things right is becoming the norm—not changing systems or practice solely due to regulatory requirements or intervention. In an organization that is truly encompassing patient safety, everyone knows that everyone else is and will be responsible for achieving a unified goal—safety.

Patient safety is also a primary focus of the US government relative to healthcare. As a result, systems such as Veterans Affairs have made necessary changes to access and care. A national news release in April 2014 (Bronstein & Griffin) revealed at least 40 veterans died while waiting for appointments. Alleged secret lists of patients waiting to be seen were not entered into the computerized scheduling system. Subsequently, the patients never received provider appointments. In addition, no official records existed to indicate a delay in care. Clearly, equal responsibility for patient safety was not infused nor adopted throughout the organization. Transparency was not valued; all realms of the organization, including the operators and receptionists, were not empowered or held accountable to ensure quality and safety were paramount. And unfortunately, organizational support to reduce medical errors may compete with other priorities and resource allocation (Keepnews & Mitchell, 2003).

The Agency for Healthcare Research and Quality (AHRQ, a federally funded US government program) has a number of resources to assist care providers and organizations in improving their quality and safety systems, which can be found here: https://www.ahrq.gov/patient-safety/index.html.

The American Nurses Association's Code of Ethics holds the nurse accountable for their nursing practice, which includes making decisions to provide optimal care. The latest version can be found here: https://www.nursingworld.org/practice-policy/nursing-excellence/ethics/code-of-ethics-for-nurses.

## MANAGE THE PATIENT HANDOFF

An additional area of practice risk is the patient handoff process. It is a very important element of patient care designed to deliver intimate details of a patient's situation and care requirements and to drive communication between caregivers. Patient care may transition from one provider to another in a variety of situations. Typical handoffs include receptionists, clerical personnel, nurses, medical providers, diagnostic personnel such as laboratory and radiology, and consultative personnel such as a dietitian or a specialist of another discipline. Handoffs may occur either inside an organization or outside to other clinics or facilities. It is incredibly important that handoffs be standardized, pertinent to individual patient needs, and include safety and quality concerns relevant to their care. The use of SBAR (situation, background, assessment, recommendation) in patient handoffs provides a standardized tool that helps to ensure pertinent information is shared. You can learn more about SBAR here from ASQ: https://asq.org/quality-resources/sbar.

### PRACTICE PEARLS

- Be transparent.
- Follow organizational policy.
- Use unique patient identifiers and include the patient in handoffs.
- Share information the next provider needs to know.

## BEDSIDE REPORTING

Nursing report is a type of handoff or communication process that has historically been in place between nurses. Other clinical care providers use a similar process. When viewing old movies with hospital scenes, medical records are often seen hanging on the footboard of the hospital bed; this promoted bedside conversations about care and report from nurse to nurse. Since that time, a variety of options for more confidential nurse reporting has evolved, whether in person, by audiotape, or in writing. More recently, report has changed location (moved back to the bedside), includes the patient, and puts information on a whiteboard in the patient room (much like the old movies). Including the patient in the handoff can be a valuable process for them to learn about their care, understand what the care plan is, know their role in the plan, and make personal introductions between caregivers.

Publications outlining the specific benefits of bedside reporting have been prevalent since the early 1980s. In 1995, Minick published a qualitative study identifying bedside report as a means for critical care nurses to identity potential problems earlier in the care of the patient. Bedside report also resulted in what Minick (1995) deemed "making a connection" with the patient when patients are included in the process.

The Joint Commission published Sentinel Event Alert 58 in 2017, which relates to inadequate handoff communication. It promotes the support needed for effective handoff communication between caregivers. Poor transitions from one nurse or care provider to the next (accepting the patient's care transition) have shown a relationship to medical errors. Too often the handoff falters, and pertinent details specific to the patient's care are not well-communicated to the receiving provider. Conversely, effective handoffs support a formalized transition of care from one nurse or care provider to the next. Implementing bedside reports in an organization that has utilized alternative methods can be quite challenging. It requires a different type of thinking from nurses and new skills in communication. Nurses who have not experienced this style of open communication with patients and family members may be unsure of themselves, uneasy with the honest dialogue, and fearful of potential questions. There is no definitive conclusion as to why resistance to bedside reporting exists, but it does (AHRQ, 2015). The AHRQ has a number of tools for caregivers related to beside reporting you can find here: https://search.ahrq.gov/search?q=bedside+report.

Challenges for nurses to overcome when using bedside report include how to deal with sensitive information in front of a patient, potential violations of confidentiality and privacy, fearing change, and not wanting to disturb the patient (AHRQ, 2015). Changing the process for nurse reporting can be complex. It is very important for nurses and nursing leadership to be jointly involved in planning the change process. The end product must ensure delivery of pertinent information and allow time for quality conversations. Measurement milestones to follow up and evaluate the new process are necessary in order to achieve a successful change in reporting practices. In addition, other pertinent confidential patient information can be shared in a more private setting for a complete and accurate picture of the patient's status.

The literature is rife with studies of organizations implementing bedside report, the challenges of doing so, the processes used, and the benefits reaped. The AHRQ published an implementation handbook for bedside report in conjunction with the US Department of Health and Human Services (2015). The step-by-step guide gives clear direction for organizations to begin the implementation process and provides case studies from hospitals that have achieved successful implementation. It also summarizes the benefits of bedside shift report including improved patient satisfaction and less time required to complete the shift report. You can find the *Nurse Bedside Shift Report* at: https://www.ahrq.gov/sites/default/files/wysiwyg/professionals/systems/hospital/engagingfamilies/strategy3/Strat3_Implement_Hndbook_508.pdf.

Anderson and Mangino (2006) reported improved relationship building among nurses and improved patient satisfaction; most patients want to know more about their health status and the plan for their care. Caruso (2007) found nurses doing bedside report were frustrated with the repetition of history in front of the patient. Caruso (2007) suggested using Lewin's change theory (unfreezing-change-refreezing model) when presenting and promoting the concept of bedside report. This process allows for controlled trial and error (you can re-read or review more about it in Chapter 7). A new reporting template using only pertinent and current information (with follow-up via mentoring and accountability) worked well for a remodeled bedside report. As a result of the study, nurses continued their improvement work and designed a pre-report that reviewed the patient's history followed by a bedside report for verification of care requirements, as well as the plan for the shift or day. The revised model provided efficiency for nurses and patients.

Many hospitals that try to implement bedside report find frustration among nurses. Because it is a radical change, it is easy to revert to what is more commonly known: nursing station report. Generally, nurses fear failure and especially failure in front of a patient. But is it really fear of the organizational change or the consequences? Whatever the reason, bedside report is best for patient outcomes (Sigma Theta Tau International, 2012). Both patients and families have reported it improves their understanding of the hospital process and considers needs the patient will have after hospitalization.

The Joint Commission made the second National Patient Safety Goal (NPSG) of 2006 this: *improve the effectiveness of communication among caregivers* (The Joint Commission, 2007). The 13th goal of 2006 was: *encourage the active involvement of the patients and their families in the patient's own care* (Patient Safety Net, 2015). Although The Joint Commission has not specifically listed bedside report as a national patient safety goal, the objectives can be easily met by using the method of bedside report for improved communication. You can read the latest version of The Joint Commission's publication *America's Hospitals: Improving Quality and Safety—The Joint Commission's*

*Annual Report 2017* at https://psnet.ahrq.gov/issue/americas-hospitals-improving-quality-and-safety-joint-commissions-annual-report-2017. And communication still remains one of The Joint Commission's listed NPSGs for 2022.

## RELIABILITY SCIENCE AND THE PREVENTION OF HARM

Sheridan-Leos (2014) discussed the premise of *reliability science* as a platform to ultimately improve quality and safety. Historically, reliability science has been commonly used in high-risk industries. The principles are designed to compensate for limitations in human performance, with a movement toward zero defects. Defects in healthcare can be defined as medical mistakes, lapses in service, omissions, and other measurable metrics demonstrating quality, safe systems, and operational success. The goals of patient safety intersect with reliability science because they are both intended to prevent harm. Healthcare must develop a laser focus on anticipation of what might go wrong (somewhat predictably) and subsequently design stop gaps to eliminate errors from occurring. The anticipation of error prevention uses systems thinking and change theory; while both concepts are somewhat familiar to nurses and other healthcare providers, this may be a paradigm shift for some in the ability to see interdependent relationships in complicated processes rather than linear cause and effect (Sheridan-Leos, 2014).

Nurses and other healthcare providers are vital participants in preventing errors and defects. They are at the "sharp point," or at the point of service delivering care (with the customer). Being at the bedside caring for incredibly sick people in trying circumstances is not without risk. However, examples of nursing work processes designed to prevent error include independent verification, individual double checks, a review of medication side effects, mediation reconciliation, consultation with colleagues regarding policy or procedure standards, and so on. Nurses and organizations that embrace safety science have an opportunity to decrease or eliminate associated organizational stressors resulting from mistakes. Organizational stress often leads to personal stress, which launches the reiterative cycle of stress, fatigue, and burnout. The challenges in the work environment of the COVID-19 pandemic certainly showed us how work-related stressors can spill over into our personal lives.

One of the hallmark characteristics of reliability, as described by Sheridan-Leos (2014)—in the modified definition of Berwick and Nolan's (2003) application of reliability to healthcare—is the measurable capacity of health-care processes, procedures, or services to perform the intended functions in the required time. Most medical care must be delivered in a timely fashion. Delays and omissions in care should be considered a defect. Delays also have the potential to disrupt care delivery and optimal healing as well as the potential to affect outcomes.

Nursing specifically has typically been silent when errors occur in practice. There is an overwhelming fear of litigation and public humiliation of both organizations and individuals who make errors. Honesty takes work. Children do not have to be taught how to lie; they have to be taught how *not* to lie. Natural instincts facilitate protection; protecting ourselves and others is human nature. Living with knowledge that an error occurred is just as stressful as reporting an error and fearing the consequence. Stress, fatigue, and burnout frequently occur more quickly for nurses in organizations where honesty and transparency are not supported, appreciated, or encouraged.

### *Case 1*

In 2011, the media reported a story about a nurse in Seattle, Washington named Kimberly Hiatt who made a serious medication error (Aleccia, 2011). Nurse Hiatt recognized the error and immediately reported it to the nurse in charge. The child who received the inaccurate dosage of medication had been a frequent patient at the healthcare facility due to a heart defect. The patient did eventually die, but it was never clear if the medication error contributed directly or indirectly to a further decline of the patient's heart function.

As sad as this death was, another unnecessary death occurred subsequent to the investigation. Nurse Hiatt had been an employee and worked in her specialty for 24 years and had never knowingly made a critical medication error. After this error, she was thoroughly investigated, terminated from her position at her hospital, and fined by the Washington State Board of Nursing. In addition, the Board of Nursing required her to complete 80 hours of medication administration coursework, and as an additional sanction, she received a four-year probationary period that required regular reporting. Unfortunately, the shame of the error, the fear of never working again as a nurse, and the guilt of the harm she may have inflicted led to her death by suicide. Nurse Hiatt's suicide was just one week after the State Board's ruling.

***Case 2***

In Ohio, also in 2011, pharmacist Eric Cropp was sentenced to six months in jail for the death of a 6-year-old cancer patient. In Cropp's case, he was obligated to supervise a pharmacy technician who inadvertently used the wrong percent of saline while mixing a medication in solution. Unfortunately, Cropp is now a convicted felon and lost his license to practice pharmacy (Lebowitz & Mzhen, LLC, 2011). Healthcare is serious business; inadvertent mistakes can result in unintended harm or death.

***Case 3***

A temporary nurse was working in an intensive care unit (ICU) and assigned to a critically ill patient. The nurse was new and unfamiliar with the unit and also with many of the hospital's unique protocols. In the absence of an intravenous (IV) pump, standard practice was to use a tube feeding pump to infuse the medication (incidentally, this was in the late 1980s—long before the global focus on patient safety). Against her better judgment, the nurse hung a 250cc bag of dopamine to be used to augment the patient's blood pressure. Unbeknownst to the nurse, shortly after initiation, the tubing became dislodged inside the tube feeding pump. Later, as the nurse was performing an assessment of the patient, she noticed the arterial line wave form had become very large and accentuated on the monitor, as well as a change in patient condition—the patient had become very restless. As the nurse proceeded to investigate the cause for a change in condition, she looked up and noted that the entire bag of IV medication had run in (through the patient's central line) in a "free-flow" fashion. She was mortified! She immediately notified the nurse in charge and the medical provider. Fortunately, the patient did not suffer any long-term ill effects and was treated with other supportive medications until the dopamine's effects were diminished. However, as for the nurse—she had a very difficult time with the fact that she had made such a potentially grave error. She took a break and went to a private area. There, she had a complete breakdown. She then requested to leave her shift for the rest of the day. The leaders obliged. She had never made a medication error before to her knowledge. The next 15 hours were agonizing for the nurse replaying the scenario in her head, asking herself what she could have done differently. This story had a happy ending—the medical director of the ICU asked the hospital and the nursing agency for the nurse's contact information. He made a call to the nurse to console her and asked her to come back to work later that day (the call was on the day following the error). He assured her that she could do it and that this mistake should not deter her confidence in her ability to practice nursing in the future! The nurse did go into the hospital that day to find a very supportive group of clinical colleagues waiting for her return—they allowed her to help them care for patients that day and not be assigned a patient or patients of her own. This compassionate and caring approach made all the difference in her own "recovery" by allowing time to process and finally accept the error. Fortunately, she was able to continue her practice working in this and other ICUs.

> She has never forgotten the error, and overall, it has made her a better nurse—more present and aware.

No professional curricula adequately prepares future healthcare practitioners with all the competencies necessary to deliver quality healthcare (Morris et al., 2013). Nurses and other healthcare providers must take special care to remain vigilant to prevent errors. Strategies for safe practice must include following organizational policy, delivering patient-centered care in an interdisciplinary team, knowing the standards of practice, utilizing available technology, staying current with medical and nursing evidence (practicing evidence-based care), being present and aware, and caring for their own well-being. The COVID-19 pandemic was sudden, severe, and has left an indelible mark on all practicing providers' well-being in healthcare. Many have suffered mental and physical conditions related to the stress; others found both positive and negative ways to cope with what they experienced in the work environment. And for those who experienced similar war-like conditions on the front lines of healthcare, it will be a time they will never forget but must process how to deal with it.

Providers in healthcare are diligently working to bridge the gaps in the care continuum for improved quality of care. The comprehensive care continuum now includes what happens before an episodic office visit or hospital encounter; those activities that take place inside a hospital, clinic, or provider office; as well as those that encompass the home environment of patients to ensure care is consistent and meets the patient's needs. The rise in homelessness has only complicated the healthcare continuum further in delivering quality services to those who do not have a permanent place of residence. You can read more about the National Health Care for the Homeless Council's work here: https://nhchc.org/understanding-homelessness/health-care-for-the-homeless-a-vision-of-health-for-all/part-three-impact.

Organizational transparency is necessary to forge optimal safety, quality, and legal reform. Public reporting has removed the veil of secrecy organizations have enjoyed; no longer is there an impenetrable shield when errors occur.

Smart organizations have begun to open their private world to the public by bringing together patients, family, healthcare providers, and community members as collective advocates for system change. The objective is to allow those whom healthcare is designed to serve to participate in setting organizational policy and decision-making.

## PRACTICE PEARLS

- Learn about reliability science.
- Apply the principles of reliability science to improve quality and safety in the work environment.
- Attend to your own well-being to be able to provide safe care.
- Design or redesign care systems to be safer, innovative, and more patient-focused.

---

## PROMOTING ACCOUNTABILITY

Promoting accountability is a difficult and somewhat ambiguous task. As people, we often link the words *accountable* and *guilty;* if you are accountable, you are the one to blame. Nurses are generally altruistic people who honor the truth. Telling the truth means reporting errors and catching near misses. Unfortunately, nurses and other healthcare providers cannot eliminate human error and are all subject to error potential with even the most well-designed processes and systems. Making any kind of mistake causes stress. Depending on the gravity of the error, the stress can be extreme, as evidenced by the earlier professional practice examples in this chapter.

Lyons and colleagues (2004) reviewed a variety of levels of human errors in healthcare, from the most unintentional of absent-minded errors to the intentional maleficent causes of harm. One rare example of intentional harm has been serial killers who happened to be nurses and their victims were patients. Fortunately, intentional harm is uncommon in healthcare.

Typically, human reliability assessment and process improvement efforts within an organization can prevent unintentional errors from recurring. Dr. Lucian Leape from the Harvard School of Public Health first briefed the US Congressional Subcommittee on the management of human error in healthcare on October 12, 1999 (Marx, 2001). Dr. Leape reported that only 2% to 3% of major medical errors are reported through hospital reporting structures. He stressed the urgency of finding ways for healthcare organizations to prevent errors, eliminate punitive error-reporting responses, and use the errors to improve the chances that they would not be repeated.

A recent, high-profile case involving Radonda Vaught, a Tennessee nurse, sparked a great deal of controversy surrounding the charges filed against her and the failure of her hospital to report the error. In this case, multiple system safeguards were *overridden,* which allowed the error to occur in late 2017. The investigation concluded with judicial sentencing in early 2022.

Read more about the Radonda Vaught case here: https://nurse.org/articles/nurse-radonda-vaught-trial.

Marx (2005) described *disciplinary system theory* as a way to define categories of error based on historical court cases, jury decisions, and penal codes. Errors are then categorized as one of "four evils":

1. **Human error**—The one committing the error should have done something other than what they did
2. **Negligent conduct**—Failure to exercise expected care and should have been aware
3. **Reckless conduct**—Conscious disregard of substantial and unjustifiable risk
4. **Knowing violations**—Knowingly violated a rule or procedure

Similarly, categories of error are used in the decision-making process called Just Culture. The visual model shown in Figure 9.1 outlines the types of error, considerations resulting from investigation of the error, and appropriate follow-up behavior.

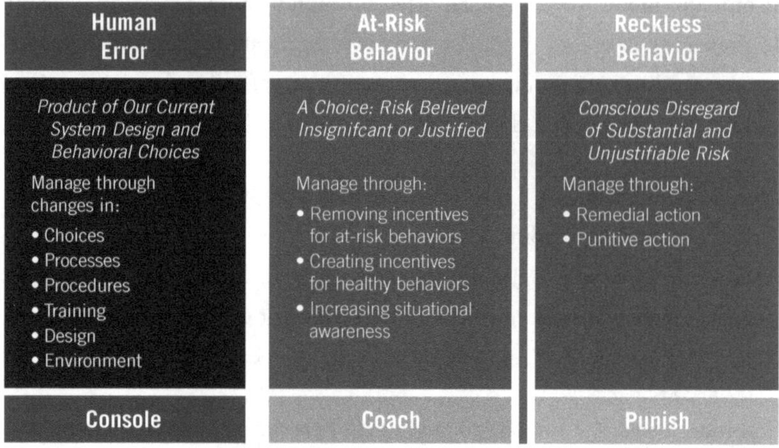


**FIGURE 9.1** The types of error, considerations resulting from investigation of the error, and appropriate follow-up behavior.

*Copyright © 2015 Just Culture. Used with permission.*

*Just Culture* is a process by which organizations can evaluate errors and determine appropriate responses. The organizational enticement to such a process is that by using the well-designed tools, leaders can encourage more reporting, learn from mistakes without blame, and appropriately identify those who behave recklessly and need to be removed from the organization. Brunt (2010) described how using Just Culture pushes organizations to make six major changes:

1. Move from looking at errors as individual failures to realizing they are often caused by system failures.
2. Move from a punitive environment to a Just Culture.

3. Move from secrecy to transparency.
4. Move from provider-centered care to patient-centered care.
5. Move from models of care that rely on independence to models of care that encourage interdependent, collaborative, and interprofessional teamwork.
6. Move from top-down accountability to universal and reciprocal accountability.

The visual model shown in Figure 9.2 is supported by learning systems, justice, and accountability. It outlines a cycle of improvement, based on values and expectations, that drives system design and behavioral choices, resulting in good or bad outcomes.

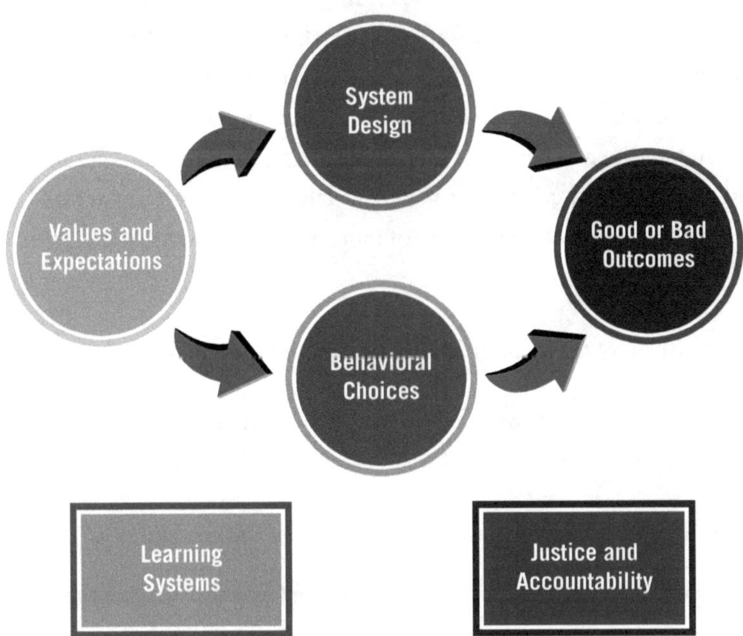


**FIGURE 9.2** The cycle of improvement is based on values and expectations that drive system design and behavioral choices.



You can learn more about Just Culture here: https://www.justculture.com.

## REPORTABLE QUALITY MEASURES

Using reportable quality measures to drive successful change is something healthcare organizations should strive for. Providers across the nation are being held responsible for reportable quality metrics such as clinical core measures, state-initiated quality indicators, and national patient satisfaction percentile rankings. Additional measurement schemes relative to patient experience and outcomes (e.g., patient satisfaction with care, hospital readmission rates, procedural complications, and infection rates for organizations by cause) complicate complex payment and reimbursement systems.

Decisions have become arduous for patients when selecting healthcare providers. Organizations that are able to convey their quality, safety, and excellent patient experiences will have clientele. Those with poor results will struggle in the marketplace. Organizations that can teach nurses and other care providers how their individual practice affects fiscal health will be successful. Nurses and other healthcare providers must learn about and understand reportable and reimbursement-dependent indicators. Organizations of the future must build team-oriented cultures with creative talent and use proactive plans to drive quality outcomes. You can learn more about the variety of performance measures at these two websites:

> https://www.jointcommission.org/measurement/measures/
>
> https://www.cms.gov/Medicare/Quality-Initiatives-Patient-Assessment-Instruments/QualityMeasures/Core-Measures

Healthcare organizations must eliminate blaming and eliminate sayings such as, "If the physician would only…" or, "If the nurse had…" and, "It was the cardio-pulmonary staff's fault for not…" Studies show open-ended and honest discussion about errors not only improves communication among the members of the healthcare team, but also improves patient care and does not lead to increased litigation (Stewart et al., 2006). Organizational stress, fatigue, and burnout are less likely to occur in transparent organizations, where all levels of healthcare providers know what to expect from each other and from the organization.

# LEADING INNOVATION AND IMPROVEMENT

Nurses, as the nation's largest healthcare profession (American Association of Colleges of Nursing, 2022), must take the lead to guide healthcare to a better future. Nurses provide the preponderance of care in most if not all types of healthcare organizations. Nurses spend the most time with patients and families. Nurses have significant influence with patients and families in care planning, accepting and translating treatment recommendations, and understanding the intricacies of their healthcare encounters.

Nursing leadership plays a significant role in the outcomes of patients. Nurse leaders control the resources—the people, places, and things that provide care. The role of a nursing leader, at whatever level, is to "set the tone." Nursing leaders must lead by example. Leaders might be in formal positions to set policy, design or collaborate in creating a philosophy for practice, or determine how a shift might operate; they may also have more informal influence as evidenced by everyday dealings with colleagues.

Clinical nurses need to take every opportunity to present themselves as leading the care team: taking charge of care coordination, rounding with other clinical and non-clinical disciplines, thinking of better ways to do things, and monitoring all patient-education initiatives. While medical providers determine the plan of treatment or appropriate procedures for a medical condition, nurses are the communication conduit among the entire clinical team and the patient for understanding the "what" and the "why."

Participating in evidence-based practice councils and shared governance committees allows nurses to be a part of important decision-making. Nurses can build the confidence needed to lead innovation and care improvement from these types of activities. Nurses need to be active in the profession and knowledgeable about their chosen specialty. The best patient advocates are informed.

While this section focused on the role of nursing in leading innovation and improvement, the intent is not to belittle or downplay the role and importance of other care providers. The best patient outcomes require an entire team of committed providers.

## PRACTICE PEARLS

- Volunteer for learning opportunities—stretch yourself.
- Participate in organization-sponsored knowledge-building programs.
- Become an expert.
- Collaborate with other care providers to design the best care strategies.

---

A healthy culture is critical for both employee and provider satisfaction, as well as patient experience. In 2013, Sheryl Sandberg (former COO of Facebook/Meta Platforms) went on a crusade to educate women in leadership roles. The vast majority of nurses are women. Sandberg described learned detrimental behaviors by women in corporate culture: They tend to sit in the second row of a meeting room, lack confidence, and are quiet and do not interrupt "testosterone driven" conversations. Women favor being pleasers, kind hearts, and servants (Sandberg, 2013). The same could be said for nurses, and it is time for change. It is also favorable that nursing is becoming more diverse both in ethnicity and gender to better match the overall population.

Nurse leaders, in particular, must be well educated, experientially prepared, and use their expertise by having a voice. It is time to "sit up and lean in," as Sandberg described, to become part of the decision-making body. As stated before, nurses represent the largest profession in healthcare. Nurses do have influence, and we need to use it as a force for good. Nurses can guide organizations to achieve desired outcomes. It is time for nurses to stand up, take charge, and be a positive force in the healthcare industry.

Nurses must also share their good work. Best practices are routinely discovered in nursing units within organizations every day. Many nurses provide exceptional care and do extraordinary things. Informal research is conducted by daily experimentation to achieve solutions to common problems. Nurses want to practice with high standards. Differing models of care are explored, knowledge is shared between novices and experts, and leadership is abundant. Knowledge is power, and communication is the only way to unleash it.

Most nurses are required to obtain pertinent continuing education to relicense or recertify. However, studying what is new in the literature related to healthcare economics, policy, or innovative methods of care provision can be difficult. The amount of information can be overwhelming. Streamlining subjects or sharing information among colleagues can be effective methods to stay current. Communication among care providers is very important for patient care, and it is also important for good practice.

Patients are also encouraged to speak up and be involved in their care for their own safety. You can read more about The Joint Commission's Speak Up campaign at this website: https://www.jointcommission.org/resources/for-consumers/speak-up-campaigns.

## PRACTICE PEARLS

- What kind of communicator are you? Do you speak up when it's important and helpful to do so?
- Do your colleagues think you are a valuable participant?
- Are you able to understand the preferences of different generations, cultures, ethnicity, gender, and religions?
- Are you able to understand the finite nuances of disease?
- Can you apply the latest knowledge and research to patient situations?

# CREATING A BETTER WORKPLACE

Research shows employee satisfaction can be linked to customer satisfaction or, in healthcare, to the patient experience. Improvements can be low or no cost. The patient experience is a critical component to the assessment of quality. Folkman (2013) listed seven ways one company found to increase employee satisfaction without giving raises:

- Consistent core values exhibited by the leadership that do not disappear during times of stress
- Long-term focus promoting a positive and bright future
- Local leadership accepting feedback and driving change
- Continuous communication in good and bad times
- Collaboration with others to maximize resources and teamwork
- Abundant opportunities for development
- Speedy and agile decision-making

Nurses are the backbone of any healthcare operation; the influence they possess must not be wasted. Nurses must be active participants in improvement activities and take full advantage of the perks associated with employment, such as tuition reimbursement, certification pay differentials, and educational offerings. Being a good employee requires give and take for all healthcare providers. More than two decades have passed since the first report by the IOM regarding the status of safety in healthcare. *We can do better*. Being an involved employee in an environment devoted to quality and safety provides a buffer from organizational stressors.

Staying connected to purpose buffers stressful conditions. In Pistorius's 2013 book *Ghost Boy,* he described a nurse who loved her job. She performed her duties with passion and commitment every day. As a result, she saw life in the boy who was truly alive inside his prison of a body. The patient, named Martin, had a mysterious illness causing him to be comatose. He lost all bodily functions, including speech. However, one day his mind woke up, but he couldn't let anybody know. Virna, his nurse, took time to relate to the boy as if he were awake. She didn't know if he was actually "in there" or not. In doing so, she found life in a boy and gave him a great gift (Pistorius, 2013). Virna was not stressed by the patient's condition or the environment, but instead provided him with care, compassion, and human kindness. Be a Virna.

### PRACTICE PEARLS

- Why did you become a healthcare provider? Passion and purpose provide amazing individual and professional rewards.
- Stay involved and contribute by sharing what you know.
- Always give your best.

## INFLUENCING STATE AND NATIONAL POLICY

Nurses are ideal advocates for healthcare change. Their knowledge and expertise of what is best for patients cannot be matched. Nurses must remain abreast of current issues to be informed and vote on amendments and healthcare laws with conviction. Be a promoter of health and the prevention of illness. Use nursing and non-nursing related venues as a platform to share expertise. Consider volunteering to speak about nursing and healthcare in the community. Be knowledgeable about the impact of changing healthcare law. The political arena offers a number of opportunities for nurses to get involved in driving change: testifying, lobbying, providing credible input for a legislative bill, voting, or running for public office.

Nurses occasionally find themselves in situations of distress. These situations commonly challenge their patience, integrity, and values. It can be morally distressing to seek justice or what you believe to be the best care for a patient without having the plan supported or agreed upon by the patient, the family, or in some cases even the medical provider. Worldwide challenges remain. Impoverished people or communities with no means of obtaining or growing their own food are not likely to have healthy food choices. Religious communities with strict conviction about immunizations may require specialized provisions to help fend off viruses. And the global COVID-19 pandemic exposed a host of social and economic challenges within the healthcare system.

Many social issues still exist in nursing and healthcare both inside and outside of the United States. Often, these types of challenges are shared with care providers and can be a source of stress. Conflicts arise in healthcare as they do in any other industry on a regular basis, but in healthcare and nursing, the conflict may have a direct impact on someone's life. Thus, a stronger focus on quality and safety must be included in all plans for the future of nursing and healthcare.

# CONCLUSION

What is nurtured is what will flourish. O'Reilly (2009) pronounced that healthcare was slightly improving 10 years after the IOM report on errors. The progress has been *slow,* and experts in the industry would give the effort toward safety and quality a grade ranging from a B- to a C+ (O'Reilly, 2009; Wachter, 2010). We can do much better. We can manage patient risk, improve safety, and become more reliable in what we do. Ask yourself these questions:

- What are you nurturing in your practice?
- What are your organization's leaders nurturing?
- What is your community nurturing?
- What can you do in your practice to make a difference?

The next chapter discusses strategies to reduce stress and fatigue in an effort to move beyond burnout and to promote a healthy work-life balance.

# REFERENCES

Agency for Healthcare Research and Quality. (2015). *Nurse bedside shift report implementation handbook.* http://www.ahrq.gov/professionals/systems/hospital/engagingfamilies/strategy3/index.html

Aleccia, J. (2011, June 27). *Nurse's suicide highlights twin tragedies of medical errors.* NBC News. https://www.nbcnews.com/health/health-news/nurses-suicide-highlights-twin-tragedies-medical-errors-flna1C9452213 http://www.nbcnews.com/

American Association of Colleges of Nursing. (2022). *Fact sheet.* https://www.aacnnursing.org/News-Information/Fact-Sheets/Nursing-Fact-Sheet

American Nurses Association. (2017). *Magnet model.* https://www.nursingworld.org/organizational-programs/magnet/magnet-model/

American Nurses Association Enterprise. (n.d.). *Find a magnet organization.* https://www.nursingworld.org/organizational-programs/magnet/find-a-magnet-organization/

American Nurses Credentialing Center. (n.d.-a). *ANCC Magnet Recognition Program.* https://www.nursingworld.org/organizational-programs/magnet/

American Nurses Credentialing Center. (n.d.-b). *Why become Magnet?* https://www.nursingworld.org/organizational-programs/magnet/about-magnet/why-become-magnet/

American Society of Quality. (2022). *What is the Malcolm Baldrige National Quality Award (MBNQA)?* https://asq.org/quality-resources/malcolm-baldrige-national-quality-award

Anderson, C., & Mangino, R. (2006). Nurse shift report: Who says you can't talk in front of the patient? *Nursing Administration Quarterly, 30*(2), 112–122. https://doi.org/10.1097/00006216-200604000-00008

Bronstein, S., & Griffin, D. (2014, April 23). *A fatal wait: Veterans languish and die on a VA hospital's secret list.* CNN. https://www.cnn.com/2014/04/23/health/veterans-dying-health-care-delays/index.html

Brunt, B. (2010, May 18). *Developing a just culture.* Healthleaders Media. https://www.healthleadersmedia.com/nursing/developing-just-culture

Caruso, E. (2007). The evolution of nurse-to-nurse bedside report on a medical-surgical cardiology unit. *MedSurg Nursing, 16*(1), 17–22.

Dweck, C. (2016). What having a growth mindset actually means. *Harvard Business Review.* https://hbr.org/2016/01/what-having-a-growth-mindset-actually-means

Epstein, A. (2007). *Introducing intentional teaching: Choosing the best strategies for young children's learning.* National Association for the Education of Young Children.

Folkman, J. (2013, November 27). Seven ways to increase employee satisfaction without giving a raise. *Forbes.* http://www.forbes.com/sites/joefolkman/2013/11/27/seven-ways-to-increase-employee-satisfaction-without-giving-a-raise

Health Quality Council of Alberta. (2021). *What is a just culture?* https://justculture.hqca.ca/what-is-a-just-culture/

The Joint Commission. (2007). *National Patient Safety Goals.* https://www.jointcommission.org/standards/national-patient-safety-goals/-/media/b35ba0b4b9754c6dbafdb1f86e152e5c.ashx

Jon M. Huntsman School of Business at Utah State University. (2021, August 10). *The Shingo Model.* Shingo Institute. https://shingo.org/shingo-model/

Keepnews, D., & Mitchell, P. H. (2003, September 30). Health systems' accountability for patient safety. *Online Journal of Issues in Nursing, 8*(3), Manuscript 2. https://doi.org/10.3912/OJIN.Vol8No03Man02

Kohn, L., Corrigan, J., & Donaldson, M. (2000). *To err is human: Building a safer health system.* The National Academies Press.

Lebowitz & Mzhen, LLC. (2011, November 16). *Pharmacist jailed for fatal medication error.* https://www.pharmacyerrorinjurylawyer.com/pharmacist_jailed_for_fatal_me_1/

Livingston, G. (2009). *Too soon old, too late smart: Thirty true things you need to know now.* Da Capo Lifelong Books: Hachette Book Group.

Lyons, M., Adams, S., Woloshynowych, M., & Vincent, C. (2004). Human reliability analysis in healthcare: A review of techniques. *The International Journal of Risk and Safety in Medicine, 16*, 223–237.

Marx, D. A. (2005, March 27). *Patient safety and the "just culture": A primer for healthcare executives.* PSNet. https://psnet.ahrq.gov/issue/patient-safety-and-just-culture-primer-health-care-executives

Minick, P. (1995). The power of human caring: Early recognition of patient problems. *Scholarly Inquiry for Nursing Practice: An International Journal, 9*(4), 303–317.

MLB Advanced Media. (2022). *Batting average (AVG).* https://www.mlb.com/glossary/standard-stats/batting-average

Morris, S., Otto, C. N., & Golemboski, K. (2013). Improving patient safety in healthcare quality in the 21st century: Competencies required of future medical laboratory science practitioners. *Clinical Laboratory Science, 26*(4), 200–204.

Nance, J. (2008). *Why hospitals should fly: The ultimate flight plan to patient safety and quality care.* Second River Healthcare Press.

O'Reilly, K. B. (2009, December 28). *Patient safety improving slightly, 10 years after IOM report on errors.* American Medical News. http://www.amednews.com/article/20091228/profession/312289980/6

Patient Safety Net. (2007). *The role of the patient in safety.* US Department of Health and Human Services; Agency for Healthcare Research and Quality.

Pistorius, M. (2013). *Ghost boy.* Nelson Books.

Reason, J. (2000). Human error: Models and management. *British Medical Journal, 320,* 768–770. https://doi.org/10.1136/bmj.320.7237.768

Rodziewicz, T. L., Houseman, B., & Hipskind, J. E. (2022). *Medical error reduction and prevention.* StatPearls Publishing.

Sandberg, S. (2013). *Lean in: Women, work, and the will to lead.* Knopf.

Sheridan-Leos, N. (2014). Highly reliable healthcare in the context of oncology nursing: Part 1. *Clinical Journal of Oncology Nursing, 18*(2), 151–153. https://doi.org/10.1188/14.CJON.151-153

Sigma Theta Tau International. (2012). *Nursing handoff at the bedside: Does it improve outcomes?* Sigma Repository.

Stewart, R. M., Corneille, M. G., Johnston, J., Geoghegan, K., Myers, J. G., Dent, D. L., McFarland, M., Alley, J., Pruitt, B. A., & Cohn, S. M. (2006). Transparent and open discussion of errors does not increase malpractice risk in trauma patients. *Annals of Surgery, 243*(5), 645–651. https://doi.org/10.1097/01.sla.0000217304.65877.27

Stulberg, B. (2017, December 14). *Mood follows action.* Medium. https://medium.com/personal-growth/mood-follows-action-3d3f651c60e3

Wachter, R. M. (2010). Patient safety at ten: Unmistakable progress, troubling gaps. *Health Affairs, 29*(1), 165–173. https://doi.org/10.1377/hlthaff.2009.0785

Warren, R. (2002). *The purpose driven life: What on earth am I here for?* Zondervan.

World Health Organization. (2022). *Patient safety campaigns.* https://www.who.int/campaigns/world-patient-safety-day

# 10

# BEYOND BURNOUT: PROMOTING OPTIMAL HEALTH AND WELL-BEING

## OBJECTIVES

- Explore the state of the nursing and healthcare professions in terms of stress and burnout.
- Consider what you can do to mitigate stress and burnout at your place of work.
- Consider how your choices affect your stress level, good and bad.
- Learn healthy coping strategies from the experts.
- Consider whether stress really is harmful or not.
- Adopt intentional practices to improve your overall health and well-being.

# A REVIEW OF BURNOUT

Maslach and Leiter (2005) have both studied and measured burnout in numerous populations and settings over the last several decades; burnout is a chronic problem. In order to reverse the trend, researchers believe burnout is not a problem for individuals to solve; rather, *burnout is a problem of the social environment in which they work.* Furthermore, when organizations do not recognize the human side of work in workplace interactions, including how work is completed, and do not assess if mismatches exist between the nature of the jobs and the people, there is a greater risk of burnout (Maslach & Leiter, 2005). Healthcare should understand this best since we are a caring people business.

The paramount risks of burnout are both professional and personal. Maslach and Leiter (2005) describe six areas for person-job mismatches:

- **Workload:** Too much work and/or not enough resources
- **Control**: Micromanagement, lack of influence, and accountability without power
- **Reward**: Not enough pay, acknowledgment, or satisfaction
- **Community**: Isolation, conflict, and disrespect
- **Fairness**: Discrimination and favoritism
- **Values**: Ethical conflicts and meaningless tasks

They describe personal consequences that may include a detriment to health and strained private lives. Professional consequences may include absenteeism, job hopping, poor relationships with others, and a tendency to be distracted. One's commitment to work will most likely wax and wane, and in a nurse's or other healthcare provider's case, patients may suffer.

The true cost of burnout in nursing and other healthcare professions is unknown. Ceridian (2019) cited "the sea" of articles when doing an internet search for "burnout" in healthcare workers. The majority described ways for individuals to identify early symptoms and find ways to better care for themselves. This assumes it is solely an individual problem. Also exposed by Ceridian (2019) was the two-thirds of physicians (recently surveyed) who said they've experienced burnout, and only 25% of their organizations are effectively addressing it. They believed the real cost of burnout in healthcare workers is found in these outcomes:

1. **Higher absence rates and lower productivity:** Healthcare organizations have one of the highest absence rates of any industry, which translates to a hefty financial burden. The Centers for Disease Control and Prevention (CDC) estimates lost productivity for US companies at over $225 billion per year. There are both direct costs for absentees and the indirect cost of those who must cover for the absentee (usually at a higher cost).
2. **Higher turnover of employees and increased contract labor:** As Ceridian described (2019), losing highly trained employees is costly. For those who stay, there is more work than can feasibly be done at times and may necessitate adding contract labor resources. There are also record numbers of healthcare workers (baby boomers) in nearly every sector retiring and causing the need for health services to rise. Others are changing jobs or leaving the industry altogether.
3. **Lower care quality and patient safety:** Patients may be at risk when being cared for by burned out healthcare workers. Leveraging technology and analytic tools may be able to reduce some of the stress in the work environment. Employers must be informed about engagement and gain an understanding of their employees' emotional status regarding the work to lessen the burden of burnout.

Their final recommendation: Make employee well-being and engagement as high a priority as patient care and finance, and fix the issues that arise to successfully navigate the evolving world of healthcare.

In addition, the six areas highlighted by Maslach and Leiter (2005) in the Stanford Social Innovation Review also provide valuable organizational insight. An assessment by healthcare entities and their leaders may raise awareness to lessen or eliminate the potential for burned-out workers.

Modern nursing (and healthcare) is plagued by increasing professional stressors (Smith, 2014). Smith (2014) as well as McCloskey and Taggart (2010) described that the modern world of healthcare and tightening budgets are resulting in additional work-related stressors such as barriers to providing care, increasing complexity of patient needs, shorter acute episodic lengths of stay, the need for increased knowledge of ever-changing technology, nursing shortages, poor staffing, long work hours, limited resources, and feelings of a lack of control. Much of the research in the literature, as well as anecdotal practice findings, are consistent with this description. And sadly, little has changed in recent years.

Each of the areas described by Maslach and Leiter (2005), when applied to nursing and/or healthcare, could be remedied as follows:

- **Workload:** Reasonable, achievable, and safe
- **Control:** An engaged and involved workforce
- **Reward:** Adequate compensation and recognition for a job well done
- **Community:** A sense of true teamwork and meaningful relationships
- **Fairness:** No discrimination or tolerance of favoritism
- **Values:** An ideal match of aligned passion and purpose

Could enlightened and engaged nurses, healthcare workers, nursing leaders, nursing educators, and other leaders in healthcare solve the current dilemma in the social environment of healthcare? The task seems somewhat daunting on a global scale. However, what if one-by-one or entity-by-entity, we began making small changes? Could these changes affect a single department, a single division, a single organization, a single health system, and eventually a region, county, state, or country? By working together we can eliminate one of the most common stereotypes in nursing, the presumption that "nurses eat their young." We must become welcoming and supportive to new practitioners.

## PRACTICE PEARLS

- Does your workplace seem to know about or be concerned about burnout? If so, how does your workplace discourage burnout?
- Is your workplace engaged and interested in your well-being?
- Does your workplace promote health?
- Could you do one thing differently to increase your job satisfaction?

# THE VALUE OF TIME

All too often in our quest for success, we jostle our way through life, juggling priorities as best as we can. We try to balance all the competing activities in our personal and professional lives. However, in the hustle and bustle of life, we frequently neglect what matters most—to take time to think or to intentionally plan our lives. One of life's lessons learned as people age is that time is finite—there is only so much of it. It is a habitually overlooked valuable resource to be savored and nurtured.

For example, if you live to the age of 80, that is nearly 22,000 days of adult life. There are approximately 20 to 22 workdays per month, leaving about 8 to 10 days of "free time." During the "free" days, all other home or personal life related activities must be accomplished, which often leaves little time for rest and recovery. This estimate of days doesn't really take into account that not much else gets accomplished on a nurse's or other healthcare worker's designated workday (due to the abnormally long hours like a 12 +/- hour shift).

Our personal free time to relax and recover is imperative for fighting stress, fatigue, and burnout. While a common suggestion is to take regular breaks at work, the value of intentional personal time should not be underestimated. And, in taking personal time it is important to do activities that are enjoyable to facilitate a "reset."

Setting intentional personal goals for good health and well-being in your lifetime is maybe more important than setting work and career goals. Intentional time sets goals for dedicated personal time with friends and family, exercising, reading, traveling, and hobbies. Intentional time is also proactive rather than reactive. It leverages the healthcare worker's locus of control. This shifts the old paradigm of the individual recharging based on chance to one where there is a higher likelihood due to intentional planning of activities. This does not mean that an individual must have a plan that includes a checklist of action items to complete when away from work. The act of simply being still, reflecting, practicing mindfulness, or meditating can all help recharge you as long as it is part of a personal time plan.

If examined from the perspective of a weekly routine, there are 168 hours of total time available per week. If you work 40 hours per week, sleep 56 hours per week, and spend 10 hours per week on activities related to daily grooming, this leaves a balance of 62 hours per week for commute time, life's activities, and free time. This amounts to a mere 8.86 hours per day. If any of the listed activities encroach on your allocation of time, this 8.86 hours per day suffers and shrinks.

## PRACTICE PEARLS

- Consider a time analysis or "work sampling" project of your life. What do you spend your available time doing?
- Assess if the time spent is doing what you want to do.
- If the exercise shows a gap in what you want for your life, spend some time brainstorming ways you can begin to make small changes.

# THE SIGNIFICANCE OF INDIVIDUAL ACCOUNTABILITY AND ACTION

Frequently, others make choices for us. We choose to allow people to guide our future, steal our present, and unearth the past. Much of what causes stress comes from the environment or situations in which we place ourselves, including poor personal relationships, bad work cultures, difficult friends or family, and other life stressors. Consciously, we often think we do not have choices. But don't we? Have we really lost the ability to choose what we do and with whom we spend our time? Can we not make changes to our current circumstances?

Indecision is a decision—good, bad, or otherwise. Of course, sometimes there is value in not deciding. Some conditions change, and some problems really do solve themselves. Being thoughtful and present, intentional in your thinking, grounded or centered enough to appraise the options, able to manage emotions, and be objectively self-aware are all learned skills that require practice.

Society teaches us that being busy equals success—too much so at present. Frequently, there is not adequate time to prepare healthy meals, walk the dog, and participate in other enjoyable activities that provide moments of stress relief. Successful people always seem to be busy.

However, being too busy can lead to stress, fatigue, and eventually burnout. What are successful people busy doing? How do they balance it all? Is what they are doing really making a difference for themselves? Is it making a difference for others? Is their contribution truly of value? We, as a society, need to slow down and take stock of what is important. A wise hospital chaplain once said, "Do you ever see a U-Haul behind a hearse?"

There will almost always be more shifts or time one can spend at work or time for other people's priorities. The question is, are you spending time on what is important to you? For your health? Are you prioritizing your intentional personal time? Nurses and other care providers are often caretakers at both work and home. Spending time on or with yourself may seem selfish, but it is actually an integral part of who you are.

## PRACTICE PEARLS

- Think of a person who many people consider successful. What do they do differently?
- Successful people have limitations and clear boundaries that surround their time.
- Choose wisely—relationships, work, and time spent.
- Think about the daily choices you make.
- To learn more about the upside of regret and how you might leverage it for good, check out Daniel Pink's new book (2022), *The Power of Regret: How Looking Backward Moves Us Forward,* here: https://www.danpink.com/.

---

# THE FOUR-LEGGED STOOL OF PHYSICAL, EMOTIONAL, MENTAL, AND SPIRITUAL WELL-BEING

What is *well-being?* It is defined as "a good or satisfactory condition of existence; a state characterized by health, happiness, and prosperity" (Merriam-Webster, n.d.). As previously noted in Chapter 7, Seligman's (2011) positive psychology movement described well-being in terms of "flourishing." Pertaining to healthcare, to *flourish* might be defined as the ability to grow, develop, and/or attract health.

Notably, as people age, well-being tends to improve. Aging is associated with a positive change in attitude, a greater acceptance of one's physical limitations, contentedness with past accomplishments, reduced preoccupation with peer pressure, and a more realistic appraisal of one's strengths and weaknesses

(Jeste & Oswald, 2014). This is excellent news for the majority of practicing nurses, as the median age of nurses was 52 in 2020 (National Council of State Boards of Nursing [NCSBN], 2020). Every two years a new study is conducted. The latest study is now underway. In addition, most leaders in healthcare are even older (sometimes by a decade or more), with a large percentage approaching retirement or have already retired as a result of COVID-19.

Well-being is also reported to be high for those embarking on adult life (Jeste & Oswald, 2014). Jeste and Oswald (2014) reviewed a multitude of studies that commonly show after the beginning of adult life, well-being seems to decline until about mid-life; hence the mid-life crisis. Mid-life is often fraught with a multitude of challenges: raising children, aging parents, increasing work and home life responsibilities, financial struggles, etc. Then, well-being continues in an upward trend toward positive well-being on the way to the end of life. A number of academic sources define spiritual well-being as being very personal; it encompasses values and beliefs that lead to purpose and meaning. Meaningful work does provide purpose.

Work is central to most people's lives because it provides income, a sense of meaning and purpose, a place to build important relationships, and a sense of belonging. Thus, job satisfaction is seemingly a relevant aspect for well-being (Gurkov et al., 2014). Although research about work satisfaction has been conducted in a multitude of industries, the authors found little evidence in this study to support research related to satisfaction and well-being in nursing or other health-related disciplines. While nurses are generally accustomed to setting aside their own needs for others, the COVID-19 pandemic exposed many cracks in the current healthcare system, increasing stress, fatigue, and burnout.

Shortages of both personnel and equipment, fear of a new disease, increased environmental stress, and fear of the many unknowns only potentiated underlying stress. In addition to the usual stressors, there are now concerning troubles with expanding homelessness, crime and violence in society, increased substance abuse, food insecurity, the waning global COVID-19 pandemic, and unstable public health guidance. Each of these is seen in a different light for healthcare providers than for the wider population.

Often, the phrase is stated that you should "never define who you are by what you do for a living." Do we, as nurses and other healthcare providers, actually take stock of who we are as *people,* or do we only look at ourselves through the lens of our professional role? Separating our personal selves from our professional selves can be difficult. The first question we often ask someone we meet outside of work is what they do for a living. We jump to what they do rather than ask questions about who they are. Turning off our "work mode" in our personal life can be quite a challenge at times. It's a challenge that requires a conscious decision to value our intentional personal time over other pursuits.

The tool Gurkov et al. (2014) selected for satisfaction/well-being measurement contained the following elements important to nurses (and relevant for other healthcare workers):

- Satisfaction with their work
- Scheduling practices
- Work-life balance
- Relationships with coworkers
- Interactions at work
- Professional opportunities
- Praise and recognition
- Control and responsibility

Interestingly, the researchers' findings did not support the idea that subjective well-being is influenced by job satisfaction; rather, satisfaction with life comes from meaningful interactions and extrinsic rewards. This study reinforces the importance of culture, relationships, and extrinsic rewards. Nurses, as well as all other healthcare providers, have the ability to effectively contribute to the development of a positive and healthy work culture and build rewarding relationships, and they possess some ability to influence or affect organizational extrinsic rewards.

Think of all the personnel who left organizations during COVID-19 to join the temporary workforce to work at other organizations. Money provided an extrinsic reward to those feeling as if their value had been compromised and their emotional connection with their employer had been broken. Now the questions are: How do we rebuild the workforce? Or do we? Are there alternative models that haven't been explored? Who will decide what the right model might be and how it is implemented?

For centuries, in a multitude of cultures, age has been associated with wisdom. Jeste and Oswald (2014) defined collective characteristics of wisdom to include social reasoning and decision-making, emotional regulation, insight, contributions to common good, tolerance of diverse value systems, acknowledgement of uncertainty, spirituality, sense of humor, and openness to experiences. Nurses are often wise due to their vast experience directly caring for others. No other healthcare profession spends as much time with patients. This collective definition describes a nurse's role in the promotion of health and healing. Harnessing this wisdom and using it in practice can be the challenge.

Loehr and Schwartz (2003) posited that every one of our thoughts, emotions, and behaviors has an energy consequence, for better or worse. The ultimate measure of our lives is not how much time we spend on the planet, but rather how much energy we invest in the time that we have. Their prescription for success is simple: Performance, health, and happiness must be grounded in the skillful management of energy. Nurses should thoughtfully develop approaches to conserve, preserve, and appropriately allocate portions of energy in the practice of nursing. Stress consumes more energy. Rest consumes less energy. Proper assessment of physical and mental energy, as well as taking stock of emotional and spiritual well-being, is crucial to preventing the detrimental effects of stress, fatigue, and burnout.

## PRACTICE PEARLS

- Don't be a victim of learn, earn, and burn.
- Design and implement new strategies to become "burnout-proof."
- Live empowered; begin by taking care of yourself first.
- Make your own well-being a priority.

---

# HEALTHY COPING STRATEGIES

Common knowledge and learned wisdom reveals what we don't schedule doesn't get done. When people get busy, they sacrifice sleep, healthy food, self-care, downtime, and exercise for other pursuits. Intentional time must be taken for planning actions related to good health: exercise, diet, sleep, and more. Health, well-being, and wellness must become a concern for people earlier in their lives to allow for healthy aging. As nurses and other healthcare providers also age, rest time or recovery becomes increasingly necessary to recharge from the inherent demands of the stress-laden workplace and a busy life. We just don't have as much energy as we used to when we were younger.

Without recovery, the job and life's responsibilities become more difficult; stress causes fatigue, fatigue may cause more stress, physical and mental tolerance weaken, and these can all lead to a host of negative health conditions. Time for respite must become the norm, and scheduling downtime to recover must become crucially important for both mental and physical health.

In addition to the usual recommendations of getting adequate rest and sleep, eating a balanced diet, and obtaining the recommended amount of physical exercise for optimal health, you should also consider adding deliberate "mental" respite or mindful exercises along with a reduction in electronic screen time. Stress and screen time are now closely linked (Lejtenyi, 2019). The relationship to technology has become increasingly complex in recent years. Lejtenyi (2019) outlined that while the majority of us love using technology with screens, millions have become totally emotionally and mentally absorbed, suffering real-life health consequences as a result. Researchers found that those who are more screen addicted are more likely to suffer stress (Lejtenyi, 2019); they also posited that screens could be used for mental health interventions in the future to decrease stress.

Learning to build adequate coping strategies with a healthy body and mind can help individuals learn adequate appraisal of stressors and determine an appropriate response. Numerous studies have investigated the defining characteristics of nurses who ineffectively cope with stress. These include sleep disturbances, interference with relationships, an inability to focus, more illness, and progression to burnout (McCloskey & Taggart, 2010). In addition, negative coping strategies (overeating or substance abuse) were found to be more common than healthy coping strategies (exercise or self-care) by Waddill-Goad (2013) in a national survey of nurse leaders.

## RESILIENCE AND HARDINESS

*Resilience* and *hardiness* are two concepts related to an individual's response to stress. Why can some people become hardy and resilient to life's demands and stressors? The answer: their thinking. Foureur et al. (2013) described an evolution of inquiry relative to resilience that has been organized into three "waves" of study:

- The first wave focused on resilience as a set of characteristics such as hardiness, coping, self-efficacy, optimism, and adaptability.
- The second wave involved the study of resilience as a dynamic process where adversity was met with adaption, secondary to learned behavior or gained experience.
- The third and most recent wave of study defines resilience in terms of an innate energy or a motivating life force within individuals that enables adequate coping via a change in thinking.

The first wave relates to lived experience. If a nurse or other healthcare provider learns positive coping skills, they can become more hardy, are instinctively optimistic when adversity strikes, are more adaptable, and essentially become more resilient. The second wave showed those who are more adaptable to adversity have naturally developed the skills of hardiness and resilience over time. The third wave explores the possibility that some people may be innately hardier, and thus resilient, due to their mindset or patterns of thinking.

In a cross-section of varying individuals with differing points of view, Kay (2017) found resilience is a mindset of awareness and practice. Ways cited to build resilience include:

1. Increase sense of control in areas of your life of which you have control. Much of our lives are beyond our control. However, once that is accepted and focus is placed on the areas within our control, we can become more at peace (with less stress).
2. Maintain perspective when faced with challenges. Adequate appraisal of situations is important. This requires skill and the ability to not overreact.
3. Develop a positive self-concept and be kind to yourself. Compassion for self can be difficult, as we are often more critical with ourselves than others.
4. Consider a faith practice; it has been shown to enhance resilience (especially when in a crisis).
5. Meditation is well-researched and provides numerous benefits for improving health and well-being.

According to Cooper et al. (2021, para. 1): Resilience enables nurses to positively adapt to stressors and adversity. It is a complex and dynamic process which varies over time and context and embodies both individual attributes and external resources. Sustaining nurse resilience requires action and engagement from both individuals and organizations.

*Hardiness* is defined as "the capacity for enduring or sustaining hardship and building the capability to survive under unfavorable conditions" (Dictionary.com, 2022). This is the crux of the current condition for all healthcare providers continuing to battle the global COVID-19 pandemic. At present, we have an aging healthcare workforce, battling the daily unknowns of this disease for the last three-plus years. It has been incredibly trying at times, and there doesn't seem to be an end in sight. The public at large have also been experiencing new stressors from COVID-19—unique in their lifetimes. No one has escaped the sequelae of the last three-plus years of uncertainty.

Bartone and Stein (2020), in the *Harvard Business Review,* explained that hardiness needs to be built into organizational culture. They described how hardy leaders have a strong sense of work and life commitment, a greater feeling of control, and are more open to change and challenges in life. In turbulent times (which are inevitable), it makes sense to strengthen your ability to adapt and be resilient (Bartone & Stein, 2020).

Bartone's individual research found four ways to develop hardiness for leaders and their teams:

1. Demonstrate a strong sense of commitment, control, and challenge when responding to stressful circumstances. Stressful situations always present an opportunity to learn and grow.
2. As a group, discuss lessons learned (mistakes and failures) in a positive way. There's always an upside to stressful conditions. Bartone and Stein concluded that "sense making" influence can occur in day-to-day interactions or more formal after-action reviews.
3. Provide opportunities for constructive performance feedback on a fairly regular basis.
4. Provide opportunities for socializing and interacting on the job and outside of work to build relationships for organizational cohesion and social commitment. Constructive coping with stress needs to become the norm.

For today's nurses and other healthcare providers, they will need to build hardiness to buffer their daily stressors from both their work environments and life in general. The uncertainty of today, or the next pandemic or public health emergency, may bring the same or similar volatility. The best strategy: Prepare yourself now.

## MINDFULNESS

The origin of "mindfulness" and most meditative methods can be historically traced back to Eastern Buddhist practices (Hardy, 2015). Sources in the literature describe an emergence in the late 1970s where study and practical application began to surface about mindfulness in Western medical and psychological practices. The origin of much of the early research in the United States was in patient populations and was meant to reduce stress; today's multitude of scientific evidence supports this notion.

In recent years, the study of mindfulness has gone mainstream and has become more prevalent in non-clinical populations, including with nurses. Mindfulness training utilizes a variety of meditative practices. *Meditation* encompasses mental exercises and the cultivation of awareness by training the mind to be present (DuVal, 2009, p. 5). Mindfulness training also teaches a set of active regulation skills that patients (or others) practice by themselves in order to cope with medical or stressful conditions (Wylie, 2015).

White (2013) described key findings from her research about the connection of mindfulness to nursing. The concept of mindfulness encompasses intricately connected attributes: it is a transformative process, where one develops an increasing ability to experience being present with awareness, acceptance and attention. Mindfulness can support improving physical, emotional, psychosocial and spiritual well-being, and can help translate holistic health promotion from theory to practice. Integrating mindfulness into education and practice can enhance therapeutic nursing qualities and support a shift from a purely theoretical way of knowing to one that is more embodied and holistic (White, 2013).

The American Holistic Nursing Association (AHNA, 2018) described how they are growing their influence in healthcare by collecting members who are highly educated nurses and healthcare providers who share a unified mission to advocate for holism in healthcare and work to bring holistic, complementary, and integrative care to diverse practice settings. In addition, they welcome the various nursing specialties (e.g. oncology, pain management, pediatrics, community health, acute care, chronic care, long-term care, etc.) to become members and gain access to a variety of services including holistic education, research, nutrition counseling, and mind-body-spirit therapies. Nurses and other healthcare providers could greatly benefit from a more holistic approach to health for both themselves and their patients versus the current system of healthcare focused mostly on illness and treatment.

You can learn more about the AHNA here: https://www.ahna.org/About-Us/What-is-Holistic-Nursing. They also have a number of resources to enhance practice that can be found here: https://www.ahna.org/Resources. You can find a number of toolkits from the AHNA for self-care and resilience here: https://www.ahna.org/Home/Resources/Self-Care-and-Resilience.

Dr. Jon Kabat-Zinn is known to be one of the first Western adopters of mindfulness (Wylie, 2015). Kabat-Zinn's idea, when introduced, was that mental and emotional acceptance could generate an inner shift in experience that often resembled a cure (Kabat-Zinn, 2013; UMass Memorial Health Center for Mindfulness, 2014). Over time, his agenda evolved into what is known today as the *mindfulness based stress reduction* (MBSR) program, and he has written a number of associated books over the last 35 years to convey his thoughts.

What if nurses and other healthcare providers could apply the same principle in changing their thought patterns or perceptions of the work environment, difficult relationships, and the current system of health? In Smith's (2014) review of the literature (to assess the state of science) relative to MBSR as a potential intervention to improve the ability of nurses to effectively cope with stress, she concluded that utilizing MBSR in the practice of nursing has plentiful benefits.

Lamothe and colleagues (2015) found 14 of 39 studies demonstrating positive outcomes for healthcare providers regarding emotional competence (scarcely defined or studied in the literature) and MBSR. Evidence regarding the effects of MBSR in healthcare professionals suggested this intervention is associated with improvements in burnout, stress, anxiety, and depression. They concluded that the question of what is emotional competence relative to empathy and how to assess it remains unanswered. This crucial answer could identify targeted interventions that could be implemented and tested in the future.

We know mindfulness can be trained and is positively associated with measures of psychological well-being and quality of life (Schoormans & Nyklicek, 2011). Self-improvement seems to be the single golden key to successfully navigating the troubled waters of stress, fatigue, and the potential for burnout in all aspects of life. In addition, *meditation* refers to a family of techniques shown to decrease anxiety and depression by a conscious attempt to focus attention in a non-analytical way and to avoid discursive, ruminating thoughts (Schoormans & Nyklicek, 2011). Practicing mindfulness and meditation can both be part of an intentional personal time plan to fight stress, fatigue, and burnout.

Schoormans and Nyklicek (2011) summarized a simple procedure that nurses and other healthcare providers can follow by engaging in eight sequential steps. This procedure was designed via a working definition of meditation formulated by a collection of experts:

1. Utilize a defined medication technique.
2. Use logic relaxation (letting go of logical thought).
3. Enter a self-induced "state."
4. Move into an aura of psychological relaxation somewhere in the process.

5. Master this self-focused skill or use it as an anchor.
6. Obtain an altered state or mode of consciousness, mystic experience, enlightenment, or suspension of logical thought processes.
7. Embed the context of meditation in a spiritual/religious/philosophy context.
8. Experience mental silence.

Most importantly, taking time for self-reflection can provide a sense of peace and healing for improved well-being. The ability to decrease or change the perception of stress, resulting in less stress and fatigue, may lessen the potential to burn out. This can yield an enhanced overall sense of well-being and a higher quality of life.

## PRACTICE PEARLS

- Learn to be mindful in order to change your thinking.
- Consider learning meditation.
- Become hardy—hardiness neutralizes stress and buffers reactions to adverse conditions.
- You can learn more about hardiness and making stress work for you from Bartone and Stein's book here: https://hardinessmindset.com.
- Consider taking mini-mental breaks to focus on breathing or "checking in" with yourself about how you feel or find things.

## EXERCISE, SLEEP, AND NUTRITION

A number of resources are available for healthy coping strategies for all of the stress life can bring. Here are just a few related to exercise, sleep, and proper nutrition.

The multiple benefits of exercise for both physical and mental health can be as simple as walking for 30 minutes three to five times per week. However, what works for one person may not for another based on lifestyle, work hours, etc. There is also conflicting information about what type, how long, how many times per week, etc. for what is needed for optimal health. It is best to use trial and error to find out what works for your individual body and lifestyle.

Here are a few relevant sources for ideas to boost mental and physical health with exercise:

- https://www.helpguide.org/articles/healthy-living/the-mental-health-benefits-of-exercise.htm
- https://www.healthline.com/health/depression/exercise
- https://www.mayoclinic.org/diseases-conditions/depression/in-depth/depression-and-exercise/art-20046495
- https://health.gov/our-work/nutrition-physical-activity/physical-activity-guidelines

Sleep science has been growing in recent years. Multiple sources recommend that adults get seven to nine hours of sleep per night. The impact to health may be more important than you think, and sleep must be a priority to achieve optimal health. Here are few sources citing the importance of sleep and its connection to health:

- https://health.clevelandclinic.org/sleep-and-health/#:~:text=A%20good%20night%E2%80%99s%20rest%20benefits%20your%20health%20and,awake.%20Sleep%20also%20helps%20your%20brain%20regulate%20emotions

- https://healthysleep.med.harvard.edu/need-sleep/whats-in-it-for-you/health

Even the CDC (n.d) is weighing in on the importance of sleep in early life:

- https://www.cdc.gov/healthyschools/sleep.htm

There are myriad sources for information on proper nutrition. Here are a few of the basics from my perspective:

1. Eliminate as much processed or packaged food from your diet as you can! Challenge yourself to find packaged food with five or fewer ingredients (that you can pronounce and know what they are).
2. Eat farm fresh and local as much as possible: This mean fruits, vegetables, dairy, bakery, and locally raised, grass-fed meat. You'll know where your food came from, and you also won't be as dependent on nationally distributed food supply chains (especially when there are shortages).
3. Consider adding other forms of protein to your diet besides meat, such as beans, lentils, legumes, seeds, nuts, etc.
4. Eat less sugar or sugary foods.
5. Pay attention to the amount and type of salt in your food by reading labels. Natural sea salt is best if you must add it (for additional flavor).
6. Drink water: It is essential for good health. Read more here to figure out what is best for you: https://www.mayoclinic.org/healthy-lifestyle/nutrition-and-healthy-eating/in-depth/water/art-20044256
7. Try to eat as much organic food as possible. This eliminates the added pesticides, fungicides, and other growth-related chemicals (fertilizer).

8. Much of our food today is nutritionally deficient due to changes in the soil from growth-related additives over the last few decades. You can learn more here: https://www.scientificamerican.com/article/soil-depletion-and-nutrition-loss/. Talk to your healthcare provider about testing and supplementation with quality vitamins and minerals.
9. Reduce inflammatory foods from your diet as much as possible. Dairy, gluten, and other allergens may also be harmful for some people based on food sensitivities or true food allergies. Researchers are learning that many of the major disease categories are caused by chronic inflammation. Some examples of inflammatory foods include: red or processed meat, refined carbohydrates, French fries and other fried food, soft drinks and other sugary beverages, and oils (margarine, shortening, and lard). You can read more about what is best to eat and not eat here: https://www.health.harvard.edu/staying-healthy/foods-that-fight-inflammation-guide
10. In general, a serving size should be approximately the size of the palm of your hand, your fist, or a deck of cards.

Positive coping strategies offer a long-term solution to most of life's difficulties and can be learned over time. However, they are usually not an immediate source of "relief" from whatever problem we are experiencing in real time. A few examples of positive coping strategies include taking a time out, deep breathing, exercise, asking for help or seeking support, confronting fears or worries, and more. The area of positive psychology has been a growing industry by focusing on character strengths of individuals and behavior that result in a good life (*Psychology Today*, 2022).

## NEGATIVE COPING HABITS

We would be remiss in this chapter if we didn't also mention the number of negative coping strategies often used to numb the sequelae of stress: avoidance, compulsive or harmful behaviors, smoking, alcohol or drug use (prescription or illicit), over-eating or drinking harmful substances, poor dietary habits, poor sleep habits, and little to no exercise. Each of these has the potential to lead to a path of destruction in health and well-being. I also found the same—more nurse leaders used negative coping skills to manage stress—in my own research about leadership fatigue in 2013.

Many times, negative coping strategies are just easier: skip the gym, grab fast food on the way home from work, don't process negative feelings, etc. And some of these are learned behavior over a lifetime. Making mindful choices about health and well-being takes *time* and *intention.*

Health-intended behaviors may also require a substantive change in our lifestyle. In the fast-paced world of rewarding a hustle culture, taking time for meaningful health assurance activities hasn't really been valued or rewarded. Think about health insurance coverage: Do the rewards outweigh the costs for being a healthy person? How many sick people (or patients) have you heard say they wished they had made different choices earlier in their life and/or lived their life differently?

Health coverage from insurance has not been allocated or accessible based on health status in the US. In contrast, think about car insurance (coverage and cost) and how it is somewhat priced based upon individual action and accountability (in addition to geographic area, years as a customer, history, etc.). Consequently, if you choose to speed, take risks, or have too many accidents, the price reflects it. I often wonder if healthcare insurance was similar, would people take more responsibility and accountability for their individual health?

Learning Mind (2022) describes how negative coping habits can have an *immediate effect* despite being unhealthy, detrimental, or destructive, and this is why people choose them:

1. Avoiding the problem.
2. Smoking.

3. Compulsive spending.
4. Drinking too much caffeine.
5. Escaping.
6. Binge drinking (alcohol).
7. Sleeping all day.
8. Becoming promiscuous.
9. Stopping eating or starting over-eating.
10. Emotional eating.

Here's a California healthcare system that has posted helpful stress-related information to assist their employees: https://www.sutterhealth.org/for-employees/employee-assistance-program/stress-relief-gone-wrong.

Even the mainstream media and magazines have advice for better ways to cope with stressors: https://www.realsimple.com/health/mind-mood/unhealthy-coping-strategies.

The point is, everyone feels stress. The difference is how one deals with it. Can it be capitalized on? Is there an upside? Can you actually learn something? Is all stress harmful? Here's a handy resource comparing positive and negative coping mechanisms and skills for life's stressors from positive psychology: https://positivepsychology.com/coping/.

## ASKING FOR HELP

Healthcare is a team sport, and we must look out for one another. We must become better at caring for ourselves and those around us who are doing the work (despite our intensive training in putting patients first). If we don't take care of ourselves now, there won't be anyone to care for patients. And we must also become more present and aware to notice when one of our team members is struggling.

One upside of the pandemic has been an increasing interest in learning about the unprecedented mental health effects of healthcare workers. Sovold and colleagues (2021) found that for too long, the burden of recognizing and dealing with healthcare stressors has been placed on the *individual worker* to resolve. They determined it is imperative that *psychological first aid* be offered. Jean (2022) promotes the idea of mental health days for healthcare workers, especially nurses. The most significant benefit of mental health days would be to give nurses and other healthcare workers permission to put themselves first and drop the "hero" mentality.

> Unfortunately, no measures to prevent burnout or other mental health issues will be effective unless attention is paid to enhancing a positive work environment, defined as one 'that attracts individuals into the health profession, encourages them to remain in the health workforce and enables them to perform effectively to facilitate better adaptation' (89). Healthcare leaders and decision makers should seek to lead by example and work toward reducing the stigma associated with mental health issues among healthcare staff, and foster a work culture of transparency, trust, respect, openness, equality, empathy, and support. Healthcare leaders should especially be mindful of promoting a culture of inclusion, collaboration, and support, instead of comparison and competition. (Sovold et al., 2021, p. 7)

The National Alliance on Mental Illness has produced a video for the "10 common warning signs of a mental health condition" you can see here: https://www.youtube.com/watch?v=zt4sOjWwV3M&ab_channel=NAMI. Even on our best days at work, it can still be overwhelming, with too much to do and too few resources. But, when the circumstances persist for an extended period of time (like with the global COVID-19 pandemic), feelings of anxiety, a sense of uneasiness, and learned helplessness can build up (and potentially result in depression).

Here's an analogy I was taught growing up to process feelings, which may help you. Think of feelings as if each one is a color on a painter's palette. If they aren't individually dealt with and become tucked away, they will slowly combine into one color, resulting in a "big blog" of black paint. And that's what happens with stress. It can insidiously develop over time into a bone-deep fatigue and then progress to burnout before you even realize it.

There's no shame in asking for help or directing others to get help, and it might just save a life. And we know historically there has been a stigma associated with speaking up and asking for help; so many have suffered in silence. There are a number of professional resources available for help at work: employee assistance programs, human resources personnel, medical providers, and mental health practitioners.

Unfortunately, COVID-19 has stretched the limitations for many in healthcare to the breaking point, and it has been painful to watch. That's why it is vitally important to know your limits and when you need to ask for help. Here are a few other resources from the 988 National Suicide and Crisis Lifeline, the National Alliance on Mental Illness, and the Substance Abuse and Mental Health Services Administration:

- 988: https://www.fcc.gov/988-suicide-and-crisis-lifeline
- NAMI: https://www.nami.org/Home
- SAMHSA: https://www.samhsa.gov/

Read on for an innovative and alternative approach to thinking about and managing stress.

# THE IMPACT OF MINDSET ON STRESS

Is it possible that stress is actually not bad for us? Could it be positively channeled for a different impact? New information has recently become available that suggests that not all of the effects of stress can be categorized as detrimental. Stress does not necessarily have to be viewed as the enemy. And it is not always a negative antidote to adequate human performance. Many people report feeling as though they are more effective in getting things done when they have too much to do or are down to the wire on a timeline.

There is developing research about mindset, the positive effects of stress, and enhanced performance secondary to a healthy dose of stress in a variety of situations and settings. Mindset science is emerging, and one of the best-known young researchers is Dr. Alia Crum, whose work at Columbia University in New York was revolutionary. Her research focused on how changes in subjective mindsets—the lenses through which information is perceived, organized, and interpreted—can alter objective reality through behavioral, psychological, and physiological mechanisms. Her work is, in part, inspired by research on the placebo effect, a notable and consistent demonstration of the ability of the mindset to elicit healing properties in the body (GoodThink, Inc., 2015).

Dr. Crum has continued her work in her position as an Associate Professor at Stanford University and is interested in understanding how mindsets affect important outcomes outside the realm of medicine, in the domains of behavioral health and organizational behavior. More specifically, Crum aims to understand how mindsets can be consciously and deliberately changed through intervention to affect organizational and individual performance, physiological behavior and well-being, as well as interpersonal effectiveness (GoodThink, Inc., 2015; Stanford University, n.d.).

You can see a video here of Crum explaining how to "change your mindset, change the game": https://www.youtube.com/watch?v=0tqq66zwa7g.

Could there be a gap in healthcare and healthcare professionals related to mindset? Do healthcare providers have the right thinking about harnessing stress in order to do good in the world in inherently stressful environments? Were they adequately prepared in their formal education programs about how to leverage the consequences of stress? Could their thinking be reframed?

In Crum's revolutionary research, she utilized samples of regular people and showed drastic changes of improvement in mindset based on the very same circumstances. Her experiments were designed to show results only secondary to a change in mindset, with no other behavioral or lifestyle changes.

There is the potential if nurses and other healthcare providers could change their mindset, they could decrease stress, fatigue, and the potential to burn out. Similarly, world-class adventurers adopt a "no-barriers" mindset; this type of mindset encourages community thinking by sharing ideas to achieve challenging goals (Rowden-Racette, 2013). A day in a nurse's or other healthcare provider's life is often like an extreme adventure: fraught with unpredictability, uncertainty, and inherent stress. Doing difficult things can challenge your beliefs, and this often requires a change in your mindset in order to be successful. The global COVID-19 pandemic tested everyone's ability to change their mindset. What we all knew as normal was upended in a matter of days, weeks, or months depending on your profession and geographic setting. Creating a "new" normal as the pandemic wanes over the last three-plus years has not been easy. Many things are still uncertain. Many things and people that we knew and loved are gone. Other things that we don't really like may be here to stay. So, how do we cope? Changing our mindset, accepting the lack of control, and building hardiness will all lead to increased resilience in the face of adversity.

Mindset is also interconnected with quality and safety. If quality is inherent to doing good work, and healthcare providers want to do good work, why does healthcare not have better results? Sherwood and Zomorodi (2014) described the new science of quality and safety shifting away from the prevailing models focused on individual action to a focus on team and system improvements. They also recognized the need for changes in how nurses are educated (trained thinking) to meet the new practice demands. The same could be said for other healthcare disciplines. For example, the Quality and Safety Education for Nurses' (QSEN) six areas of competency include knowledge, skills, and attitudinal competencies woven into them.

The QSEN competencies encompass all of nursing practice: patient-centered care, teamwork and collaboration, evidence-based practice, quality improvement, safety, and informatics (Sherwood & Zomorodi, 2014). Full engagement and proactive inquiry to develop safe practices are evidenced by a mindset of mindfulness and focused attention. Nurses, as well as other healthcare providers, need to have a calm and confident demeanor or mindset as described by Robotham (2014). This mindset entails learning mind-changing or brain-transformation skills that result in greater mental clarity, physical vitality, and whole-of-life balance.

In the book *The Upside of Stress,* McGonical (2015) outlined how stress might actually be good for us and explains how people can get good at using it. Also in 2015, Epstein reminded us that correlation does not imply causation. This is a fundamental lesson in psychology, and violating this principle can lead to serious misconceptions and maybe even dangerous practices. It is easy to draw incorrect conclusions about the causes of stress and the resulting consequences.

Hall (2015) described six phases to discovering the upside of stress:

1. Be honest about self-talk (acknowledge it, accept it, and move on).
2. Catch it before it starts (identify the stress early).
3. Reframe challenges as opportunities (a change in mindset).
4. Think about what works and does not work for you (identify triggers).
5. Change your surroundings (make lifestyle or work-related changes).
6. Ask for help (use available resources).

In addition to the personal consequences of stress, professional penalties may surface. Misperceptions of attitude or capability or incorrect assumptions about motives may limit work-related opportunities. Generally, people like to work with other people they know and like and who are similar to them. Fitting into the right organizational culture and being perceived as positive, enthusiastic, and competent is far better than being seen as negative, burned out, and questionably competent.

Many of the prevalent and most significant health-related conditions today's workers suffer are not caused solely by workplace hazards but result from a combination of work and non-work factors. These include genetics, age, gender, chronic disease, obesity, smoking, alcohol use, and prescription drug use (Schulte et al., 2015). Nurses and others in healthcare must consider the individual and organizational impact of stressful work. Only then can effective strategies be designed to mitigate the consequences of stress.

## PRACTICE PEARLS

- Study the effects of stress, both positive and negative.
- Assess yourself on the Perceived Stress Scale (10 items) at https://www.mindgarden.com/documents/PerceivedStressScale.pdf.
- Learn more about mindfulness-based stress reduction (MBSR) at http://www.umassmed.edu/cfm/stress-reduction.
- Find mindfulness meditation tools with Dr. Jon Kabat-Zinn at http://www.mindfulnesscds.com.
- Review the cutting-edge research by Dr. Richie Davidson, who says that well-being is a skill, and the more we understand ourselves and our emotions, the more we can do to create a kinder, wiser, more compassionate world: http://www.investigatinghealthyminds.org.

- You can read more about Davidson's latest work in global healthcare here: https://centerhealthyminds.org/news/new-research-grant-explores-programs-to-improve-the-well-being-of-healthcare-professionals-in-mexico.
- And don't forget to have fun—life is short, and it seems to pick up speed as we age.

---

# CONCLUSION

What if the stress in nursing and healthcare could be reframed and harnessed as positive? What if we could become "superhero-like" stress-proof and hardy practitioners? Could people be trained in hardiness as a buffer for stress to become more resilient? Could the challenges in the work environment be viewed differently, and thus reduce the feelings of stress, fatigue, and burnout?

A positive view of stress could possibly change our perceptions of the work environment. If nurses and other healthcare providers did not interpret the daily stress in the same way, there may be less resulting fatigue and the propensity to burnout. This radical change in thinking is monumental but may just be what healthcare now needs most. This isn't to say that the systems driving much of the stress should be ignored—they also need to be fixed.

Healthy living is certainly an intentional choice. Not an easy choice at times, but it is a choice. There are many factors in our control, especially with lifestyle related choices. This means everything from chosen vocation, geographic area to live, type of living situation, type of work, work location, relationships, exercise, diet, sleep, and more. Placing a higher priority on yourself and your overall health, with a more reasonable work-life balance, yields a much more satisfying life.

# REFERENCES

American Holistic Nurses Association. (2018). *About us.* https://www.ahna.org/About-Us/What-is-Holistic-Nursing

Bartone, P. T., & Stein, S. J. (2020, March 9). Build "hardiness" into your organizational culture. *Harvard Business Review.* https://hbr.org/2020/03/build-hardiness-into-your-organizational-culture

Centers for Disease Control and Prevention. (n.d.). *Sleep and health.* https://www.cdc.gov/healthyschools/sleep.htm#:~:text=Children%20and%20adolescents%20who%20do,poor%20mental%20health%2C%20and%20injuries.&text=They%20are%20also%20more%20likely,poor%20academic%20performance%20in%20school

Ceridian HCM, Inc. (2019). *What's the real cost of burnout in the healthcare workforce?* https://www.ceridian.com/blog/cost-of-burnout-healthcare-workforce

Cooper, A. L., Brown, J. A., Rees, C. S., & Leslie, G. D. (2020). Nurse resilience: A concept analysis. *International Journal of Mental Health Nursing, 29*(4), 553–575. https://doi.org/10.1111/inm.12721

Dictionary.com. (2022). *Hardiness definition.* https://www.dictionary.com/browse/hardiness

DuVal, M. (2009). *Mindfulness based stress reduction handbook.* The Mindful Center.

Epstein, R. (2015, July 1). MIND reviews "The upside of stress." *Scientific American, 26*(4). http://www.scientificamerican.com/article/mind-reviews-the-upside-of-stress

Foureur et al. (2013). Enhancing the resilience of nurses and midwives: Pilot of a mindfulness-based program for increased health, sense of coherence and decreased depression, anxiety and stress. *Contemporary Nurse, 45*(1), 114-125.

GoodThink, Inc. (2015). *Dr. Alia Crum* [Biographical sketch]. http://goodthinkinc.com/speaking/alia-crum

Gurkov, E., Harakova, S., Dzuka, J., & Ziakova, K. (2014). Job satisfaction and subjective well-being among Czech nurses. *International Journal of Nursing Practice, 20*(2), 194–203. https://doi.org/10.1111/ijn.12133

Hall, A. (2015, February 2, updated 2017, December 6). *6 simple steps to discovering the upside of stress.* Huffpost. http://www.huffingtonpost.com/2015/02/02/turn-bad-stress-into-good-stress_n_6524954.html

Hardy, S. (2015). Mindfulness: Enhancing physical and mental well-being. *Practice Nursing, 26*(9), 450–453. https://doi.org/10.12968/pnur.2015.26.9.450

Jean, J. Y. (2022, August 29). Why nurses need more mental health days. *NurseJournal.* https://nursejournal.org/articles/why-nurses-need-more-mental-health-days/

Jeste, D. V., & Oswald, A. J. (2014). Individual and societal wisdom: Explaining the paradox of human aging and high well-being. *Psychiatry: Interpersonal & Biologic Processes, 77*(4), 317–330. https://doi.org/10.1521/psyc_2014_77_3_1

Kabat-Zinn, J. (2013). *Full catastrophe living: Using the wisdom of your body and mind to face stress, pain and illness.* Random House.

Kay, M. F. (2017, November 7). Resilience is a mindset of awareness and practice. *Forbes.* https://www.forbes.com/sites/michaelkay/2017/11/07/resilience-awareness-practice/?sh=41e5779a775b

Lamothe, M., Rondeau, E., Malboeuf-Hurtubise, C., Duval, M., & Sultan, S. (2015, November 27). Outcomes of MBSR or MBSR-based interventions in healthcare providers: A systematic review with a focus on empathy and emotional competencies. *Complimentary Therapies in Medicine, 24*, 19–28. https://doi.org/10.1016/j.ctim.2015.11.001

Learning Mind. (2022). *10 negative coping mechanisms people use to hide from their problems.* https://www.learning-mind.com/coping-mechanisms/

Lejtenyi, P. (2019, August 27). *Stress and screen time are closely connected, new Concordia research shows.* Concorida University. https://www.concordia.ca/news/stories/2019/08/27/stress-and-screen-time-are-closely-connected-new-concordia-research-shows.html

Loehr, J., & Schwartz, T. (2003). *The power of full engagement: Managing energy, not time, is the key to high performance and personal renewal.* Free Press.

Maslach, C., & Leiter, M. P. (2005). Reversing burnout: How to rekindle your passion for your work. *Stanford Social Innovation Review*, 43–49. http://ssir.org/articles/entry/reversing_burnout

McCloskey, S., & Taggart, L. (2010). How much compassion have I left? An exploration of occupational stress among children's palliative care nurses. *International Journal of Palliative Nursing, 16*(5), 233–240. https://doi.org/10.12968/ijpn.2010.16.5.48144

McGonical, K. (2015). *The upside of stress: Why stress is good for you, and how to get good at it.* Penguin Books.

Merriam-Webster. (n.d.). Well-being. In *Merriam-Webster.com dictionary.* http://www.merriam-webster.com/dictionary/well-being

National Council of State Boards of Nursing. (2020). *National Nursing Workforce Study.* https://www.ncsbn.org/research/recent-research/workforce.page

Psychology Today. (2022). *Positive psychology.* https://www.psychologytoday.com/us/basics/positive-psychology

Robotham, J. (2014). How to create a calm and confident mindset. *Australian Nursing & Midwifery Journal, 22*(4), 30.

Rowden-Racette, K. (2013). The no-barriers mindset. *ASHA Leader, 18*(10), 56–57.

Schoormans, D., & Nyklicek, I. (2011). Mindfulness and psychologic well-being: Are they related to type of meditation technique practiced? *The Journal of Alternative and Complementary Medicine, 17*(7), 629–634. https://doi.org/10.1089/acm.2010.0332

Schulte, P. A., Guerin, R. J., Schill, A. L., Bhattacharya, A., Cunningham, T. R., Pandalai, S. P., Eggerth, D., & Stephenson, C. M. (2015). Considerations for incorporating "well-being" in public policy for workers and workplaces. *American Journal of Public Health, 105*(8), e31–e44. https://doi.org/10.2105/AJPH.2015.302616

Seligman, M. E. P. (2011). *Flourish: A visionary new understanding of happiness and well-being.* Free Press.

Sherwood, G., & Zomorodi, M. (2014). A new mindset for quality and safety: The QSEN competencies redefine nurses' role in practice. *The Journal of Nursing Administration, 41*(10), S10–S18.

Smith, S. A. (2014). Mindfulness-based stress reduction: An intervention to enhance the effectiveness of nurses' coping with work-related stress. *International Journal of Nursing, 25*(2), 119–130. https://www.jstor.org/stable/26813186

Sovold, L. E., Naslund, J. A., Kousoulis, A. A., Saxena, S., Qoronfleh, M. W., Grobler, C., & Munter. L. (2021, May 7). Prioritizing the mental health and well-being of healthcare workers: An urgent global public health priority. *Frontiers in Public Health, 9*(679397).

Stanford University. (n.d.). *Alia Crum.* https://profiles.stanford.edu/alia-crum

UMass Memorial Health Center for Mindfulness. (2014). *History of MBSR.* http://www.umassmed.edu/cfm/stress-reduction/history-of-mbsr/

Waddill-Goad, S. (2013, December). *The development of a leadership fatigue questionnaire* [Dissertation, American Sentinel University].

White, L. (2013). Mindfulness in nursing: An evolutionary concept analysis. *Journal of Advanced Nursing, 70*(2), 282–294. https://doi.org/10.1111/jan.12182

Wylie, M. S. (2015, January 29). How the mindfulness movement went mainstream—and the backlash that came with it. *AlterNet, Psychotherapy Networker.* https://www.alternet.org/2015/01/how-mindfulness-movement-went-mainstream-and-backlash-came-it/

# 11

# BURNOUT AND THE NURSING OR HEALTHCARE STUDENT

## OBJECTIVES

- Define academic burnout and its components.
- Discuss the impact of burnout in all healthcare students.
- Review the data related to burnout in all healthcare students.
- Explore the impact of burnout from a student perspective.
- Determine the consequences of prolonged burnout.
- Consider practical solutions to decrease burnout in healthcare students.

The last semester of a nursing program, or any program related to healthcare, should be a time when students are looking forward to starting their career. However, in the current healthcare environment, students are questioning their choice of careers. Academic burnout, and its relation to clinical experiences, is one reason for this ambivalence. *Academic burnout* is defined as a psychological symptom associated with excessive academic burden and ongoing academic stress (Hwang & Kim, 2022).

## ACADEMIC BURNOUT IN NURSING STUDENTS

Hwang and Kim (2022) identified the components of academic burnout related to nursing students. These components may apply to all other types of healthcare students as well. Components of academic burnout include:

- Apathy
- Incompetence
- Emotional exhaustion

### APATHY

In the context of academic burnout, *apathy* is a cynical and detached attitude toward study. This can occur when students are not able to take the information presented and put it into context. Students are given an exorbitant amount of information in any academic program yet are unable to "put it all together" in a more practical sense. Students are used to memorizing information to pass exams, and they frequently struggle to apply the knowledge. Application of knowledge in a clinical setting is where education meets applicable practice.

## INCOMPETENCE

Academic incompetence may manifest itself in many forms. A student may have failed an exam, committed an error in a simulation, or simply answered a question incorrectly in class. When required to complete a case study or participate in an in-class simulation, the student may be unable to "piece the puzzle" together utilizing critical thinking. Unfortunately, this may lead a student to develop an "I don't care" or "What is the use?" mindset versus one of taking responsibility for their own learning.

## EMOTIONAL EXHAUSTION

Emotional exhaustion is present in many instances and may result from a plethora of sources. More often than not, students are also working, may have family obligations or other drivers of stress, and are taking classes that demand time both in the classroom and clinical setting. Competing priorities force students to try to juggle all the responsibilities in their life. It can lead to feelings of stress, fatigue, becoming overwhelmed, not being a success at any one of the competing priorities, and burnout. It is crucial that students master skills in prioritization; once they enter the healthcare workforce, the balancing act doesn't become any easier with competing work and life priorities.

## STUDENT BURNOUT SYNDROME

Albuquerque et al. (2021) defined *student burnout syndrome* as emotional stress related to academic demands and direct contact with other human beings. They also identified two other components: depersonalization and low personal accomplishment.

*Depersonalization* can be compared to the emotional exhaustion identified by Hwang and Kim (2022). Students have an insensitivity to those that they are closest to and often feel that those around them do not understand the rigor and time demands of their academic obligations. Thus, students limit their communication with those they feel do not understand their circumstances and consequently neglect those relationships.

*Low personal accomplishment* includes feelings of inadequacy related to academics along with low self-esteem (Albuquerque et al., 2021). Limited communication with only those who share the student's frustration (peers) can provide some synergy and validation to the student's frustration, and this also eliminates feeling like they are alone in their perception of the stress. Nursing programs, in particular, are based on a required progression from one course to the next to be successful in a program. If a student fails a course, they are not able to continue in the program and may have to wait an entire calendar year until that course is offered again. This puts a great deal of stress on the student to be successful. Thus, an underlying fear of failing can be found in many students in nursing and other healthcare programs.

*Burnout* has been defined as previously described by Maslach and Leiter (2016) as being a psychological syndrome in response to prolonged stress over time, without relief, and includes feelings of emotional exhaustion, insufficiency, and detachment from work. The symptoms of burnout have been studied in healthcare professionals in the work setting during the last couple of decades. More recently, it has been suggested that burnout is now prevalent and rising in the nursing student population (Wei et al., 2021).

Often, students are working in the healthcare industry while attending nursing or other healthcare programs. For example, students may be practicing licensed practical nurses, nurse aides, or paramedics. Due to their non-school-related occupation, students who are working in healthcare may suffer from a degree of professional burnout along with academic burnout. This presents a recipe for disaster because burnout from dual sources many only escalate the signs and symptoms.

Healthcare students often witness conflict between their chosen education program versus their work environment. There may be differing approaches in policy and practice. There is also often a gap between what the student learns in school based on evidence compared to actual practices they observe in the clinical setting. The student can be disillusioned by what they are taught compared to what they see as being practiced in the "real world" by nurses and other healthcare providers.

If burnout goes unidentified in academic programs, it may place students at an increased risk for work-related stress and professional burnout in their new career (Wei et al., 2021). Given this, nursing along with other healthcare programmatic leaders should consider the impact of burnout on both the academic and professional levels for students.

In the spring of 2022, a graduating class of 53 nursing students in a community college's associate degree program was asked to complete the Maslach Burnout Survey prior to graduation from the program. Several students chose to study the impact of burnout and the associated consequences in their final project for the course, "Transition to Practice." The survey identified the degree of burnout based on 22 questions, which were placed into three categories: occupational exhaustion, depersonalization, and personal accomplishment. Those categories were broken down further into low, moderate, and high degrees of burnout within each category. The results of the survey were revealing and simultaneously disheartening (see Figure 11.1).

Fifty-one percent of respondents reported suffering from a high degree and 36% a moderate degree of occupational exhaustion. Only 13% reported a low degree. Depersonalization also affected a majority of the students: 40% reported experiencing a high degree and 36% a moderate degree. In terms of personal accomplishment, only 4% said they felt a high degree of personal accomplishment and 21% a moderate degree. An astounding 75% of those surveyed felt a low degree of sense of accomplishment.

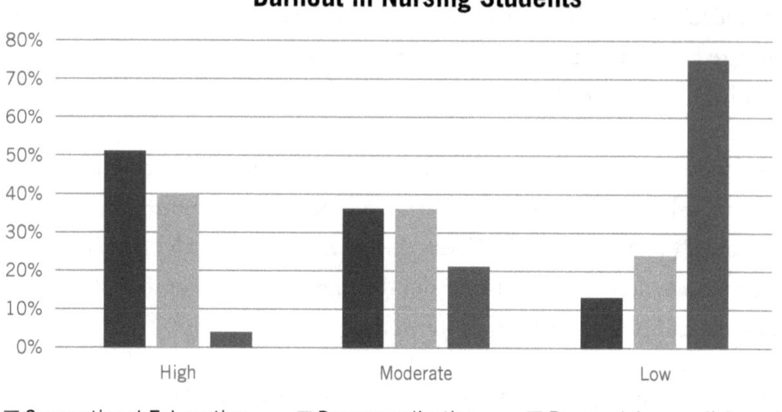


**FIGURE 11.1** Burnout in nursing students.

Based on these results, Albuquerque et al.'s (2021) academic burnout component of low personal accomplishment became glaring. The degree of burnout, when combined with low personal accomplishment, has an additional impact on the individual and may cause them to ultimately question their career choice.

## PRACTICE PEARLS (FOR ACADEMIC AND HEALTHCARE INSTITUTIONS)

- Have a credible measurement tool in place to identify burnout in nursing and healthcare students.
- Develop "destress" resources for students to access throughout their program.
- Conduct periodic program reviews to identify ways to assess and decrease stress.
- Implement stress management and resilience skills throughout nursing programs.

- Eliminate the historical practice of nurses (in particular) "eating their young."
- Offer multiple methods for stress relief through colleges (for students) and employers (for employees) that are accessible and at no cost.
- Decrease the stigma attached to mental health diagnoses and treatment.

---

# FACTORS THAT CONTRIBUTE TO STUDENT BURNOUT

Healthcare students, particularly nursing students, have the desire to help people. They feel a distinct "calling" to become a member of the healthcare community. The giving of oneself is a noble endeavor, while at the same time it can be destructive if one gives too much.

Reith (2018) looked at the history of burnout and discussed its origins. Burnout was originally defined (Reith, 2018) by the psychologist Freudenberger in 1974 as "exhaustion that resulted from excessive demands in the workplace." Freudenberger worked in a free clinic in a drug-ridden area of New York city. He noticed the effects of long hours and the impact it had on the people who worked alongside him in the clinic. They seemed to work more and more hours but accomplished less and less. They became short-tempered and cried easily, and over time they lost friends and their relationships suffered.

Nursing students frequently share experiencing similar symptoms with faculty and peers. The loss of social experiences and time with their family and friends impacts students' well-being. They verbalize that they study more, for longer hours, and cover the material presented over and over. Yet, some are not successful in courses and are required to repeat them to be able to complete their program of choice. Many programs allow a specific number of attempts for a course. If a student is not ultimately successful, they are not able to continue. This forces them to seek other programs to complete their modified career trajectory or alter their career path altogether.

## THE CHALLENGE OF TOO MANY DEMANDS

Students in healthcare programs are often juggling many different obligations and may suffer from the symptoms noticed by Freudenberger. The symptoms include frustration, malaise, cynicism, fatigue, and inefficiency (Reith, 2018). Many nursing students, in particular, work part- or full-time, have families, and are attending school on a part- or full-time basis. During the COVID-19 pandemic, many were mandated additional hours at their places of work, which limited their amount of time for study. Students also witnessed the helplessness and inability of nurses and other care providers to care for patients as they feel they should.

To combat the multidirectional "pulls" felt by students, instructors, preceptors, and peers, each needs to realize that communication is key; this is especially important as academic and clinical demands are expected to increase in any given course (especially in the latter days of education) depending on the schedule and planning. It's easy to look at a syllabus and course schedule one assignment or one obligation at a time, which is what many students have done to survive and achieve in past endeavors. However, instructors should spend more time at the beginning of a course to review the syllabus and identify increased times of intensity or rigor. Students should be encouraged to have open dialogue with their social support network and significant others about what the future will bring. Populating a shared calendar, on paper or via electronic means, may be helpful to avoid conflict, gain collective support from those who may not be aware of how healthcare students must learn, and allow the proper time for practice to achieve clinical and operational excellence.

## CLINICAL ROTATIONS DURING COVID-19

During the global COVID-19 pandemic, nursing and other healthcare students were exposed to a higher rate of mortality than had been witnessed in the past. Exposure to work-related stress on a personal level and observed in their peers severely impacted the students beyond their education experience. They also were exposed to COVID-19, cared for family members that contracted COVID-19, and/or contracted the COVID-19 virus themselves. This rendered many students unable to work, thus limiting their income. This compounded their stress and added to the symptoms of burnout.

In addition to the work and personal experiences with the COVID-19 pandemic, students also had their program experiences altered significantly. Time spent at the bedside decreased. Students were transitioned quickly from the traditional classroom with clinical experience to an online environment. This only exacerbated the level of stress that students had experienced previous to the COVID-19 pandemic. Further stressors were added as the pandemic languished, controversy surrounding mandates of the COVID vaccine ensued, and reliable guidance from government sources was questioned. Many students, when returned to the clinical setting, did not want to take the vaccine. This put their program completion in jeopardy. Students verbalized frustration over the unending stress surrounding constant change with few solid and reliable answers.

The clinical setting is another area where students not only witness the impact of burnout but may become secondary victims. Nursing and other healthcare students are generally assigned clinical instructors and, in some courses, preceptors in the clinical setting. Clinical instructors are hired on a per diem basis and often work in a clinical setting at the bedside. The instructors have a desire to pass on information to assist the students in their success as future nurses or other types of clinicians. Clinical groups assigned to an instructor may include up to 10 students each. The students are also free to interact with staff in the clinical unit they have been assigned.

In some cases, the units use the students to answer call lights, provide personal care, or perform simple procedures for patients, and they come to rely on the extra help. Often, the students remark that they are performing nurse aide work and are not learning anything pertaining to nursing practice. However, much can be learned by providing personal care to a patient. This allows time for listening to patient concerns; the care provider may assess clinical and functional status; they can educate a patient regarding their diagnosis and treatment; engage a patient in their care plan, etc. The clinical instructor is responsible for the oversight of students and often finds themselves needed in multiple places at once, thus limiting the total learning experience for all the students.

In a different clinical model, a preceptor and clinical instructor are assigned to the student. The preceptor has oversight of the student with the clinical instructor being responsible for the education requirements of the college. This model can be much more advantageous for the clinical site, as it may feed the pipeline for future nurse hires. It is also a great learning experience for nurse preceptors and for the student. Students are able to witness what a practicing nurse does—throughout an entire shift. The student may acquire their own preceptor or be assigned by the school or organization where their clinical rotation or experience is assigned. It is crucial for both that they are a "match" to work together. They must build rapport and learn to trust one another.

It is best when the preceptor has some specialized training about how to work with students. Students need a supportive individual to "show them the ropes" who has a positive attitude and is an excellent practitioner. Students don't want to feel they are a burden to the assigned preceptor but an equal learning partner. At times, there are miscommunications about who can and should be assigned as a preceptor, which may cause students to feel unwanted. It is the department's leadership who must outline the process for assigning students to learn in their unit.

Clearly, some people are not cut out to be a preceptor for helping others learn. And students don't want to feel they are being taken advantage of or not learn what they need to accomplish for their academic requirements. The learning environment needs to be inclusive and comfortable. If a staff member is overburdened, they should not be assigned to precept new employees or students. Leaders in both academia and practice need to take responsibility and accountability for the preceptor-student-new employee system of learning to prevent feelings of low personal accomplishment for all parties, as identified by Albuquerque et al. (2021). Simple system design can prevent potential conflict.

## FACULTY BURNOUT

The final area of burnout that may impact students is that of healthcare faculty burnout. Thomas et al. (2019) conducted a literature review looking at the causes of nursing faculty burnout. They identified interpersonal relationships, professional stress, and incivility from peers as well as students. One study indicated that peer-to-peer incivility occurred 80% of the time. Student to faculty incivility may have a lasting impact, leading to faculty resignations and retirements. This is not unlike their counterparts who work in practice.

Nursing faculty are somewhat more difficult to replace due to the high education requirements and lower salary. New faculty with a master's degree may have a starting salary of $70,000 per year, while a nurse practitioner, with the same degree, may start at $95,000 per year or more. Salary discrepancies only add to the level of burnout experienced by faculty, which is mostly related to how they feel they are valued (or not).

### PRACTICE PEARLS

- Educate nursing and healthcare students on the impact of burnout in their formal academic programs.
- Provide education on the impact of burnout in orientation programs.
- Review a course syllabus and study/practice implications in class and with social support networks to communicate when acuity/intensity of study and time requirements will ebb and peak during a course.
- Encourage educators in the clinical setting to evaluate their personal level of burnout and impact on students.
- Advocate for more salary equity with the level of required education at all levels.

# STACKED BURNOUT

In a consensus study published by the National Academy of Medicine (NAM, 2019), personal consequences related to burnout were identified from both a student and professional perspective. Burnout in students may be associated with less-than-optimal clinical experiences, poor support, grading rules, and behavior of peers and instructors. Other personal impacts, according to the study, may include injury in the clinical setting, problematic substance use, and the increased risk for suicide (NAM, 2019). These factors have an impact on the professional development of a student and the subsequent transition to a novice clinician.

Rudman et al. (2020) reported that burnout symptoms were identified by 20% of newly graduated nurses, with 27% of them intending to leave the profession after the first year and 45% after three years. Reith (2018) noted that the consequences of early burnout in nursing lead to an increase in hospital-acquired infections, reduced patient safety, and increased mortality. Rudman et al. (2020) looked at symptoms surrounding burnout in a group of nurses who were early in their career. One of the symptoms was that of cognition problems. Clear cognition is essential in critical thinking and clinical reasoning, which lead to an increase in positive patient outcomes and decrease in failure to rescue. Physicians and other providers were also identified as victims of burnout by Reith (2018). Reith termed these providers as being unhappy and demoralized.

In looking at the consequences of burnout over time, it is important to consider all aspects of the healthcare continuum. According to the Consensus Study Report (National Academy of Medicine, 2019), personal consequences of burnout may include risk for suicide (specifically among learners), occupational injury, and an increase in alcohol abuse. Regret of career choice and less than optimal professional development were also identified.

# SUICIDE PREVENTION

The National Institute of Mental Health identified suicide as the 10th leading cause of death in 2019 (McGuinness, 2021). McGuinness (2021) also cited previous studies by Davidson et al. reporting female nurses have a significantly higher rate of suicide than other women. Patrician et al. found the same for men in nursing having a higher likelihood of suicide than in the general population.

## ONE NURSE'S STORY

A recently shared example of stacking the symptoms of burnout from nursing school to career highlights the dire consequences. A young nurse recently took on the role of house supervisor in a small, rural hospital. The nurse had graduated from nursing school just prior to the COVID-19 pandemic. She had worked on a medical-surgical unit throughout the pandemic and was offered the house supervisor position. The schedule worked better for her as she was enrolled in an RN to MSN program with the goal of becoming a nurse practitioner at a clinic in her community.

Shortly after taking on the new role, the nurse's peers noticed she was losing weight. When asked about her recent weight loss, she commented that it was intentional to get in better health. The weight loss became more pronounced, and when questioned, she told her friends that she was just really busy and often "forgot to eat." As time went on, the nurse became more withdrawn, and her peers noticed she was "not herself." Her peers asked if she was OK and were reassured that she was fine.

One morning she did not show up for her shift and did not answer her phone. The police were called for a welfare check. When they arrived at her home, she was found unresponsive. She died shortly after arriving at the hospital. She had overdosed on insulin, knowing that most people would not figure out soon enough to reverse the effects, if she was found. The note she left behind outlined the stress that she could no longer manage. The death and despair of her patients, prolonged work hours, and the effects on her peers became unbearable. This is just one story. How many more are there?

Guille (2021) in the context of the COVID-19 pandemic stated that the highest level of psychological distress was found in nurses, female workers, frontline workers, and younger medical staff. Those who had higher work-family conflict were also identified as being at higher risk for burnout, depression, and leaving their chosen profession. Guille (2021) also noted that suicide among nurses exceeded that of the general population, and female nurses were at twice the risk of those in the general population. According to Lee and Friese (2021), female nurses are not only twice as likely to die by suicide over women in the general population, but they are 70% more likely than a female physician to die by suicide.

### PRACTICE PEARLS

- Burnout has lasting effects across the continuum.
- Efforts to combat burnout need to be addressed beginning within education programs.
- Share your challenges with others and don't hide your problems.
- Remember it is OK to ask for help when feeling overwhelmed.

## CONCLUSION

Healthcare education, particularly in nursing, has a tremendous challenge to combat the symptoms of burnout and the subsequent consequences if left untreated. The global pandemic brought many untoward subjects to the forefront. Many of the subjects most likely would have remained in the dark related to stress and its impact on the mental and physical well-being of students, nurses, and other healthcare providers. Organizations and individuals must be willing to come together with a collective voice to combat burnout. We must end the devastating consequences of daily stressors to our professions. The healthcare industry must address how the work environment negatively impacts the lives of those we love and care about. An unknown author said it best: "Decisions will be made for you if you are not in the room." Nurses and other healthcare providers need to pull up a chair now more than ever.

# REFERENCES

Albuquerque, R. N., Barbosa, A. F., & Pacheco, G. B. F. (2021). Burnout syndrome in nursing students. *Cuidado é Fundamental, 13,* 1596–1602. https://doi.org/10.9789/2175-5361.rpcfo.v13.10547

Guille, C. (2021). Rate of suicide among women nurses compared with women in the general population before the COVID-19 global pandemic. *JAMA Psychiatry*, *78*(6), 597–598. https://doi.org/10.1001/jamapsychiatry.2021.0141

Hwang, E., & Kim, J. (2022). Factors affecting academic burnout of nursing students according to clinical practice. *BMC Medical Education*, *22*(346). https://doi.org/10.1186/s12909-022-03422-7

McGuinness, M. (2021). *Suicide: A dark cloud over nursing.* AACN. https://www.aacn.org/blog/suicide-a-dark-cloud-over-nursing

National Academies of Sciences, Engineering, and Medicine. (2019). *Taking action against clinician burnout: A systems approach to professional well-being.* The National Academies Press. https://doi.org/10.17226/25521

Reith, T. P. (2018, December 4). Burnout in United States healthcare professionals: A narrative review. *Cureus, 10*(12), e3681. https://doi.org/10.7759/cureus.3681

Rudman, A., Arborelius, L., Dahlgren, A., Finnes, A., & Gustavsson, P. (2020). Consequences of early career nurse burnout: A prospective long-term follow-up on cognitive functions, depressive symptoms, and insomnia. *The Lancet,* 27. https://papers.ssrn.com/sol3/papers.cfm?abstract_id=3627244

Thomas, C., Bantz, D. & McIntosh, C. (2019). Nurse faculty burnout and strategies to avoid it. *Teaching and Learning in Nursing, 14,* 111-116. https://doi.org/10.1016/j.teln.2018.12.005

Wei, H., Dorn, A., Hutto, H., Webb Corbett, R., Haberstroh, A., & Larson, K. (2021). Impacts of nursing student burnout on psychological well-being and academic achievement. *Journal of Nursing Education, 60*(7), 369–376. https://doi.org/10.3928/01484834-20210616-02

# 12

# LOOKING TOWARD THE FUTURE

## OBJECTIVES

- Explore how to succeed as a nurse or other healthcare provider in the rapidly changing landscape of healthcare.
- Consider how increasing your education and knowledge or learning new skills has the potential to increase your job satisfaction.
- Learn how technology advances your professional goals.
- Look realistically at how stress affects your job and your life.
- Understand that a career change is not a failure.

Every nurse and healthcare provider should be familiar with the Institute of Medicine's (IOM) 2010 report, *The Future of Nursing: Leading Change, Advancing Health.* This report was generated as a response to the recognized need to transform the profession of nursing. Four key messages were identified in the report (IOM, 2010):

- Nurses should practice to the full extent of their education and training.
- Nurses should achieve higher levels of education through a seamless system.
- Nurses should become equal partners with all members of the healthcare team to redesign healthcare in the United States.
- Data collection and information systems should improve to support policy-making and workforce planning.

It's now been more than a decade since this report was written. How much has really changed? The most radical changes came as a result of the global COVID-19 pandemic. Recently retired practitioners were recalled, the Great Resignation of those currently practicing began, students were banned from entry at their clinical learning sites (drastically changing their learning experience), and more. The first writings of this text (in 2015, for a 2016 release) have only been exacerbated by what has happened since that time. Are healthcare settings any less stressful? Not likely, and in fact, I think it has only worsened.One of the same questions remain unanswered: Could implementation of the recommendations in this text radically change the practice of nursing and healthcare to decrease stress, fatigue, and the potential for burnout? The only way for nurses and other healthcare providers to know is to do something different than before. Each person practicing in healthcare must learn where change can make a difference and take action.

# SAVING THE NURSING AND HEALTHCARE WORKFORCE

To consider how practice might change to allow nurses to work at the height of their license, and for companies to begin encouraging higher education, we first need to consider if there are—and will be—enough nurses in the workforce to create space for such improvements.

Even before the COVID-19 pandemic, the US Bureau of Labor Statistics (2022) projected that the employment of registered nurses will grow 9% from 2020 to 2030, providing approximately 195,000 jobs. Most likely, this number has grown due to the number of nurses leaving both the bedside and healthcare.

In 2021, hospitals lost 2.47% of their bedside nursing workforce, and the turnover rate for staff nurses increased by 8.4% (compared to 2020); turnover currently stands at 27.1% on average (Colosi, 2022). This loss of nurses, exposed by Colosi (2022) in a report of hospitals from 32 states, results in the average hospital losing between $5.2 million to $9.0 million per year in turnover costs (each RN at ~$46k). In general, experts agree the reasons nurses are leaving include feeling burned out, unappreciated, or not valued; low wages (many left to pursue more lucrative traveling nurse jobs); and feeling "locked in" due to diminished opportunities for growth. Many other professions provide more flexibility to create a better balance between work and personal responsibilities. In addition, the average lead time or "time to fill" to recruit and onboard an experienced RN is 87 days—essentially three months (Colosi, 2022). Historically, RN turnover has trended below the hospital average.

Abating this evident exodus will require creativity, flexibility, and probably even some humility on the side of employers. Becker's Hospital Review reported efforts in 2021 that included wage increases and appreciation bonuses, referral bonuses, pay-on-demand (pay received following worked shifts), retention bonuses, financial academic assistance, and even housing assistance where costs of living were exponentially increasing (Plescia & Gooch, 2021). These transactional efforts have proven to be a variable utility in the past; however, longer-term, engaging solutions are needed. Two strategies nurses and all healthcare providers in every role can help move forward are: 1) restoring a sense of mission and purpose; and 2) ensuring a safe, supportive, and positive culture across and between all hierarchies in the organization.

Creating a new or reinvigorating an old purpose begins with employers being transparent about how the work is being done by individuals, groups, and departments. Who is benefitting from that work is key. With this transparency must come two-way dialogue that enables, empowers, and responds to the voice(s) of the workforce just like the voice of the customer. The platform to enable people to use their voice and leaders to hear their pleas must be genuine. Action must be demonstrable and more immediate than the surveys and town halls of days passed.

It's likely many pro-nursing organizations already have some platform for this in "practice" or "shared-governance" councils. However, leaders will have to go deeper and wider to align with the values of every employee and to allow space for people to work on real problems. Albert et al. (2022) asserted that a strong focus on mission and purpose leads to ensuring that all workers in the system are motivated and committed to achieving positive organizational outcomes and improving the success of the organization.

## MENDING THE FENCE—CULTURE

Today, leaders of healthcare organizations are facing tremendous financial and delivery challenges. Depending on their level of experience, they may be used to a command-and-control style of leadership from managing through COVID-19 and its prolonged effects. Burnout on the front line and among leadership has only compounded the challenges that now need to be faced head on. Many cultures have become too competitive and overly toxic. This further exacerbates turnover both by staff and leaders.

The signs of a toxic workplace culture include: broken communication lines, hyper-competitiveness, pressure to assimilate, and a resulting unnatural or uncomfortable workplace presence. The absence of open communication, discouragement to speak up (overt or implied), and lateral or horizontal shame and blame ultimately erode trust, which is the bedrock of a functional team.

"Healing and hope are the responsibility of the clinicians who practice in the healthcare organizations, and organizations are responsible for living their values, which must include respect, justice, ethical practice, compassion, and inclusivity" for both their workforce and community (Albert et al., 2020, p. 461).

Fortunately, caring with a focus on purpose and cultivating a positive work culture can go hand in hand.

### PRACTICE PEARLS

- Hear and respond to nurses' and other healthcare workers' concerns.
- Adjust work assignments to meet standards of care and ideal workflow while accommodating the skill level of available personnel.
- Support nurses and other clinicians with new and "out of the box" ideas.

## WORKFORCE—ACADEMIC RECRUITMENT

Also contributing to the growing nursing (and other personnel) shortage is a significantly reduced supply of new and energetic clinicians into the healthcare professions. Though interest in baccalaureate and graduate nursing programs is strong, thousands of qualified students are turned away from community colleges and universities each year. In 2021, a total of 91,938 qualified applications (not applicants) were not accepted at schools of nursing nationwide (Rosseter, 2022). Historically, this trend has been on the rise due to an insufficient number of qualified and interested faculty, diminishing clinical sites and willing preceptors, a lack of classroom space, and budget constraints. Barriers cited by multiple experts summarize low pay, retirement outpacing recruitment of new educators, and low interest of nurses with advanced degrees to step out of the practice and entrepreneurial spaces they now occupy.

Dean Emami, of the University of Washington School of Nursing, adds that federal funding for nursing education continues to lag far behind demand; federal and state funding for nursing school facilities has also trailed the need, and funding from tuition is not adjusted for the higher cost of nursing education that results from mandated faculty-to-student ratios for clinical and laboratory settings (2021). Inevitably, industry, academia, and policy-makers will have to partner to expedite and build sustainable nursing education programs and workplaces that serve to retain talent across the span of their professional careers.

Some examples include schools that increasingly engage with health systems to deploy clinical staff in teaching roles (Bakewell-Sachs et al., 2022). In some states, like Oregon, senior nursing students are being granted licenses to practice under the supervision of licensed registered nurses, where they can earn wages and get credit for working in nursing departments (Stites, 2022). Retired nursing staff are being recalled to be part-time instructors, new care models are being developed, and innovative approaches to offload tasks that don't require nursing assessment and diagnosis may be delegated to other licensed or unlicensed personnel.

## AN INTERNATIONAL PERSPECTIVE

Most of the opportunities and challenges discussed in this text have applied to the healthcare system in the United States. However, we believe the same challenges exist for nurses and other healthcare providers worldwide—especially related to the global COVID-19 pandemic. A nurse colleague of one of the contributors was kind enough to give us her perspective.

Siew Lee Grand-Clément is a global healthcare executive in clinical and quality operations, patient advocacy and safe health design, the Vice President of Nursing & Quality for UPMC International, and the Acting Chief Operation Officer of China's Chengdu Wanda UPMC International Hospital. Here is what she said (S. L. Grand-Clément, personal communication, September 2, 2022):

> The Great Resignation phenomenon is not solely due to the pandemic effect. Societal, economic, and political issues have often made their way into our healthcare settings that challenge our safe staffing, morale distress, and workplace violence. Healthcare workers and nurses have been facing threats of mental health and anxiety from burnout that is now exacerbated—by waves of the pandemic—from infections and capacities surges to emergent threats of monkeypox to climate impacts to health conditions. As a nurse executive integrated into multi-countries operation spanning from North America, Europe, and Asia, the common themes are universal of these unsustainable burnout and shortage of resources to escalating demands.
>
> Nursing and healthcare executives are faced with coming up with many quick fixes while developing sustainable strategies that can help us get ahead of the curve of crisis after crisis. Developing a balanced solution requires global thinking that also accounts for ethical and social responsibility approach. In the midst of the pandemic, we have seen in the United States the negative impact of robbing Peter to pay Paul of states or health systems competing for nurses with incentives paid, resulting in worsening gaps of care in deprived areas. Patient experience and clinical quality outcomes were also impacted by poor integration of temporary workers that further exacerbates clinicians' burnout, which in turn harms patients' experience. Similarly, high-income countries that are members of the Organisation for Economic Co-operation and Development deploying international nurse migration resources is also leading to poorer and deprived countries losing their last defense in healthcare resources to

care for their own population and the inability to offer better wages to their own nurses. In 2022, the International Council of Nursing highlighted this issue in its Global Nursing Workforce call for action report, that we need to consider a more self-sufficient solution in the nursing resource supply chain.

There is no easy way out of this with solely reactions to the current crisis without paralleled strategic investment of resetting the nursing workforce and pipelines of resources that can mitigate further damage of the workforce burnout and supply. Our current priorities ought to evaluate if we are making time to address these:

- Partnership with local school of nursing and health sciences program to evaluate and pilot test new skills mix and care model can be an effective approach and a medium-term solution to the ongoing shortage of resources.
- Redesigning the care delivery approach to offer more diverse care opportunities in the value stream of health promotion to disease management for nurses is essential for the longevity of the profession. Deploying community care centric model from recruitment to deployment is all of our social responsibility to population health.
- Finally, attention to how we care for one another as nurses are critical to instill the sense of radical belonging. Investment in effective wellness and well-being programs should no longer be nice to have versus must have and accessible to all.

## THE CHALLENGE OF PRACTICING TO THE FULL EXTENT OF YOUR LICENSE

The first message from the IOM's (2010) recommendations for nurses was to practice to the full extent of their education and training, implying that nurses are not doing this now (or then). Here we are 12-plus years later and the question still remains: Why not? What barriers prohibit nurses from utilizing their knowledge and skills to the fullest extent?

Ward (2014, p. 1) identified nine common problems in the "very rewarding but equally challenging" practice of nursing:

- **Staffing:** Inadequate resource allocation
- **Interprofessional relationships:** Produce conflict
- **Patient satisfaction:** Many have unrealistic expectations
- **On-the-job hazards:** Related to safety
- **Mandatory overtime:** Due to insufficient resources or high patient acuity
- **"Ask a nurse":** Everyone wants to ask nurses questions about their health issues
- **Patient relationships:** Can cause stress, pain, and feelings of loss
- **Advances in technology:** Require changes in duties and skill
- **Certifications and other demonstrations of competence:** Now a must

Similarly, during a BSN completion program titled "Nursing Research" (Buck, 2014), practicing nurses were asked about barriers to implementing evidence-based practice and conducting nursing research. The primary impediment nurses cited was time. The nurses stated that their workload did not allow time for any other activities outside of direct patient care. The nurses verbalized an understanding of the importance of conducting research, and many had taken courses, yet they found it difficult to utilize what they had learned. Barriers to implementing best practice evidence from relevant research in practice is not new. Wallis (2012) wrote about how in most cases, time is a barrier, and the majority of organizational cultures don't support it. It's often difficult to get past resistance, especially with those who think, "What's wrong with the way we've always done it?"

It might just be time for nursing work to be revamped in the age of pay-for-performance. Analysis of nursing work, just as in building a business case, could yield novel yet drastic recommendations. For example, does each nurse know the impact of their practice? Are they making a positive contribution? It is plausible there could be greater returns on investment, better utilization of resources, and improved patient outcomes by radically changing how nurses work and are compensated? Could a practice scorecard, similar to a business balanced scorecard, yield the knowledge to make substantive changes? Nursing's work is subsumed in the room charge for an inpatient stay and has been this way for our lifetime; it's time for change.

The second issue prohibiting nurses from practicing to the full extent of their education and training is inconsistency in practice regulations along with inconsistency in educational programs from state to state. Some states allow a wide scope of practice, with full prescriptive authority for the advanced practice nurse (APN), while others do not. Some states require a specified number of clinical hours to achieve and maintain licensure, while others are laxer. In addition to the variability in the scope of practice, there are also variations in required supervision. In some states, APNs can practice independently; in others, they must be either directly or indirectly supervised by a physician as specified in the state's Nurse Practice Act.

If nurses are going to practice to the full extent of their education and training, scope of practice, and supervision, wider standardization must occur. The future of nursing rests with the profession to promote the importance of nurses as equal and valuable members of the healthcare team and be properly rewarded for it. Through the use of research, nurses will be able to quantify substantive activities as opposed to referring to common successful practices (we have always done it this way). Thinking needs to change. In addition, adopting nursing best practices from research findings will add credibility to nursing practice with other practitioners in the healthcare professions.

## STREAMLINE HIGHER EDUCATION FOR NURSES

The second message presented in the IOM report (2010) was that nurses should achieve a higher level of education and training. This can easily be structured via a seamless system that promotes academic progression. The report called for 80% of the nursing workforce to have the minimum preparation of a bachelor of science in nursing degree (BSN) by 2020. The Campaign for Action report (AARP, 2020) reported that as of 2018, 57% of nurses in the United States had a bachelor of science in nursing degree. Here's a link to the most recent report: https://campaignforaction.org/wp-content/uploads/2022/03/r4_CCNA-0029_2022-Dashboard-Indicator-Updates-copy-1.pdf.

Although there are many patient-care outcomes that support an all-BSN staff, there are still many nurses working in the US who possess either an associate degree or have graduated from a diploma program. You can read more here about the most recent nursing statistics in a fact sheet from the American Association of Colleges of Nursing (AACN): https://www.aacnnursing.org/News-Information/Fact-Sheets/Nursing-Fact-Sheet.

This change in the required educational standard presents an interesting dilemma. Due to industry financial pressures, many healthcare entities are decreasing or eliminating education reimbursement for those seeking an advanced degree. At the same time, many healthcare entities have decreased or eliminated financial incentives or pay differential for advanced education. There is also salary/compensation compression between nursing roles (staff, manager, director, chief, etc.), which has only been worsened by the COVID-19 pandemic. Unfortunately, with little salary separation between staff and leadership roles, it can be difficult to attract qualified and interested nursing leadership candidates.

Concurrently, some healthcare entities have espoused a course of action requiring a BSN for associate and diploma degree nurses to be completed within "x" years of hire. Given the current climate in nursing and the decrease in reimbursement for education by employers, achieving an advanced degree may become more difficult. Many nurses are being mandated to work extra shifts due to the decrease in available personnel, which only adds to the stress of completing coursework and balancing personal lives.

An additional hurdle for nurses to return to school is the requirement to repeat courses they may have already taken in entry-level training to meet newer graduation requirements; unfortunately, some coursework has an expiration date. Education must be easily accessible and streamlined for nurses and other healthcare providers to pursue the achievement of a higher degree. Employers must be supportive, with flexible schedules and judicious use of financial resources for support. Education should be viewed as an investment versus a cost, and the interested parties must be committed to obtaining new skills and education regardless of financial support. Education in nursing does have a return on investment with new opportunities, obtaining a set of qualifications for a higher role, and so on. Grants, loans, and scholarships should all be explored in addition to personal and employer resources. Some organizations still offer tuition reimbursement after a defined number of years of service have been completed.

The IOM report further recommended that the number of nurses prepared at the doctoral level double by the year 2020. In 2010, fewer than 1% of nurses held a doctorate degree in nursing or a nursing-related field; to double this would merely be 2%. In 2018, 1.9% of nurses held a doctorate degree as their highest level of educational preparation in nursing or a related field (AARP, 2020). In order to continue this forward movement, nurses must be vocal regarding their educational needs to be able to complete a higher degree. In addition, a number of APN practice programs are transitioning from a master level entry to a doctoral degree just as they have in other healthcare professions such as pharmacy, physical therapy, etc. In 2018, the National Organization of Nurse Practitioner Faculties, the leading organization for nurse practitioner (NP) education, called for moving to the doctor of nursing practice degree as the entry-level preparation for NPs by 2025 (AACN, 2022).

Fortunately, schools of nursing have become creative in offering varying methods of attaining an advanced degree. This has come largely from the objective of meeting numerical targets for students and consumer demand. Increasingly, registered nurse (RN) to master of science in nursing (MSN) programs, and RN to doctor of nursing practice (DNP) programs are much more accessible as online offerings. As we move into the future, we must emphasize the value of an advanced degree and provide support for those seeking such degrees. Even more importantly, we must ensure that nurses as well as other healthcare providers can actually utilize and apply their learned knowledge. The current demand for master- and doctoral-prepared nurses for advanced practice, clinical specialties, teaching, and research roles far outstrips the supply (AACN, 2015), and this challenge continues seven years later. Effective collaboration between nursing schools and healthcare organizations is crucial. The need for nurses at the bedside compared to the number of nurses needed overall in healthcare organizations demands a strong professional relationship between nursing schools and nursing leadership in these organizations. The relationship between these two groups can help prepare tomorrow's nurses for their careers and as a lifelong learners who seek to continue their formal nursing education via an advanced degree.

## BECOME AN EQUAL PARTNER IN PROVIDING PRACTICE EXPERTISE

A third message from the IOM report (2010) stated nurses should collaborate with physicians and other healthcare professionals as full partners to redesign healthcare in the US. This is an immense opportunity for collective collaboration and for nurses to have a voice in healthcare's future. This recommendation provides a platform for change in healthcare that can ultimately be even more patient-focused.

The Affordable Care Act of 2010 (or Obamacare as it is commonly referred to) radically changed the delivery of healthcare, shifting a greater out-of-pocket expense to many US citizens. Although more people have access to care, costs are still unaffordable for many citizens. This leaves a large void for those who remain either uninsured or under-insured. Healthcare spending has risen around the world, but none as fast as the US; costs for healthcare in the US now account for 40% of global spending (Morabito, 2022). Morabito (2022) also cited comparative costs from 1960 listing healthcare as consuming only 5% of the gross domestic product (GDP), and in 2020 the spending hit almost 20% of the GDP. In addition, more than 54% of Americans access healthcare coverage through their employer, who sets the price to be paid by negotiating with large insurance carriers.

Utilizing APNs to provide primary care, as well as other mid-level providers, standardizing treatment for patients with similar diagnoses, changing the focus to prevention of illness, and including the patient in the care and decision-making process can revolutionize healthcare as we know it. Nurses have and can continue to champion many of these changes in healthcare due to the fact that they outnumber physicians by three to one (AACN, 2022). But are they always invited to the table where healthcare policy is set?

## IMPROVE DATA-COLLECTION METHODS

The fourth and final message put forth in the IOM report (2010) identified that effective policy-making and workforce planning related to healthcare requires improved data-collection methods along with an improved information infrastructure. One of the greatest challenges that nurses and other healthcare clinicians face is the potential to make an error. Patient deaths due to medical errors ranked third in the top five causes of death, only surpassed by heart disease and cancer (McCann, 2014). In 2016, Johns Hopkins Medicine reported medical errors had moved to the third spot on the top listing for causes of death in the US. As expected, many have challenged the data and its accuracy. You can find the CDC's most recent listing of leading causes of death in the US here (COVID-19 now stands in the number three spot on this list): https://www.cdc.gov/nchs/fastats/leading-causes-of-death.htm.

Nurses' fear of repercussions when reporting an error is one of the most commonly cited reasons for not reporting medical errors (Haw et al., 2014). And quite honestly, they are most likely underreported for all care providers. In addition, reporting systems can be complicated, many do not allow for accurate near-miss reporting, and some are difficult to navigate.

Unfortunately, a culture of blaming an individual for a medical error is still prevalent, if not dominant, in many traditional organizations. For these organizations, there is an assumption that the care provider is to blame based on poor performance. Thus, the automatic response is to blame the caregiver rather than look at policy, process, and structures that may have caused or contributed to the error. More organizations are adopting a culture that seeks to overcome barriers to improve safe care for patients by advancing the error reporting process.

Self-actualized organizations understand caregivers must be held accountable, as warranted. However, poor systems from bad policy or practice must also be accountable. Leaders must identify and address policy, systems, work processes, and structure (along with caregiver performance) to reduce medical errors. When using this approach, organizations clearly define the difference between human error and reckless behavior.

In the future, it will be essential to identify more efficient ways for nurses and other healthcare providers to capture real and potential errors. Some organizations have taken steps to internally publicize information about "lessons learned." This is a substantial change in thinking and past practice but critically important for patient safety and clinician awareness. Nurses often know patients the best of all other healthcare providers, and they should be leading the way toward enhanced quality and safety initiatives. In addition, it is the nurse's responsibility to be an active participant in making care improvements, which lead to safer care and ideally reduce medical errors.

In one example of collaboration with other healthcare professionals, the Robert Wood Johnson Foundation took a leap of faith by bringing together a diverse group of people to clarify the role of the APN (Iglehart, 2013). This is what nursing and healthcare needs: teams of experts solving complex and longstanding problems. Maybe some of the team should even be *outside* of healthcare. Much of the business world does not run similar to healthcare, and experienced individuals could add a valuable perspective (so too could consumers of healthcare).

Nurses must step up and have the confidence to share their expertise with others related to care delivery, the practice of nursing, and in the legislative arena.

### PRACTICE PEARLS

- Be a team player and recognize the strengths in others.
- Share expert knowledge (gained over time) for improvement initiatives and best practice.
- Be willing to learn from others.
- Speak up and lead to change healthcare from within.

## SPEAK UP AND LET YOUR VOICE BE HEARD

In recent times, interpersonal interactions in healthcare settings have become more challenging for nurses and some other healthcare providers. The social environment has been profiled as a source of stress. With a laser-like focus on customer experience and satisfaction, operational performance, and publicly reported metrics, nurses often feel trapped in tough interpersonal situations. A balance must take place with realistic expectations, achievable outcomes, and a safe process to get there.

Customer experience or satisfaction is important. However, care must be taken to meet customer requests without compromising the nurse's or other health-care provider's better judgment. These caregivers are on the front line, taking heavy responsibility for meeting patient, family, and provider needs. In some healthcare settings, if customer needs are not met, the nurse is to blame. Nurses also blame each other. Both of these make no sense since caregiving is a team effort. A culture of blaming by peers only adds to workplace stress, fatigue, and burnout.

Cipriano (2015) referred to these types of issues as "emotional labor" in nursing. She defined *emotional labor* as emotions that nurses are required to exhibit such as a smile, a comforting gesture, deference, or scripting when they do not truly feel the emotion. This takes a tremendous toll on nurses, and they often release their stress via frustration and anger with those around them. Peers and subordinates are easy targets. The global COVID-19 pandemic only heightened the frustration with system issues and intensified the stress that was already present in many workplaces.

Frequently, there are no obvious repercussions in general for this type of behavior. But there should be. We must all be respectful and professional with each other. There is an old saying, "Physician, heal thyself." Nurses also need to consider healing themselves; they are the only ones capable of changing the circumstances in the *profession* of nursing. It's time to speak up and step out. There won't be a better time in our lifetimes where an external force created such an opportunity by making a significant impact on the way things used to be done.

Disruptive or bad behavior should no longer be tolerated. It can take various forms that can be subtle or openly aggressive. These behaviors include blaming others for safety issues, sarcasm, not offering assistance when the need is obvious, not helping a coworker when asked, and not serving as a resource to others by sharing their knowledge.

In a recent exchange with an ED (emergency department) nurse, she shared a brief conversation that took place between her and an administrator. The nurse had taken care of a patient in the ED who was a member of a local gang. She shared her concern related to the safety of the staff in the ED based on a recent string of gang shootings in the city. The patients were brought to her hospital, and the gang member told her that the biggest safety concern the hospital should have is the ED waiting room windows.

He described that gang members often drive through the parking lot to see who is in the waiting room. The waiting room's windows allowed anyone sitting in the area to be seen, especially at night. The nurse was shocked and immediately took this information seriously by reporting it to the hospital administration as a safety concern. The response from the administrator a few days later was, "the interior decorator did not feel it would be aesthetically pleasing to frost the glass," so they had no intention to further address the issue.

Safety needs to be at the highest level of concern in healthcare, including work safety, patient safety, and healthcare-provider safety. Nurses need to assess and report areas of risk—understanding fully that others may not see an immediate need for change. Be persistent, convincing, and follow the chain of command! Job safety includes injuries that occur secondary to lifting; slips, trips, and falls; the escalating threat of violence in the workplace from either internal or external sources; a lack of proper equipment; and long hours and rotating schedules. Nurses, as well as other healthcare providers, are at risk for injury, so supplies and equipment need to be operational and readily available to provide care.

Lachman (2014) described how The Joint Commission issued a Sentinel Event Alert (in 2008) that addressed behaviors undermining a culture of safety:

> Intimidating and disruptive behaviors can foster medical errors, contribute to poor patient satisfaction and to preventable adverse outcomes, increase the cost of care, and cause qualified clinicians, administrators and managers to seek new positions in more professional environments. (The Joint Commission, 2009)

Yet, these types of behaviors are still tolerated in a number of healthcare settings. Research shows an increase in lateral violence; bullying; violence in the nursing work environment from patients, visitors, and physicians; as well as increasing mental and emotional demands by the plethora of information available in the literature. *Lateral violence* refers to acts that occur between colleagues, where *bullying* is described as acts perpetrated by one in a higher level of authority and occurring over time; the acts can be verbal or non-verbal aggression (American Nurses Association [ANA], 2011). *Horizontal violence* refers to a relationship in a reporting structure where one person is subordinate to another and may experience these types of unprofessional behavior.

In one case during a seven-day period, 12.1% of ED nurses experienced an act of physical violence, and 42.5% experienced verbal abuse (Emergency Nurses Association [ENA], 2011). The acts of violence were committed by patients and visitors. Perpetrators of verbal abuse included peers and medical providers, as well as patients and visitors. The ENA also noted that organizations with reporting mechanisms related to these types of incidents have significantly lower numbers of acts of violence within the organization (2011). Training for nurses (and all other healthcare providers) to recognize, dissuade, and prevent violence in health settings is crucial.

Nurses' idealism and professionalism can be undermined by individuals who create unhealthy or even hostile work environments (Lachman, 2014). This type of work culture is problematic to survive and causes a great deal of stress. Lachman (2014) cited a range of examples of disruptive behavior including throwing objects, banging down the telephone receiver, intentionally damaging equipment, exposing patients or staff to contaminated fluids or equipment, bullying, and lateral or horizontal violence.

Lateral or horizontal violence can be overt, covert, or both. Stanton (2015) described how nurse leaders must take an active role to eradicate it. There is no place for this type of behavior in healthcare settings, and zero tolerance should be the mantra of the future. In addition to leadership, all nurses and other healthcare providers must be educated on the signs of lateral violence and be assertive in their ability to communicate to intervene (Ceravolo et al., 2012). Behaviors include gossiping, withholding information, and ostracism (ANA, n.d.). Sometimes job stress is the result of the overall culture of an organization. This is especially stressful for the nurse leader (or any leader) who strives to be a role model for staff while at the same time not being supported in their own role by their upline leader or leaders. Aries (2017), in *Forbes,* described five signs of a toxic job:

1. Narcissists at the top of the hierarchy for management
2. Commiserating coworkers
3. Management's lack of transparency
4. Management applies the rules to some but not all employees equally (equality)
5. Coworkers call in sick

This stress is compounded by the outcomes from a toxic work environment, which includes problems with morale, employee job satisfaction, nursing turnover and vacancies, patient satisfaction, complaints, clinical outcomes, and medical errors.

The nurse leader can evaluate management's likelihood for change and make a choice. What are the key drivers that will help support the nurse leader to move from a toxic environment to one that is healthy? Meet with your team members and discuss the drivers by framing the conversation in a solution-oriented way. Proposing new solutions may allow the nurse leader to take back their "agency" and change their and others' perspective by regaining control over what they are able to influence. Understanding what parts of your role bring you fulfillment, happiness, and joy are key to survival. If the pros don't exceed the cons on your comparative list—make a change.

Positive mentoring is an underutilized role in nursing and some other healthcare roles. The potential benefits are well documented in the literature (Green

& Jackson, 2014). Having a "wingman/woman/person" or a "buddy" to support newbies, those changing specialties, those learning new roles, and so on can be invaluable. Mentoring can have a strong impact in peer-to-peer interactions. In the medical system of education for physicians, they call this *proctoring*. Providers aren't allowed to practice in high-risk areas (on their own) until their proctor assures the organization they are safe and competent to practice. Too often the competencies used to verify a nurse's skill and critical thinking are not seen as an important verification of ability in the same way as physician proctoring.

Novice nurses need to see good examples of excellent practice, interpersonal relations, and leadership to mold their own style. Mentors serve as a guide. In some organizations, mentors take on the role without recognition or additional compensation. They are frequently asked to work with others in addition to maintaining their own workload, which may not be the best approach. Some incentive for those who are qualified and interested in mentoring others shows value and rewards the mentor.

Exercise caution to avoid burning out those interested in mentoring or becoming leaders. Public recognition for a job well done, as well as highlighting positive work contributions of expert nurses, is a must; nursing must serve as an example to others both inside and outside the profession to continue to attract qualified, talented, and dedicated people to healthcare. Caring for each other is an important aspect in nursing and other healthcare professions that needs heightened awareness. An example is described in the sidebar on the next page, where multiple incidents affect nurses, yet they receive little if any support.

In today's chaotic and stressful healthcare environment, it is vital to recognize the ramifications for nurses and other healthcare providers of inherent stress, the physical and emotional toll, and the potential for burnout. Caregivers can always be counted on to do what is necessary under almost any circumstance despite their personal feelings or emotional turmoil. Educating the public is an essential piece of nursing and healthcare's responsibility and helps those outside the profession gain a realistic understanding of the role. Fortunately, the global

COVID-19 pandemic has done some of that for us—under the worst of circumstances.

## DEALING WITH PERSONAL LOSS IN THE ED

An ambulance is dispatched to a call for a shooting victim. A radio call immediately comes into the emergency department (ED) with situational details. The nurse learns that the patient is a detective from the local police department who is in full cardiac arrest. The ED staff know most members of the police force well due to the small geographic area. Multiple police officers enter the ED as the detective is being wheeled into the trauma room. The staff on duty recognize the detective. The nurses, the physician, and the respiratory therapist take over care from the paramedics. The room is chaotic and emotions are high. After a lengthy resuscitation attempt, the detective is pronounced "dead on arrival." The ED staff leave the room in tears, all the while knowing that they must pull themselves together to continue taking care of their other assigned ED patients. There is no time for crying, taking a break, or holding a debriefing.

Later, a debriefing is held for the police officers and the paramedics who were involved. Nursing should have been included—either through an informal (immediately post incident) or formal (days after the incident) debrief. Two weeks after the incident, one of the ED physicians suddenly died at home. The staff were notified by the paramedics on scene (after permission from the physician's wife was obtained). The ED staff, once again, experienced a second and more significant loss, with no formal debriefing. The ED staff knew patient care needed to continue for the other ED patients, so the nurses pressed on.

While this case is somewhat of an extreme example, nurses' experiences are so often overlooked. Nurses are expected to carry on despite feeling grief from troubling events. The global COVID-19 pandemic brought these types of troubling situations to each shift, challenging even the most experienced providers.

Nurses and other members of the healthcare team need to support each other by advocating for resources to provide needed care at difficult times. A nurse is not just a nurse; nurses regularly take on the role of social worker, chaplain, and counselor in times of crisis. Nurses refer to their peers as "family" due to the traumatic encounters that forge tight emotional bonds. And in these types of situations, they should be supported like family.

## PRACTICE PEARLS

- Don't tolerate bad behavior.
- Recognize feelings and take the time to adapt and process them.
- Look out for each other—be a good "wingman/woman/person."
- Seek help in tough situations.

# TYING IT ALL TOGETHER

Technology is changing the world. It is one of the newest and most challenging additions to healthcare; however, it is badly needed to move nursing and the healthcare industry forward. New advances in information technology appear nearly every day. Staying current with the skills required through training, experience, and interaction with others can be daunting. Peers and patients feel the impact of constant change. The implementation of technology is testing both the art and science of nursing and other providers of healthcare. Many cite it as one of the top sources of stress. While it should be improving practice and making data acquisition more efficient, it may be causing additional stress, fatigue, and the potential for burnout due to the excessive amount of required information.

The ability to look at a machine to obtain clinical information is nothing short of amazing. However, it may also place nurses' critical thinking skills at risk. Over-reliance on technology for an accurate reading of blood pressure or heart rate, a barcode scanner or pump for medication administration, and other medical device advances may compromise a nurse's ability to effectively assess a patient's clinical status and solve problems. Critical thinkers in nursing must be skillful in applying intellectual knowledge for sound reasoning (Heaslip, 2008). Nurses especially must guard their knowledge and maintain the ability to think critically and "just know" when something isn't right.

Heaslip (2008) concluded that nurses must be adept at gathering, focusing, remembering, organizing, analyzing, generating, integrating, and evaluating information. The world is changing the ways we interact with information. More information is available now than ever before. Formal nursing training lays a foundation for critical thinking. However, education needs to focus on preparing nursing students to be the best novice nurse possible. The novice nurse must be able to utilize the foundation of critical thinking and expand it for clinical reasoning and clinical judgment.

In practice, nurses encounter increasingly more complex situations, which require expert reasoning (Heaslip, 2008). The future of nursing depends on the ability of nurses and healthcare providers in general to possess new expertise fueled by technology and rapid change; to remain devoted to quality and safety; and to be intentionally thoughtful. We must not lose sight of the human factors that allow nurses to care for themselves, their coworkers, and their patients in an empathetic way.

One of the messages in the IOM report (2010) is the need for nurses to partner with others to improve healthcare. One major way for nurses to contribute to the quality of healthcare is participating in and conducting either solo, multi-provider, or specialty research. Nurses have been practicing at the bedside by utilizing differing treatment methods and resources to provide similar care since the beginning of nursing.

One of the biggest challenges nurses of the future will face is the need for new scientific evidence to support practice. In addition, practice environments must become skilled at rapid-fire change so they are able to quickly embrace evidence-based research recommendations for improvement in systems, processes, and procedures. This could potentially change the social milieu. And the COVID-19 pandemic certainly challenged it. We must now take our lessons learned and move forward creating new and better systems.

Hockenberry et al. (2006) cited the following barriers for nurses to make improvements: limited knowledge of the nursing research process, lack of knowledge related to statistics and their use in research, time to conduct and/or implement research, and a lack of power and authority to implement change. Additionally, a lack of respect from peers, decreased resources to provide patient care, poor work environments, and job dissatisfaction continue to contribute to the limited amount of research being appropriated into practice. We must address the time factor and adequate resources to move the profession forward. The time for change has been delayed for too long; nurses and other healthcare providers can no longer accept the status quo and survive in today's stress-laden healthcare environments.

In addition to the barriers of implementing research at the bedside, there is a known lack of nurses prepared to conduct research. How many healthcare organizations support formal research and development (R&D) programs? Is it considered a core part of their healthcare business (as other industries consider R&D)? How many healthcare entities have a "learning lab" set up to test new ideas or pilot new programs? Are the best organizations innovating healthcare processes and sharing their knowledge in a broad way?

The numbers are few, unless the healthcare organization is formally aligned with an academic source. Informal research by healthcare providers, in their work environments, is taking place every day in an attempt to do things better. These systems need to be formalized, and new knowledge needs to be shared. Nursing practice settings should consider building alliances with schools of nursing in order to receive the research support they need. The schools of nursing often need populations with which to do desired research, so the partnership could be quite productive for both parties.

In 2011, the Health Resources and Service Administration estimated the number of nurses with a doctorate at 1% (Nickitas & Feeg, 2011). Doctoral programs in nursing are increasing in the US, with multiple sites and creative educational formats to allow nurses to obtain the degrees, but there are *still* not enough, as previously described (AACN, 2015).

Letourneau (2022) described how there are not enough nursing faculty to train the next generation of nurses. She explained that despite a national nursing shortage, nearly 100,000 nursing applicants were turned away from colleges due to a shortage of faculty in 2020, and there is also a shortage of APNs. COVID-19 only exacerbated the health and wellness problems with the nursing workforce (Letourneau, 2022). These projections could have a grave impact in the ability to obtain qualified faculty to train new nurses and to conduct necessary research in the future.

A further complication to increasing the number of nurses with advanced educational preparation for academic positions is the wide gap in compensation. Often, nursing researchers and faculty are paid lower salaries than nurses entering the nursing profession and practicing at the bedside. As nursing moves into the future, this needs to change. Letourneau (2022) also posited that one solution to increase qualified faculty might be to match the salaries in practice in order to recruit those with expertise for educating the next generation of nurses and other healthcare workers. Nursing must keep pace in advancing the profession and stature among other disciplines; higher education is one answer.

One of the most difficult challenges nurses and other healthcare providers face when speaking up, attempting to make improvement suggestions, or continuing to advance via educational pursuits is the negative comments by their peers. This lack of collegial support causes unnecessary stress. Alienation from peers by negative comments deters nurses and others from suggesting organizational improvements and engaging in self-improvement activities. As a profession, nurses must move to embrace compassion and care for fellow nurses and their professional colleagues. Nurses who serve in leadership positions must be committed to providing necessary support and not tolerating lateral violence or bullying behavior. This type of encouragement and a change in the culture of nursing could facilitate a revolution of positive change.

Ward (2014) identified mandatory overtime and the length of nursing shifts as concerns for nurses and patients. According to Stimpfel et al.'s research (2012), shifts exceeding 13 hours in length result in proportionately higher patient dissatisfaction. In addition, the combination of shift rotation, working overtime, and continual changes in personnel and staffing create a higher level of stress and turnover, which potentiate fatigue and burnout. Shift rotation is also not without health consequences. You can read more here:

> The health risks of shift work: https://www.webmd.com/sleep-disorders/features/shift-work
>
> The impact of shift work on health: https://www.medicalnewstoday.com/articles/288310
>
> Health consequences of shift work and insufficient sleep: https://pubmed.ncbi.nlm.nih.gov/27803010/

In an interview with Beverly Malone, the CEO of the National League for Nursing (Sullivan, 2014), she stated the future of nursing remains in flux and the following considerations must be taken seriously for nurses of the future: an aging workforce, a lack of educators, and too few new nurses entering the profession to meet patient-care demands. In addition, a lack of relevant research, multiple generations of nurses in the workforce, aging leaders in healthcare, and increasing pressure on healthcare organizations further complicate needed change. It sadly appears nothing has changed for the better in nearly a decade.

As healthcare continues to evolve, many new challenges and opportunities will surface. New roles in nursing will be discovered, care will continue to move to alternative venues, and the demand for APNs will grow. Educators and clinicians are still predicted to be in short supply. The time is now to get creative in the design and development of new strategies for nursing and all of healthcare's future.

## PRACTICE PEARLS

- Get involved—support professional practice and nursing/medical research.
- Engage in self-improvement.
- Recognize the value of advancing knowledge and skill.

# CONCLUSION

Nurses and other healthcare providers have a tremendous responsibility to promote and support a new system of healthcare. Cohesion is necessary for a single voice supporting unified policy and practice. While direct care for patients will remain a priority, supportive elements to deliver care in complex atmospheres will be required.

Hopefully, many facets of nursing practice in the future will change for the better: research to policy-making; new evidence regularly implemented in practice; a focus on health and prevention of illness; a shift from stress-laden cultures to those supporting optimal well-being; excellent leadership; and most of all, constructive interactions with each other. It is each nurse's responsibility to promote optimism and engage in mindful practice to ensure that nursing remains the most trusted profession and that we leave a progressive legacy for those who follow.

The concepts, questions, and exploration of topics throughout this book were meant to provoke thought. Not necessarily thoughts about how things got to this point, but what we can do differently going forward. Some of the information may be seen as controversial, not usually discussed, or even intentionally hidden in a veil of secrecy. But if *we* don't change, how can we change nursing and healthcare for the better?

To gather some ideas about how you might participate in changing healthcare for the better, read more about the latest trends in global healthcare at these websites:

- Top 10 Emerging Trends in Health Care for 2021: The New Normal | AHA Trustee Services: https://trustees.aha.org/top-10-emerging-trends-health-care-2021-new-normal
- 2022 Healthcare Industry Trends That Will Make a Difference | UCF Online: https://www.ucf.edu/online/healthcare/news/healthcare-industry-trends/
- The Five Biggest Healthcare Tech Trends in 2022 (forbes.com): https://www.forbes.com/sites/bernardmarr/2022/01/10/the-five-biggest-healthcare-tech-trends-in-2022/?sh=f3d009154d01
- 2022 Key Trends in Healthcare | Capgemini: https://www.capgemini.com/insights/expert-perspectives/2022-key-trends-in-healthcare/
- 10 Healthcare Technology Trends for 2022 | Philips: https://www.philips.com/a-w/about/news/archive/features/2022/20220120-10-healthcare-technology-trends-for-2022.html
- Nursing and Healthcare Trends We Can Expect to See in 2022 | NurseJournal.org: https://nursejournal.org/articles/2022-nursing-healthcare-trends/
- 2022 Healthcare Trends: 6 Defining Areas (healthcatalyst.com): https://www.healthcatalyst.com/wp-content/uploads/2022/03/2022-Healthcare-Trends_whitepaper.pdf

- 2022 Global Health Care Outlook: Are We Finally Seeing the Long-Promised Transformation? | Deloitte: https://www.deloitte.com/global/en/Industries/life-sciences-health-care/perspectives/global-health-care-sector-outlook.html
- 10 Healthcare Marketing Trends for 2022 | Cardinal Digital Marketing: https://www.cardinaldigitalmarketing.com/healthcare-resources/blog/10-healthcare-marketing-trends-2022/
- Seven Predictions for Healthcare Technology Trends in 2022 | Wolters Kluwer: https://www.wolterskluwer.com/en/expert-insights/predictions-in-healthcare-technology-2022
- Acceleration in Healthcare: Six Trends to Heed | McKinsey: https://www.mckinsey.com/industries/healthcare-systems-and-services/our-insights/the-great-acceleration-in-healthcare-six-trends-to-heed
- The Productivity Imperative for Healthcare Delivery in the United States | McKinsey: https://www.mckinsey.com/industries/healthcare/our-insights/the-productivity-imperative-for-health-care-delivery-in-the-united-states

This quote from author, speaker, consultant, and university president Nido Qubein seems apropos for healthcare:

> "Your present circumstances don't determine where you can go, they merely determine where you start."

It is time to start a revolution! Positive change is crucial for nursing and healthcare. We must strive to change the environment to *banish* stress, fatigue, and burnout. Onward!

# REFERENCES

AARP. (2020). *Campaign for Action.* https://campaignforaction.org/

Albert, N., Pappas, S., Porter-O'Grady, T., & Mallock, K. (2020). Leading constant movement: Transforming chaos and crisis. In T. Porter-O'Grady & K. Malloch (Eds.), *Quantum leadership: Creating sustainable value in health care* (6th ed.). Jones & Bartlett Learning.

American Association of Colleges of Nursing. (2015). *DNP fact sheet.* http://www.aacn.nche.edu/media-relations/fact-sheets/dnp

American Association of Colleges of Nursing. (2022). *Nursing fact sheet.* http://www.aacn.nche.edu/media-relations/fact-sheets/nursing-fact-sheet

American Nurses Association. (n.d.). *Violence, incivility, & bullying.* http://www.nursingworld.org/Mobile/Nursing-Factsheets/lateral-violence-and-bullying-in-nursing.html

Aries, E. (2017, March 7). 5 signs you're in a toxic workplace. *Forbes.* https://www.forbes.com/sites/emilieaaries/2017/03/07/5-signs-youre-in-a-toxic-workplace/?sh=798552e95134

Bakewell-Sachs, S., Trautman, D., & Rosseter, R. (2022, August 4). Addressing the nurse faculty shortage. *American Nurse.* https://www.myamericannurse.com/addressing-the-nurse-faculty-shortage-2/

Buck, D. (2014, April 5). *Evidence based practice.* Lecture presented at Leadership in Classroom, Battle Creek, Michigan.

Ceravolo, D. J., Schwartz, D. G., Foltz-Ramos, K. M., & Castner, J. (2012). Strengthening communication to overcome lateral violence. *Journal of Nursing Management, 20*(5), 599–606.

Cipriano, P. (2015, September 19). Mitigating the risks of emotional labor. *The American Nurse, 47*(3), 3.

Colosi, B. (2022, March). *2022 NSI national health care retention & RN staffing report.* NSI Nursing Solutions, Inc. https://www.nsinursingsolutions.com/Documents/Library/NSI_National_Health_Care_Retention_Report.pdf

Emami, A. (2021, February 6). *Nursing program challenges.* University of Washington School of Nursing. https://nursing.uw.edu/nursing-program-challenges/

Emergency Nurses Association. (2011, November). *Emergency department violence surveillance study.* https://enau.ena.org/Listing/2011%20Emergency%20Department%20Violence%20Surveillance%20Report

Green, J., & Jackson, D. (2014). Mentoring: Some cautionary notes for the nursing profession. *Contemporary Nurse: A Journal for the Australian Nursing Profession, 47*(1/2), 79–87. https://doi.org/10.5172/conu.2014.47.1-2.79

Haw, C., Stubbs, J., & Dickens, G. L. (2014). Barriers to the reporting of medication administration and near misses: An interview study of nurses at a psychiatric hospital. *Journal of Psychiatric and Mental Health Nursing,* 21(9), 797–805. https://doi.org/10.1111/jpm.12143

Heaslip, P. (2008, revised). *Critical thinking and nursing.* Foundation for Critical Thinking. https://www.criticalthinking.org/pages/critical-thinking-and-nursing/834

Hockenberry, M., Wilson, D., & Barrera, P. (2006). Implementing evidence-based practice in a pediatric hospital. *Pediatric Nursing, 32*(4), 371–377.

Iglehart, J. K. (2013). Expanding the role of advanced nurse practitioners: Risks and rewards. *The New England Journal of Medicine, 386*(20), 1935–1941.

Institute of Medicine. (2010). *The future of nursing: Leading change, advancing health.* National Academies Press. https://nap.nationalacademies.org/read/12956/chapter/1

Johns Hopkins Medicine, University and Hospital. (2016, May 3). *Study suggests medical errors now third leading cause of death in the U.S.* https://www.hopkinsmedicine.org/news/media/releases/study_suggests_medical_errors_now_third_leading_cause_of_death_in_the_us

The Joint Commission. (2009, July 9). *Sentinel event alert 40: Behaviors that undermine a culture of safety.* https://www.jointcommission.org/resources/sentinel-event/sentinel-event-alert-newsletters/sentinel-event-alert-issue-40-behaviors-that-undermine-a-culture-of-safety/#.Y0YdMHbMLIV

Lachman, V. D. (2014). Ethical issues in the disruptive behaviors of incivility, bullying, and horizontal/lateral violence. *Urologic Nursing, 35*(1), 39–42.

Letourneau, R. M. (2022, January 1). The US doesn't have enough faculty to train the next generation of nurses. *The Journal of Nursing.* https://www.asrn.org/journal-nursing/2684-the-us-doesn%E2%80%99t-have-enough-faculty-to-train-the-next-generation-of-nurses.html

McCann, E. (2014, July 18). *Deaths by medical mistake hit records.* Healthcare IT News. http://www.healthcareitnews.com/news/deaths-by-medical-mistakes-hit-records

Morabito, C. (2022, February 28). *Why health-care costs are rising in the U.S. more than anywhere else.* CNBC. https://www.cnbc.com/2022/02/28/why-health-care-costs-are-rising-in-the-us-more-than-anywhere-else-.html

National Council of State Boards of Nursing. (2015). *Nurse practice act toolkit.* https://www.ncsbn.org/policy-gov/npa-toolkit.page

Nickitas, D. M., & Feeg, V. (2011). Doubling the number of nurses with a doctorate by 2020: Predicting the right number or getting it right? *Nursing Economics, 29*(3), 109–110, 125.

Plescia, M., & Gooch, K. (2021, December 9). 7 efforts launched in 2021 to recruit, retain healthcare employees. *Becker's Hospital Review.* https://www.beckershospitalreview.com/hr/7-efforts-launched-in-2021-to-recruit-retain-healthcare-employees.html

Rosseter, R. (2020, September). *Nursing faculty shortage.* American Association of Colleges of Nursing. https://www.aacnnursing.org/News-Information/Fact-Sheets/Nursing-Faculty-Shortage

Rosseter, R. (2022, April 5). *Nursing schools see enrollment increases in entry-level programs, signaling strong interest in nursing careers.* American Association of Colleges of Nursing. https://www.aacnnursing.org/News-Information/Press-Releases/View/ArticleId/25183/Nursing-Schools-See-Enrollment-Increases-in-Entry-Level-Programs

Stanton, C. (2015). Action needed to stop lateral violence in the perioperative setting. *AORN Journal, 101*(5), 7–9. https://doi.org/10.1016/s0001-2092(15)00320-8

Stimpfel, A. W., Sloane, D. M., & Aiken, L. H. (2012). The longer the shifts for hospital nurses, the higher the levels of burnout and patient dissatisfaction. *Health Affairs (Project Hope), 31*(11), 2501–2509. https://doi.org/10.1377/hlthaff.2011.1377

Stites, S. (2022, February 26). *Nurses would get more support under Oregon legislative plan.* OPB. https://www.opb.org/article/2022/02/26/oregon-legislature-nurses-shortage-house-bill-4003-license-nursing-students-practice/

Sullivan, K. (2014, September 25). *The future of nursing: An industry in flux.* Fierce Healthcare. https://www.fiercehealthcare.com/special-report/future-nursing-industry-flux

US Bureau of Labor Statistics. (2022, April 18). *Occupational outlook handbook: Registered Nurses: Job outlook.* https://www.bls.gov/ooh/healthcare/registered-nurses.htm#tab-6

Wallis, L. (2012). Barriers to implementing evidence-based practice remain high for U.S. nurses. *American Journal of Nursing, 112*(12), 12–15.

Ward, J. (2014, May 14). 8 common problems in the nursing profession. *NurseTogether.* https://www.nursetogether.com/9-common-problems-nursing-profession/

# INDEX

# A

## C

# D

## E

## F



## G

## H

## I

## J



## K



## L

# M

## N

# Q



# R

## S

## W